1991
YEAR BOOK OF
CRITICAL CARE
MEDICINE®

The 1991 Year Book® Series

Year Book of Anesthesia®: Drs. Miller, Kirby, Ostheimer, Roizen, and Stoelting

Year Book of Cardiology®: Drs. Schlant, Collins, Engle, Frye, Kaplan, and O'Rourke

Year Book of Critical Care Medicine®: Drs. Rogers and Parrillo

Year Book of Dentistry®: Drs. Meskin, Currier, Kennedy, Leinfelder, Matukas, and Rovin

Year Book of Dermatology®: Drs. Sober and Fitzpatrick

Year Book of Diagnostic Radiology®: Drs. Hendee, Keats, Kirkpatrick, Miller, Osborn, Reed, and Thompson

Year Book of Digestive Diseases®: Drs. Greenberger and Moody

Year Book of Drug Therapy®: Drs. Lasagna and Weintraub

Year Book of Emergency Medicine®: Drs. Wagner, Burdick, Davidson, Roberts, and Spivey

Year Book of Endocrinology®: Drs. Bagdade, Braverman, Halter, Horton, Kannan, Molitch, Morley, Odell, Rogol, Ryan, and Sherwin

Year Book of Family Practice®: Drs. Berg, Bowman, Dietrich, Green, and Scherger

Year Book of Geriatrics and Gerontology®: Drs. Beck, Abrass, Burton, Cummings, Makinodan, and Small

Year Book of Hand Surgery®: Drs. Dobyns, Chase, and Amadio

Year Book of Health Care Management: Drs. Heyssel, King, and Steinberg, Ms. Avakian, and Messrs. Berman, Brock, Kues, and Rosenberg

Year Book of Hematology®: Drs. Spivak, Bell, Ness, Quesenberry, and Wiernik

Year Book of Infectious Diseases®: Drs. Wolff, Barza, Keusch, Klempner, and Snydman

Year Book of Infertility: Drs. Mishell, Paulsen, and Lobo

Year Book of Medicine®: Drs. Rogers, Des Prez, Cline, Braunwald, Greenberger, Utiger, Epstein, and Malawista

Year Book of Neonatal and Perinatal Medicine: Drs. Klaus and Fanaroff

Year Book of Neurology and Neurosurgery®: Drs. Currier and Crowell

Year Book of Nuclear Medicine®: Drs. Hoffer, Gore, Gottschalk, Sostman, Zaret, and Zubal

Year Book of Obstetrics and Gynecology®: Drs. Mishell, Kirschbaum, and Morrow

Year Book of Occupational and Environmental Medicine: Drs. Emmett, Brooks, Harris, and Schenker

Year Book of Oncology: Drs. Young, Longo, Ozols, Simone, Steele, and Weichselbaum

Year Book of Ophthalmology®: Drs. Laibson, Adams, Augsburger, Benson, Cohen, Eagle, Flanagan, Nelson, Reinecke, Sergott, and Wilson

Year Book of Orthopedics®: Drs. Sledge, Poss, Cofield, Frymoyer, Griffin, Hansen, Johnson, Springfield, and Weiland

Year Book of Otolaryngology–Head and Neck Surgery®: Drs. Bailey and Paparella

Year Book of Pathology and Clinical Pathology®: Drs. Brinkhous, Dalldorf, Langdell, and McLendon

Year Book of Pediatrics®: Drs. Oski and Stockman

Year Book of Plastic, Reconstructive, and Aesthetic Surgery: Drs. Miller, Cohen, McKinney, Robson, Ruberg, and Whitaker

Year Book of Podiatric Medicine and Surgery®: Dr. Kominsky

Year Book of Psychiatry and Applied Mental Health®: Drs. Talbott, Frances, Freedman, Meltzer, Perry, Schowalter, and Yudofsky

Year Book of Pulmonary Disease®: Drs. Green, Loughlin, Michael, Mulshine, Peters, Terry, Tockman, and Wise

Year Book of Speech, Language, and Hearing: Drs. Bernthal, Hall, and Tomblin

Year Book of Sports Medicine®: Drs. Shephard, Eichner, Sutton, and Torg, Col. Anderson, and Mr. George

Year Book of Surgery®: Drs. Schwartz, Jonasson, Robson, Shires, Spencer, and Thompson

Year Book of Ultrasound: Drs. Merritt, Mittelstaedt, Carroll, and Nyberg

Year Book of Urology®: Drs. Gillenwater and Howards

Year Book of Vascular Surgery®: Drs. Bergan and Yao

Roundsmanship '91–'92 A Year Book® Guide to Clinical Medicine: Drs. Dan, Feigin, Quilligan, Schrock, Stein, and Talbott

Contributing Editors

Robert A. Balk, M.D.
Associate Professor of Medicine, Section of Pulmonary Medicine, Department of Medicine, Rush-Presbyterian-St. Luke's Medical Center, Chicago, Illinois

John T. Barron, M.D., Ph.D.
Assistant Professor of Medicine, Section of Cardiology, Department of Medicine, Rush-Presbyterian-St. Luke's Medical Center, Chicago, Illinois

Thomas A. Bleck, M.D.
Associate Professor of Neurology, Department of Neurology, University of Virginia, Charlottesville, Virginia

Michael J. Breslow, M.D.
Assistant Professor, Co-Director, Surgical Intensive Care Unit Department of Anesthesiology and Critical Care Medicine, Johns Hopkins Medical Institutions, Baltimore, Maryland

Thomas A. Buckingham, M.D.
Associate Professor of Medicine, Section of Cardiology, Department of Medicine, Rush-Presbyterian-St. Luke's Medical Center, Chicago, Illinois

Robert E. Cunnion, M.D.
Head, Cardiovascular Section, Critical Care Medicine Department, National Institutes of Health, Bethesda, Maryland

Robert L. Danner, M.D.
Senior Investigator, Critical Care Medicine Department, National Institutes of Health, Bethesda, Maryland

Andrew C. Dixon, M.D.
Fellow, Section of Critical Care Medicine, Department of Medicine, Rush-Presbyterian-St. Luke's Medical Center, Chicago, Illinois

Steven M. Hollenberg, M.D.
Medical Staff Fellow, Critical Care Medicine Department, National Institutes of Health, Bethesda, Maryland

Jeffrey R. Kirsch, M.D.
Assistant Professor, Co-Director, Residency Education, Department of Anesthesiology and Critical Care Medicine, Johns Hopkins Medical Institutions, Baltimore, Maryland

Lloyd W. Klein, M.D.
Associate Professor of Medicine, Section of Cardiology, Department of Medicine, Rush-Presbyterian-St. Luke's Medical Center, Chicago, Illinois

Anand Kumar, M.D.
Fellow, Section of Critical Care Medicine, Department of Medicine, Rush-Presbyterian-St. Luke's Medical Center, Chicago, Illinois

Phillip R. Liebson, M.D.
Professor of Medicine, Section of Cardiology, Department of Medicine, Rush-Presbyterian-St. Luke's Medical Center, Chicago, Illinois

Robert W. McPherson, M.D.
Associate Professor, Chief, Division of Neurological Anesthesia, Department of Anesthesiology and Critical Care Medicine, Johns Hopkins Medical Institutions, Baltimore, Maryland

Charles Natanson, M.D.
Senior Investigator, Critical Care Medicine Department, National Institutes of Health, Bethesda, Maryland

David G. Nichols, M.D.
Assistant Professor, Director, Pediatric Intensive Care Unit, Department of Anesthesiology and Critical Care Medicine, Johns Hopkins Medical Institutions, Baltimore, Maryland

Frederick P. Ognibene, M.D.
Head, Pediatric Section, Critical Care Medicine Department, National Institutes of Health, Bethesda, Maryland

Margaret M. Parker, M.D.
Head, Critical Care Section, Critical Care Medicine Department, National Institutes of Health, Bethesda, Maryland

Gary L. Schaer, M.D.
Associate Professor, Section of Cardiology, Department of Medicine, Rush-Presbyterian-St. Luke's Medical Center, Chicago, Illinois

Anthony F. Suffredini, M.D.
Senior Investigator, Critical Care Medicine Department, National Institutes of Health, Bethesda, Maryland

Alan L. Van Dervort, M.D.
Medical Staff Fellow, Critical Care Medicine Department, National Institutes of Health, Bethesda, Maryland

1991

The Year Book of CRITICAL CARE MEDICINE®

Editors

Mark C. Rogers, M.D.
Professor and Chairman, Department of Anesthesiology and Critical Care Medicine; Professor, Department of Pediatrics; Associate Dean for Clinical Practice, The Johns Hopkins University, School of Medicine, Baltimore, Maryland

Joseph E. Parrillo, M.D.
James B. Herrick Professor of Medicine; Chief, Section of Cardiology; Chief, Section of Critical Care Medicine; Medical Director, Rush Heart Institute, Rush-Presbyterian-St. Luke's Medical Center, Chicago, Illinois

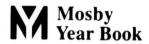
**Mosby
Year Book**

St. Louis   Baltimore   Boston   Chicago   London   Philadelphia   Sydney   Toronto

Editor-in-Chief, Year Book Publishing: Nancy Gorham
Sponsoring Editor: Rebecca A. Ede
Manager, Medical Information Services: Edith M. Podrazik
Senior Medical Information Specialist: Terri Strorigl
Senior Medical Writer: David A. Cramer, M.D.
Assistant Director, Manuscript Services: Frances M. Perveiler
Associate Managing Editor, Year Book Editing Services: Elizabeth Fitch
Production Coordinator: Max F. Perez
Proofroom Manager: Barbara M. Kelly

Editorial Office:
Mosby–Year Book, Inc.
200 North LaSalle St.
Chicago, IL 60601

International Standard Serial Number: 0734-3299
International Standard Book Number: 0-8151-7252-4

Table of Contents

The material in this volume represents literature reviewed up to July 1990.

Journals Represented

Mosby–Year Book subscribes to and surveys nearly 850 U.S. and foreign medical and allied health journals. From these journals, the Editors select the articles to be abstracted. Journals represented in this YEAR BOOK are listed below.

Acta Chirurgica Scandinavica
Acta Neurologica Scandinavica
American Heart Journal
American Journal of Cardiology
American Journal of Diseases of Children
American Journal of Emergency Medicine
American Journal of Infection Control
American Journal of Medicine
American Journal of Pathology
American Journal of Physiology
American Journal of Surgery
American Review of Respiratory Disease
Anesthesia and Analgesia
Anesthesia and Intensive Care
Anesthesiology
Annals of Emergency Medicine
Annals of Internal Medicine
Annals of Neurology
Annals of Surgery
Annals of Thoracic Surgery
Archives of Disease in Childhood
Archives of Internal Medicine
Archives of Neurology
Archives of Physical Medicine and Rehabilitation
Archives of Surgery
British Heart Journal
British Medical Journal
Chest
Circulation
Circulation Research
Circulatory Shock
Cleveland Clinic Journal of Medicine
Critical Care Medicine
Dermatologica
Electroencephalography and Clinical Neurophysiology
European Heart Journal
European Respiratory Journal
Head and Neck
Heart and Lung
Hepatology
Intensive Care Medicine
International Journal of Cardiology
Israel Journal of Medical Sciences
Journal of Applied Physiology
Journal of Burn Care & Rehabilitation
Journal of Clinical Investigation
Journal of Clinical Psychopharmacology
Journal of Emergency Medicine

Journal of Infectious Diseases
Journal of Neurology, Neurosurgery and Psychiatry
Journal of Neuroscience Nursing
Journal of Pediatric Surgery
Journal of Pediatrics
Journal of Surgical Research
Journal of Thoracic and Cardiovascular Surgery
Journal of Trauma
Journal of the American College of Cardiology
Journal of the American Geriatrics Society
Journal of the American Medical Association
Lancet
Laryngoscope
Neurology
Neurosurgery
New England Journal of Medicine
Pediatric Emergency Care
Pediatric Infectious Disease Journal
Pediatric Radiology
Pediatric Research
Pediatrics
Quarterly Journal of Medicine
Scandinavian Journal of Clinical Laboratory Investigation
Southern Medical Journal
Stroke
Surgery
Surgery, Gynecology and Obstetrics
Transplantation

STANDARD ABBREVIATIONS

The following terms are abbreviated in this edition: acquired immunodeficiency syndrome (AIDS), the central nervous system (CNS), cerebrospinal fluid (CSF), computed tomography (CT), electrocardiography (ECG), and human immunodeficiency virus (HIV).

Acknowledgment

This volume would not have been possible without the tireless dedication of Peggy Riley, Cindy Sheffield, Geri Byrd, and Katherine Swanigan, who spent countless hours coordinating this project. The editors are deeply in their debt.

Dedication

To the families of the editors of the YEAR BOOK OF CRITICAL CARE MEDICINE.

Introduction

The 1991 YEAR BOOK OF CRITICAL CARE MEDICINE features a whole new set of papers that have been carefully abstracted and commented on to reflect recent developments in critical care medicine. For those of us in the specialty, it is both exciting and disturbing to see so many of the considerations of critical care medicine revolve around ethical and financial issues. The lay press is filled with concerns about continuing or removing life support systems, expenses of medical care (particularly intensive care), and similar considerations. The financial and ethical concerns in critical care medicine are now topics for the evening news, for family discussion, and for new legislation.

As a result of these considerations, it is apparent that the tradition of having sections of the YEAR BOOK OF CRITICAL CARE MEDICINE dealing with ethical and financial issues is both appropriate and important. Along with reviewing the current areas of new treatments for infectious disease, concerns about AIDS, new modes of support for ventilatory failure, and ways to treat patients with acute myocardial infarction, the YEAR BOOK has continued to grow and develop its sections on the social and economic implications of the specialty.

Mark C. Rogers, M.D.
Joseph E. Parrillo, M.D.

1 Trauma

Trial of Normobaric and Hyperbaric Oxygen for Acute Carbon Monoxide Intoxication
Raphael J-C, Elkharrat D, Jars-Guincestre M-C, Chastang C, Chasles V, Vercken J-B, Gajdos P (Hôp Raymond Poincaré, Garches, France; Hôp St Louis, Paris)
Lancet 2:414–419, 1989   1–1

Acute carbon monoxide intoxication remains a frequent occurrence in the home. Oxygen is the usual treatment, but the indications for hyperbaric oxygen (HBO) remain uncertain. The value of HBO was studied within 12 hours of hospital admission in 629 adults who were poisoned at home. When consciousness was intact, 6 hours of normobaric oxygen (NBO) were compared with 2 hours of HBO at 2 atm absolute plus 4 hours of NBO. In those with initially impaired consciousness, 1 and 2 sessions of HBO were compared. The 2 sessions were 2–12 hours apart.

In patients with intact consciousness, treatment with NBO alone and combined HBO-NBO was similarly successful. About two thirds of the patients recovered within 1 month. In those with impaired consciousness, 1 session of HBO and 2 sessions of HBO had similar effects. All of these patients also received NBO. Just more than half of these patients recovered within 1 month. All 7 patients with neuropsychiatric sequelae and all 4 who died were comatose on hospital arrival. The type of treatment still made no difference when the outcome was stratified by the carboxyhemoglobin concentration.

Normobaric oxygen is adequate for carbon monoxide-intoxicated patients whose consciousness is unimpaired. Those with brief loss of consciousness should have 1 session of HBO. It is not likely that 2 HBO sessions have significant value, but whether more than 2 sessions are indicated remains uncertain.

▶ Definition of the proper role of HBO in the treatment of carbon monoxide intoxication has been difficult because the outcome measure depends on the resolution of subjective neuropsychiatric symptoms, and because previous studies have been uncontrolled with small numbers of patients. The large, controlled study by Raphael et al. adds important information: (1) Level of consciousness is more important than carboxyhemoglobin level in predicting outcome. In the absence of coma, there is no advantage of HBO over NBO in improving the neurologic outcome regardless of the initial carboxyhemoglobin level, even though carboxyhemoglobin levels are lowered more rapidly by HBO. (2) Two sessions of HBO do not improve serious neurologic morbidity or mortality compared to 1 session in comatose patients. In the design of this study, the authors made the assumption that coma secondary to carbon monoxide intoxication justified at least 1 session of hyperbaric oxygenation. However, their data suggest that a well-controlled, randomized study comparing

NBO with HBO in comatose patients is needed urgently if the continued use of a scarce resource such as HBO for carbon monoxide is to be justified.— D.G. Nichols, M.D.

Traumatic Rupture of the Thoracic Aorta: A Clinicopathological Study
Søndenaa K, Tveit B, Kordt KF, Fossdal JE, Pedersen P-H (Rogaland Central County Hosp, Stavanger, Norway)
Acta Chir Scand 156:137–143, 1990   1–2

The incidence of traumatic rupture of the thoracic aorta is probably underestimated, because most patients so injured die before arrival at the hospital and autopsy is often not performed. A retrospective review was performed to determine the incidence of traumatic rupture of the thoracic aorta.

During a 6-year study period, 18 males aged 7–72 years and 9 females aged 16–83 years sustained traumatic rupture of the thoracic aorta. Eighteen patients died instantly, but in 2 of them death was caused by head injuries. One patient had vital signs after the accident but died during transport to the hospital; 5 others were treated but died in the hospital. All 5 had extensive injuries other than the aortic rupture, and in 4 of them the aortic injuries were not diagnosed before death. The remaining 3 patients survived. Twenty of the 27 patients were injured in automobile accidents.

Two of the 3 survivors underwent direct cross-clamping of the aorta with Dacron interposition grafting soon after admission. The third survivor had placement of a Gott shunt and Dacron interposition graft the day after the accident. The chest radiograph demonstrated rib fractures and lung contusions on the right side and widening of the mediastinum with deviation of the trachea to the right. This patient survived but was paraplegic.

Most patients who died at the scene were in a condition that precluded any life-saving measures. A chest radiograph in survivors suspected of traumatic injury of the thoracic aorta is mandatory; it may show a number of signs that indicate aortic rupture, of which mediastinal widening is considered the most reliable. Some authors recommend that aortography be performed in all patients suspected of rupture of the thoracic aorta by virtue of the mechanism of injury. Most patients should immediately undergo left fourth intercostal thoracotomy. Several surgical techniques are available, but there is still no agreement on what constitutes the safest technique. Paraplegia remains the most feared complication of cross-clamping. The simple-clamp repair technique appears to be just as reliable as other techniques in avoiding paraplegia.

Based on a total population of approximately 240,000 inhabitants served by the present hospital, the incidence of traumatic rupture of the thoracic aorta was 1/53,000 inhabitants. Therefore, this type of traumatic injury occurs more often than is generally thought.

▶ Traumatic rupture of the thoracic aorta is a well-known complication of decelerating injuries such as "steering wheel" trauma. During the 6 years of this study, 18 males and 9 females were identified who sustained traumatic rupture of the thoracic aorta. The conditions that cause some to die instantaneously and allow others to reach the hospital alive are discussed in some detail, and it is a useful review of the subject.—M.C. Rogers, M.D.

Rupture of the Distal Thoracic Esophagus Following Blunt Trauma: Case Report

Micon L, Geis L, Siderys H, Stevens L, Rodman GH Jr (Methodist Hosp of Indiana, Indianapolis)

J Trauma 30:214–217, 1990   1–3

Rupture of the distal thoracic esophagus from blunt external trauma is uncommon because most ruptures involve the cervical esophagus. Only 5

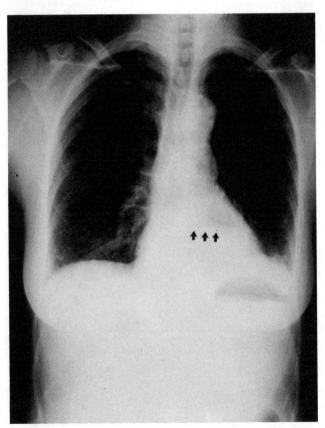

Fig 1–1.—Repeat posteroanterior and lateral chest radiograph, 90 minutes after presentation. Note air-fluid level in mediastinum (*arrows*). (Courtesy of Micon L, Geis L, Siderys H, et al: *J Trauma* 30:214–217, 1990.)

such cases have been reported in the world literature. A patient was seen who sustained a lower thoracic esophageal rupture in an automobile accident

Woman, 59, was involved in an automobile accident shortly after eating a large meal. She wore a lap belt in the rear seat of the automobile when the collision occurred. Upon arrival at the emergency department, she complained of dyspnea and substernal chest and upper abdominal pain. Anteroposterior and lateral chest radiographs revealed an air-fluid level in the mediastinum (Figs 1–1 and 1–2). A subsequent water-soluble contrast esophagram demonstrated a distal esophageal rupture. The patient was operated on approximately 5 hours after the injury occurred. A 2-cm longitudinal laceration in the right lateral esophageal wall was closed in 2 layers, and the closure was reinforced with a pedicle flap of parietal pleura. The patient had an uneventful postoperative course, and no complications occurred during 12 months of follow-up.

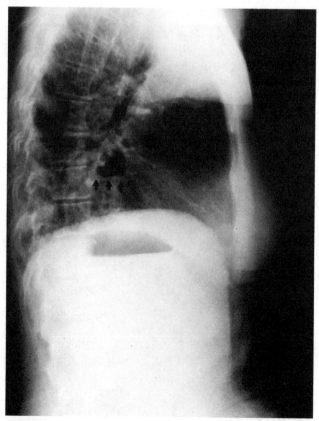

Fig 1–2.—Repeat posteroanterior and lateral chest radiograph, 90 minutes after presentation. Note air-fluid level in mediastinum (*arrows*). (Courtesy of Micon L, Geis L, Siderys H, et al: *J Trauma* 30:214–217, 1990.)

Although the beneficial effects of seatbelts have been well documented, numerous injuries have been attributed to current passive restraint systems, particularly the single lap belt. Improper positioning of the lap belt was presumed to contribute to the esophageal injury in this patient.

▶ A very uncommon finding is blunt trauma rupture to distal esophagus. This case report and discussion of the predisposing factors, as well as the management, should add to the intensivist's knowledge of this unusual but life-threatening complication.— M.C. Rogers, M.D.

Acute Tracheobronchial Injury
Flynn AE, Thomas AN, Schecter WP (Univ of California, San Francisco)
J Trauma 29:1326–1330, 1989   1–4

Experience with 22 patients seen from 1977 to 1988 with tracheal or bronchial injuries was evaluated. The 20 men and 2 women had a mean age of 28 years. Penetrating trauma caused 77% of the injuries. Sixteen injuries involved the cervical trachea and 6 were located in the intrathoracic trachea or bronchi. Thirteen patients had major associated injuries, most often of the esophagus or spinal cord. The most frequent findings were tachypnea and subcutaneous emphysema.

All penetrating injuries were explored on an emergency basis and repaired by primary suture closure. Six patients had tracheostomy as well. Intrathoracic bronchial injuries were managed by urgent thoracotomy. Two patients with blunt injuries were managed nonoperatively. Three patients died, for a mortality rate of 14%; all deaths resulted from major vascular injury. Complications occurred in 8 patients and included a chronic tracheoesophageal fistula, tracheal stenosis, pneumonia, and empyema.

Selected patients with blunt tracheobronchial injuries can be managed nonoperatively, but penetrating injuries call for early exploration and primary repair. It is necessary to take urgent measures if there is airway obstruction.

▶ This paper on penetrating tracheobronchial injuries documents that management with surgical exploration and primary repair is most appropriate. As described in another abstract in this same section on tracheal injury, however, selected patients with blunt injury may be treated nonoperatively. This is an important message for those managing the care of these patients when they are admitted to the intensive care unit.— M.C. Rogers, M.D.

Acute Epiglottitis in Children and Adults in Sweden 1981–3
Trollfors B, Nylén O, Strangert K (Univ of Göteborg, Sweden; St Göran's Hosp, Stockholm)
Arch Dis Child 65:491–494, 1990   1–5

The most common and serious manifestations of invasive *Hemophilus influenzae* type b infections are meningitis and epiglottitis. The reported incidence of acute epiglottitis in children has varied considerably. Although some studies found meningitis to be more common, an examination of cases in the Göteborg area in Sweden during 1971–1980 put the ratio between epiglottitis and *H. influenzae* at 1.44:1. The incidence of acute epiglottitis in children in all of Sweden from 1981 through 1983 was investigated using the case records of patients with hospital discharge diagnoses of acute epiglottitis.

Of the 1,101 patients identified, 485 children and 356 adults fulfilled study criteria. The children's mean age was 3.7 years. Of the 290 blood cultures obtained, *H. influenzae* was isolated in 267 (92%). All of the 139 serotyped isolates were type b. The majority of children (73%) required intubation or tracheotomy; 6 died.

Blood cultures were obtained from 185 adults and *H. influenzae* was isolated from 98 of them; 53 were type b. Adults were hospitalized slightly longer than children (a mean of 5 vs. 4 days), but fewer (19%) required an artificial airway. Two adults died.

The age-specific incidence of epiglottitis in Swedish children (10/100,000/yr) was higher than that of meningitis and differs from previous reports of *H. influenzae* meningitis. The difference may result from variations in reporting of cases or may be because Swedish children have less exposure to the infection in their early years when *H. influenzae* is more likely to manifest as meningitis than as epiglottitis. The incidence of acute epiglottitis is also high in adults (1.8/100,000/yr). Mortality is low in both groups.

▶ This paper was included for 2 reasons: First, it demonstrates the significant number of adults in whom epiglottitis develops. Interestingly, the frequency of positive blood cultures was very low in adults with epiglottitis. Second, this study indicates that some children and some adults can be observed without an artificial airway. This continues to be a very controversial area. It is my opinion that it is actually more conservative to have an artificial airway than it is to observe the patients, but I do recognize the fact that this is a field that is changing. Nevertheless, I caution all readers to be very careful about leaving patients at risk for airway obstruction without an artificial airway in place.—M.C. Rogers, M.D.

Evaluation and Treatment of Acute Laryngeal Fractures
Schild JA, Denneny EC (Univ of Illinois, Chicago)
Head Neck 11:491–496, 1989   1–6

Treatment of laryngeal fractures has advanced in recent years, and the airway can now be restored without aspiration or stenosis in most patients. However, the best treatment of injury-induced vocal cord dysfunction remains controversial. In particular, the role of CT has yet to be defined.

The symptoms, type of injury, and treatment were reviewed in 12 cases of blunt and 3 cases of penetrating laryngeal trauma. Photographs of each patient were taken during direct laryngoscopy. All patients had normal findings on cervical spine radiographs. Axial CT scans were obtained and findings were compared with clinical findings. Treatment results were evaluated for speech and for adequate airway patency.

The 15 patients were aged 16–67 years; 11 were male. Symptoms ranged from mild neck discomfort to dyspnea and hoarseness. Five patients had respiratory distress and stridor, 6 had dysphagia or odynophagia, and 3 had hemoptysis. Treatment varied according to severity of injury: 7 patients were observed only, but 8 required surgery. Endoscopic photographs were valuable in assessing patients' progress, particularly in more severe injuries. Computed tomography was reliable for defining the extent of soft tissue injury and for diagnosing the presence and displacement of fractures.

At completion of treatment all 15 patients had satisfactory airways for normal activity and normal deglutition. All patients returned to preinjury activities without dyspnea. Three of 12 patients with voice abnormalities as presenting symptoms had permanent voice changes, but none required amplification devices.

In all cases CT scans were valuable in accurately evaluating soft tissue trauma and fractures. Compared with plain films, CT also enabled better visualization of the cricoarytenoid area, where severe abnormalities produced later vocal cord dysmotility. Patients with minor injuries were accurately evaluated by CT for conservative management, and severely injured patients had better planning for surgical treatment.

▶ Acute laryngeal fractures can be life-threatening. On the other hand, they are not very common, and there is often confusion as to whether or not the patients need to be operated on immediately or simply observed. Findings in the cases reviewed in this study show that CT scans are valuable in assessing the injury and allow the separation of patients into 2 groups. The first group, patients with minor injuries, could be treated conservatively, but the second group, the more severely injured patients, required surgery.—M.C. Rogers, M.D.

Scorpion Sting-Induced Pulmonary Edema: Scintigraphic Evidence of Cardiac Dysfunction
Rahav G, Weiss AT (Hadassah Univ Hosp, Jerusalem)
Chest 97:1478–1480, 1990   1–7

A boy and a man were treated for pulmonary edema that resulted from the sting of a scorpion. The clinical findings included nausea, vomiting, profuse sweating, irritability, salivation, priapism, somnolence, and urinary retention. Both had severe dyspnea. The ECG showed sinus tachycardia and diffuse ST-T changes. Serum levels of creatinine phosphokinase were elevated. Findings on chest films were compatible with those of pulmonary edema. Pulmonary wedge pressure was normal in 1 patient. Radionuclide ventriculography performed with a mobile gamma camera (MUGA) showed reduced left and right ventricular function with abnormal hypokinesis of the anteroseptal and apical walls.

Treatment consisted mainly of specific antivenom and supportive therapy. Follow-up MUGA scans 6 months after discharge showed apical hypokinesis and reduced but improved ejection fraction in 1 patient.

Previously reported pathologic findings in fatalities caused by scorpion stings included marked changes in the papillary muscles and subendocardial tissue, including diffuse or focal myocarditis and muscle necrosis. These and the present hemodynamic findings point to myocardial failure as the cause of scorpion sting-induced pulmonary edema. In 1 patient primary pulmonary injury was probably the major determinant of the pulmonary edema in view of the normal wedge pressure.

Diagnostic Difficulties of Foreign Body Aspiration in Children
Losek JD (Med College of Wisconsin, Milwaukee)
Am J Emerg Med 8:348–350, 1990   1–8

Aspiration of foreign bodies occurs most commonly in children aged 6 months to 6 years. The most frequently aspirated objects are radiolucent organic materials. Young children cannot report the initial choking and coughing episode, which may be unobserved by caregivers. The respiratory tract can adapt rapidly to a foreign body, and the child may have no signs of respiratory distress. Chest radiographs may also be normal.

Boy, 4 years, aspirated a 22-caliber bullet. Although the bullet was large, cough, dyspnea, and wheezing were absent on presentation. The diagnosis of a radiopaque bronchial foreign body was confirmed by chest radiography (Fig 1–3). The bullet was removed successfully with the use of bronchoscopy and forceps, and the child was discharged the following day.

Forty-two additional reports of children with foreign body aspiration were reviewed. The aspirations were unwitnessed in 19% of the cases, and 57% of the children were asymptomatic when first seen by a physician. Results of physical examinations were normal in 19%, and inspiratory/expiratory chest radiographs were normal in 24%.

The diagnosis of foreign body aspiration in children can be difficult. The common presenting symptoms are often absent. Bronchoscopy should be considered for any child who has a history of possible foreign body aspiration but who is asymptomatic with normal radiographic findings.

▶ This paper was included because it demonstrates, again, the need for bronchoscopy when foreign body aspiration is suspected. The frequency with which foreign body aspiration is associated with asymptomatic presentation is the reason for my concern, and the fact that physical findings and even x-ray

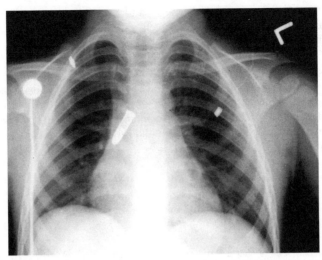

Fig 1–3.—Chest roentgenogram illustrating radiopaque foreign body (bullet) located in the right mainstem bronchus. (Courtesy of Losek JD: *Am J Emerg Med* 8:348–350, 1990.)

appearances may be normal in these patients can lead to missing the diagnosis.—M.C. Rogers, M.D.

Liver Transplantation for Severe *Amanita phalloides* Mushroom Poisoning

Pinson CW, Daya MR, Benner KG, Norton RL, Deveney KE, Ascher NL, Roberts JP, Lake JR, Kurkchubasche AG, Ragsdale JW, Alexander JP, Keeffe EB (Oregon Health Sciences Univ, Portland; VA Med Ctr, Portland, Ore; Univ of California, San Francisco)
Am J Surg 159:493–499, 1990   1–9

Mushroom poisoning is increasing in the United States, and *Amanita phalloides* is responsible for 95% of the fatal poisonings. Liver transplantation is now considered the definitive treatment for severely poisoned patients. However, patient selection criteria and the timing of transplantation have not been clearly defined. The clinical course of 5 severely poisoned patients, 4 of whom underwent liver transplantation, was reviewed.

Indications for transplantation included a prolonged prothrombin time that could be corrected only partially, metabolic acidosis, hypoglycemia, hypofibrinogenemia, and an increased serum level of ammonia after elevation of serum aminotransferase levels. Hepatocyte viability of resected liver was 0% to 30%. Complications caused by poisoning included diarrhea, gastrointestinal hemorrhage, hypophosphatemia, bowel edema, and marrow suppression with lymphopenia, thrombocytopenia, and neutropenia. All 5 patients remained well at 1-year follow-up. Patients with *Amanita* poisoning and a prolonged prothrombin time, acidosis, hypoglycemia, gastrointestinal hemorrhage, and hypofibrinogenemia after elevation of serum aminotransferase levels should be considered for urgent liver transplantation without waiting for further progression.

▶ The use of liver transplantation continues to grow, and the indications are becoming more fascinating with each passing year. These authors review 5 patients severely poisoned with *Amanita phalloides* and describe the clinical course of 4 who underwent liver transplantation. It has gradually become apparent that liver transplantation is the definitive treatment for these severely poisoned patients.—M.C. Rogers, M.D.

Lithium Toxicity and Myxedema Coma in an Elderly Woman

Santiago R, Rashkin MC (Univ of Cincinnati)
J Emerg Med 8:63–66, 1990   1–10

Thyroid diseases occur more often in the elderly than in younger adults. Hypothyroidism as a side effect of lithium therapy is a well-recognized complication. However, myxedema coma after lithium intoxication has not been reported previously.

Woman, 71, incoherent, was taken to the emergency department for evaluation. She had been treated chronically with lithium and trifluoperazine for an unspecified psychiatric condition and had recently started taking a combination diuretic of hydrochlorothiazide and triamterene to treat hypertension. The patient had also been taking naproxen for arthritis. Laboratory evaluation revealed chronic lithium toxicity and mild dehydration. The patient was placed on a monitored bed and treated with forced alkaline diuresis for 2 days. Plasma lithium values dropped gradually from 2.48 mEq/L at admission to 1 mEq/L on day 4. Her condition appeared to stabilize during the first 3 days of admission. However, on day 4 she was suddenly noted to have no spontaneous respirations, and she became bradycardiac with an undetectable pulse. After resuscitation the patient was transferred to the intensive care unit where third-degree heart block was diagnosed. A transvenous pacemaker was inserted. The patient was comatose with a Glasgow Coma Scale score of 8. Thyroid function tests drawn on admission showed a thyroxine level of 1 μg/dL and triiodothyronine resin uptake of 84%. She was given 500 μg of levothyroxine intravenously and 50 μg daily for an additional 2 doses, after which she was maintained with thyroid therapy orally. At the time of discharge, the patient was alert, oriented, and ambulatory, and she had returned to her baseline mental status.

Because the typical signs and symptoms of hypothyroidism in elderly persons may be either absent or misinterpreted as age-related changes, dementia, or depression, the diagnosis of lithium toxicity may not be recognized immediately. A careful differential diagnosis in an elderly patient with vague symptoms suggesting dementia or depression who is taking lithium for recurrent affective disorder cannot be overemphasized.

Acute Mountain Sickness at Intermediate Altitude: Military Mountainous-Training

Pigman EC, Karakla DW (Georgetown-George Washington Univ, Washington, DC: United States Marine Corps, Camp Lejeune, NC)
Am J Emerg Med 8:7–10, 1990   1–11

Acute mountain sickness (AMS) is usually produced at exposure to altitudes in excess of 3,000 m. Although it is unlikely that United States troops would be involved in warfare at such extremes of altitude, exposure to altitudes of 2,000–2,500 m is possible.

A US Marine Corps Battalion Landing Team (BLT) conducted mountainous warfare training at intermediate altitudes. The training took place in January when temperatures ranged from −10° C to −15° C at night, and from −7° C to 2° C during the day. The BLT consisted of 638 men who had been stationed at sea level and had not been deployed to any altitude greater than 400 m during the preceding 11 months. The BLT was flown from sea level to an altitude of 1,370 m and then bussed to 2,065 m. During the next 3 days there were marches of 5–8 km to altitudes ranging from 2,240 to 2,444 m. On day 4 the BLT marched 13 km to an altitude of 2,620 m and remained there for 5 days, participating in an arduous training schedule.

Nine marines (1.4%) aged 19–32 years had incapacitating symptoms consistent with AMS. All 9 patients complained of headaches not relieved by aspirin or acetaminophen, dyspnea at rest, and nausea or anorexia. Five patients had to be evacuated from the field to the base camp where they were treated with complete rest. Three of these 5 patients had resting tachypnea and 3 had hemoconcentration with a mean hemoglobin level of 16.9 g/dL (table). Two patients received supplemental oxygen and intravenous rehydration with crystalloid solution that markedly improved their symptoms. Seven patients were treated with acetazolamide and experienced relief of their symptoms within 24 hours. None of the patients had abnormal findings on chest radiography, and none was hypothermic or hyperthermic.

Presenting Signs of AMS

Patient	Heart Rate (/min)	Respiratory Rate (/min)	Hemoglobin (g/dL)	Chest X-ray	Ataxia	Where Raised
1	98	22	17.4	Normal	−	New York, NY
2	88	20	10.3	Normal	+	Philadelphia, PA
3	72	20	14.7	Normal	−	rural Kentucky
4	96	24	16.7	Normal	+/−	rural Maryland
5	Normal	Normal	—	—	−	Baltimore, MD
6	Normal	Normal	—	—	−	Newark, NJ
7	Normal	Normal	—	—	+	rural Mississippi
8	72	32	16.7	Normal	−	rural Alabama
9	Normal	Normal	—	—	−	Houston, TX

+, present; −, not present.
(Courtesy of Pigman EC Karakla DW: *Am J Emerg Med* 8:7–10, 1990.)

All 9 patients were born and raised in low-altitude areas, and 8 of them had never ventured higher than 1,000 m. Eight of the 9 patients were black and 1 was white. The same BLT participated in a 10-day military exercise 11 months later in a similar cold environment and under an equally demanding training schedule but at a maximum elevation of 500 m. Review of the sick call log showed that only 1 marine (.16%) complained of a headache without dyspnea.

Acute mountain sickness at intermediate altitudes is not uncommon. Prophylaxis with acetazolamide for subsequent altitude exposure in individuals who are susceptible to AMS is recommended.

▶ Military medicine sometime uncovers facts that are not detectable by studying the general public. When a US Marine Corps BLT was brought to intermediate altitudes, a significant number of the men experienced mountain sickness. Interestingly, blacks were the most commonly afflicted. This raises the possibility that extreme exertion may uncover sickle cell trait in blacks. Stress, as reported in military studies, may also give rise to this same observation.— M.C. Rogers, M.D.

Traumatic Occlusion of Two Radiocephalic Fistulas: Case Reports and Their Management
Highbloom RY, Koolpe H, Morris MC (Albert Einstein Med Ctr, Philadelphia; Temple Univ)
J Trauma 30:364–365, 1990   1–12

With the growing number of ambulatory dialysis patients, physicians can expect to see more traumatic injuries to arterial-venous fistulas. The salvage of radiocephalic fistulas is crucial to the continuation of dialysis. In 2 cases, nonfunctioning fistulas were able to be restored for use in hemodialysis.

Case 1.—Man, 18, had a left radiocephalic fistula placed 1 year before admission. An injury incurred in a fall left him with pain, swelling, and nonfunction of the fistula. An angiogram revealed acute obstruction to the outflow at the midforearm. Further investigation identified a large subcutaneous hematoma and complete venous laceration. A thrombectomy and reanastomosis restored good flow in the vein. Access was suitable for dialysis on the third postoperative day.

Case 2.—Man, 42, with end-stage renal disease, had a left forearm fistula that collapsed after he lifted a weight. The fistula was restored and patent venous outflow resumed by means of an arteriotomy followed by proximal and distal thrombectomy.

There are many advantages to salvaging a natural arteriovenous fistula. The fistula is preferable to a prosthetic graft with regard to long-term patency and resistance to infection. Other vessels are conserved for later use, an important consideration in younger patients. An injured extremity with an injured fistula segment should be treated aggressively soon after the traumatic occlusion.

▶ Patients who have indwelling fistulas for ambulatory dialysis are not exempt from trauma. This report of 2 such patients indicates what happens when these arterial-venous fistulas are traumatized.—M.C. Rogers, M.D.

Sensitivity and Specificity of Transcranial Doppler Ultrasonography in the Diagnosis of Vasospasm Following Subarachnoid Hemorrhage
Sloan MA, Haley EC Jr, Kassell NF, Henry ML, Stewart SR, Beskin RR, Seville EA, Torner JC (Univ of Virginia, Charlottesville)
Neurology 39:1514–1518, 1989   1–13

Vasospasm is the leading cause of death and disability in patients with aneurysmal subarachnoid hemorrhage (SAH). Transcranial Doppler ultrasonography (TCD) is a promising noninvasive test for the diagnosis of arterial narrowing in the middle cerebral arteries, but its sensitivity and specificity in a patient population with a high frequency of angiographic vasospasm has not been evaluated. Thirty-four patients with SAH had coronary angiography and TCD during the period of greatest risk for vasospasm (days 3–13) after SAH. Findings with the 2 techniques were correlated to define the sensitivity and specificity of TCD in the diagnosis of vasospasm. Vasospasm on TCD was defined as a mean flow velocity >120 cm/sec.

Twenty-nine patients had angiographically determined vasospasm. Of these, 17 were correctly identified by TCD, and there were no false positive results. Five patients who had no vasospasm were correctly identified, whereas 12 had false negative TCD examinations. The latter were frequently attributable to vasospasm in vessels that could not be adequately assessed by TCD. Overall, TCD had a sensitivity of 58.6%, specificity of 100%, positive predictive value of 100%, and negative predictive value of only 29.8%. Transcranial Doppler ultrasonography was remarkably sensitive (84%) and specific (89%) in detecting vasospasm in the middle cerebral arteries. There was a strong correlation between mean flow velocity and angiographic residual lumen diameter of the middle cerebral artery.

The findings indicate that TCD is highly specific but less sensitive in detecting angiographic vasospasm after SAH. Confirmatory angiography may be avoided if TCD findings are positive, particularly if the vasospasm involves the middle cerebral artery. However, additional tests may be necessary when the clinical syndrome is suggestive of vasospasm and TCD is negative.

▶ This paper reaffirms my general impression that TCD can be useful, but that it is somewhat limited. Basically, this study indicates that vasospasm can be detected by Doppler, but that it is commonly not sufficient to do just Doppler studies. In fact, when Doppler studies are positive, angiography can be avoided, but a negative study requires further evaluation.—M.C. Rogers, M.D.

Tracheobronchial Rupture Due to Blunt Chest Trauma: A Follow-Up Study
Taskinen SO, Salo JA, Halttunen PEA, Sovijärvi ARA (Helsinki Univ Central Hosp)
Ann Thorac Surg 48:846–849, 1989   1–14

Tracheobronchial rupture after blunt chest trauma is an uncommon complication. However, its incidence has been increasing because of an increase in traffic accidents and improved ambulance services that bring patients with major chest trauma to the hospital alive. The diagnosis of tracheobronchial rupture is often not clear because of a lack of specific findings.

Between 1970 and 1988, 9 males aged 15–50 years were treated for tracheobronchial rupture caused by blunt chest trauma. Four patients had rupture of the right main bronchus, 3 had rupture of the left main bronchus, 1 had rupture of the right intermediate bronchus, and 1 had rupture of the trachea. Six patients had been involved in a high-impact traffic accident and 3 had sustained compression trauma. All 9 patients were dyspneic on arrival at the hospital. Eight patients had subcutaneous emphysema, and 2 had flail chest. In all 9 patients pneumothorax was observed on chest radiography, as were pneumomediastinum in 6, hemothorax in 4, and rib fractures in 4. In 1 patient a pneumothorax developed on the right side 2 days after the accident, although the rupture was in the left main bronchus (Fig 1–4). Another patient had a pneumoperitoneum, but laparotomy did not show intra-abdominal damage. All patients had concomitant injuries that in 6 were life-threatening.

Four patients underwent operation within 24 hours after the accident. Indications for emergency operation were a massive air leak via the suction drainage in patients with bronchial rupture or difficulties with endotracheal intubation in the patient with tracheal rupture. Primary reconstruction was performed in all 4 patients. Operation was delayed from 9 to 89 days in the other 5 patients because of a delay in diagnosis. All 5 had good primary healing, but dyspnea later redeveloped. Bronchoscopy identified obstruction and granulation tissue as marks of rupture in the involved bronchus. The stenosed segment was resected at thoracotomy in 4 patients and lobectomy was performed in 1.

Seven patients were followed for 6 months to 18 years. One patient who had a 9-day delay in treatment required further operation because of scar obstruction. The other 6 had no evidence of stricture or reduction in pulmonary function caused by rupture, even if operation had been delayed. Although bronchial rupture can be treated successfully in the acute or the delayed phase, early diagnosis and treatment minimize the risk of infection and resection.

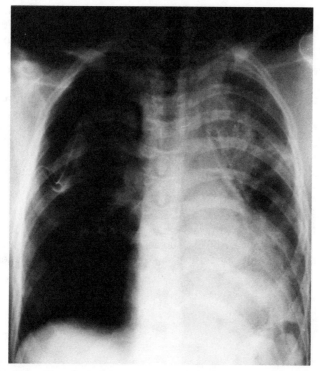

Fig 1–4.—Right pneumothorax 2 days after rupture of left main bronchus. (Courtesy of Taskinen SO, Salo JA, Halttunen PEA, et al: *Ann Thorac Surg* 48:846–849, 1989.)

▶ This review of 9 patients with lung-chest trauma who sustained tracheobronchial rupture indicates that it is possible to wait before operation. Five of these patients had surgery after 9 days to almost 3 months. Despite that, they all had a good surgical outcome. Although I do not recommend waiting for repair, it is of interest that it can be done.—M.C. Rogers, M.D.

Intraosseous Infusion

Fiser DH (Univ of Arkansas)
N Engl J Med 322:1579–1581, 1990   1–15

Immediate vascular access may prove difficult in critically ill children. Intraosseous infusion offers an alternative rapid vascular access in these cases. Such infusion has broad applicability and the few contraindications to its use include the presence of osteogenesis imperfecta or osteopetrosis and an ipsilateral fractured extremity. The risk of infectious complications is increased when a needle is introduced through an area affected by cellulitis or infected burn. Blood products, fluids, and pharmacological agents can be given by intraosseous infusion.

The proximal tibia is generally agreed to be the optimal site for needle insertion in children, although the distal tibia and femur are useful alternative sites. It is estimated that insertion can be completed within 3–5 minutes. The success rate for insertion is high, even when performed by medical personnel, and the rate of complications is low. The infusion should be discontinued preferably within an hour or 2 after conventional vascular access is established.

Presently, intraosseous infusion should be reserved for children in crisis, such as those with cardiopulmonary arrest, shock, burns, and life-threatening status epilepticus, in whom other methods of vascular access have failed. A reasonable time limitation is 5 minutes for children with cardiopulmonary arrest, preferably 5 minutes after adequate ventilation is established, because many such children respond to adequate ventilation alone without need for drug therapy.

▶ The use of intraosseous infusions is increasing in the setting of critically ill patients. It is useful for vascular access and is infrequently associated with complications. This review of the subject should be useful to any intensivist who needs to know the current thinking on this subject.—M.C. Rogers, M.D.

2 Cardiopulmonary Resuscitation

Aortic Diameter and Pressure-Flow Sequence Identify Mechanism of Blood Flow During External Chest Compression in Dogs
Guerci AD, Halperin HR, Beyar R, Beattie C, Tsitlik JE, Wurmb EC, Chandra NC, Weisfeldt ML (Johns Hopkins Hosp; Francis Scott Key Hosp, Baltimore)
J Am Coll Cardiol 14:790–798, 1989   2–1

There is controversy over the mechanism of blood flow during external chest compression. Animal studies in which external manual chest compression was used have shown that blood flow and aortic diastolic pressure are sensitive to compression duration but insensitive to compression rate, whereas studies of internal cardiac massage have indicated that aortic pressure and flow are sensitive to compression rate but not to compression duration. The dominant mechanism of blood flow during manual external chest compression was identified in 2 sets of experiments performed in 14 anesthetized large dogs. Aortic pressure, blood flow relationships, and aortic diameter were measured during sinus rhythm and internal cardiac massage, and during vest cardiopulmonary resuscitation (CPR), conventional manual CPR, and high-impulse manual CPR.

During sinus rhythm and internal cardiac massage, ascending aortic flow and ascending aortic pressure increased simultaneously, the increase in ascending aortic pressure preceded the increase in descending aortic pressure, the ratio of pulse pressure to stroke volume did not significantly increase, the ascending aortic diameter increased by 8%, and the descending aortic diameter increased by 13%. During vest, conventional, and high-impulse external CPR, aortic pressure increased before any aortic flow was detected, ascending and descending aortic pressures increased simultaneously, the ratio of pulse pressure to stroke volume increased by a factor of 5.4 to 12 for all 3 techniques, and the diameter of the ascending and descending aorta decreased by 7% and 10% during vest and high-impulse CPR. Thus blood flow with external chest compression techniques appears to result from fluctuations in intrathoracic pressure.

▶ The mechanism by which internal cardiac massage, vest resuscitation, external high impulse manual compression, and conventional external resuscitation maintain blood flow was examined. External high-impulse manual compression differs from conventional chest compression in that compression strokes are rapid and jabbing, whereas conventional compression resuscitation emphasizes slower and more sustained compression strokes. The results indicate that the

3 modalities of external chest compression (vest, high impulse, and conventional) induce the flow of blood by similar physiologic means, i.e., by fluctuations in intrathoracic pressure. It will be of interest to ascertain which technique is the most effective in resuscitation in arrest situations.—J.T. Barron, M.D., Ph.D., and J.E. Parrillo, M.D.

Improved Patient Survival After Cardiac Arrest Using a Cardiopulmonary Support System
Reichman RT, Joyo CI, Dembitsky WP, Griffith LD, Adamson RM, Daily PO, Overlie PA, Smith SC Jr, Jaski BE (Univ of California, San Diego)
Ann Thorac Surg 49:101–105, 1990   2–2

Cardiopulmonary resuscitation (CPR) techniques are widely used, but according to 1 study only 14% of patients who survive in-hospital cardiac arrest are discharged. A portable cardiopulmonary support system (CPS) was used instead of standard CPR techniques on 38 patients with cardiovascular collapse refractory to advanced cardiac life support protocol. The portable CPS system permits rapid deployment in a nonsurgical setting by using the nursing staff. Diagnoses included postcardiotomy deterioration, failed coronary angioplasty, major trauma, myocardial infarction with cardiogenic shock, and pulmonary embolus. Percutaneous or cutdown cannulation sites were individualized.

Thirty-six of the 38 patients (95%) were successfully resuscitated to a stable rhythm. Eighteen of the 36 were successfully weaned, but 12 died later in the hospital including 5 who died of CNS failure and 3 who died of multisystem failure. Eight early deaths resulted from massive hemorrhage, 10 were caused by irreversible myocardial injury, and 2 resulted from inability to cannulate. Eight diagnostic procedures, including coronary angiography, pulmonary angiography, and aortography, were performed on patients who were on the CPS system. Six long-term survivors were salvaged by using this system.

It is encouraging that 6 of 38 patients in whom standard CPR was ineffective and who had an otherwise fatal arrhythmia were treated successfully with the CPS System, providing time for diagnostic studies to be performed. Clinical trials of the CPS system for early use in selected critically ill patients are recommended.

▶ In the setting of cardiopulmonary arrest, failure to respond to advanced cardiac life support protocols usually implies the patient's death. This is not universally the case when cardiopulmonary bypass is immediately available (generally in an operating room setting or in a cardiovascular intensive care unit). Animal models of fibrillatory arrest using cardiopulmonary bypass have suggested considerable potential for the bypass technique. Human studies, although demonstrating occasional salvage, have not been equally impressive (1). This study documents the survival to discharge of 6 of 38 patients in cardiopulmonary arrest after failure to respond to standard arrest protocols associated with the use of a portable cardiopulmonary bypass system.

Although this approach has some potential in tertiary care centers where the necessary expertise and support are likely to be available, the utility of the system in broader settings is doubtful. The approach is highly labor intensive and most institutions are unlikely to be able to provide the highly trained nurses, perfusionists, and physicians required. In addition, simpler, noninvasive, nonstandard resuscitative techniques involving the use of α-adrenergic agents, new antiarrhythmics, and new compressive techniques currently under investigation may ultimately allow similar salvage of current resuscitative failures.— A. Kumar, M.D., and J.E. Parrillo, M.D.

Reference

1. Hartz R, et al: *Ann Thorac Surg* 50:437, 1990.

Increases in Coronary Vein CO_2 During Cardiac Resuscitation

Gudipati CV, Weil MH, Gazmuri RJ, Deshmukh HG, Bisera J, Rackow EC (Univ of Health Sciences/Chicago Med School, North Chicago, Ill)
J Appl Physiol 68:1405–1408, 1990   2–3

Studies of the cause of acidosis during cardiopulmonary resuscitation (CPR) have reached varying conclusions. Although such acidosis is believed to result primarily from the anaerobic production of lactic acid when oxygen transport is critically reduced, recent reports have suggested a role for myocardial CO_2 production during CPR. The aortic, mixed venous, and great cardiac vein acid-base changes were studied in 8 female, domestic pigs during cardiac arrest and CPR.

Cardiac arrest was produced in the animals by ventricular fibrillation (VF). Chest compressions were initiated after 5 minutes of VF. After 13 minutes of VF, a 300-J direct-current countershock was delivered with a conventional defibrillator until normal sinus rhythm was restored or asystole appeared. The arterial CO_2 pressure (PCO_2) was unchanged during CPR, whereas the great cardiac vein PCO_2 increased from a control value of 52 torr to 132 torr. Thus the coronary venoarterial PCO_2 increased significantly from 13 torr to 94 torr. Great cardiac vein lactate concentrations, measured simultaneously, increased from .64 mmol/L to 7.4 mmol/L. Increases in the lactate content of aortic blood were far more moderate, from .64 mmol/L to 2.56 mmol/L.

During CPR, increases in great cardiac vein PCO_2 and lactate were highly correlated. The coronary venoarterial PCO_2 gradient returned to normal levels within 2 minutes after spontaneous circulation was restored with CPR. Within 30 minutes after CPR, the lactate content was rapidly reduced and lactate extraction reestablished.

These findings may have important implications for an understanding of the primary acid-base defect that accompanies cardiac arrest as the result of VF. Despite the anaerobic production of lactate, markedly low coronary flow states such as those prevailing during cardiac arrest are associated with acidosis that results primarily from excesses of CO_2.

▶ The marked increase in the P_{CO_2} of blood from the great cardiac vein is attributable to buffering the lactic acid produced by the heart as a consequence of a switch to anaerobic glycolysis during hypoxic states. The H+ associated with the lactate anion combines with the HCO_3^- anion-forming carbonic acid. This dissociates to $CO_2 + H_2O$, thus causing an increase in P_{CO_2}. The authors argue that hypercarbia can depress myocardial contractile function. Therefore, they question the utility of administering bicarbonate buffers during arrest situations because it can lead to increased levels of CO_2, which can diminish cardiac resuscitability. If the hypothesis is correct that bicarbonate administration leads to hypercarbia in arrest situations, thereby diminishing resuscitability, it stands to reason that administration of a CO_2-consuming buffer in these situations would improve resuscitability. This group of investigators subsequently performed such a study, the results of which failed to support their hypothesis (1).—J.T. Barron, M.D., Ph.D., and J.E. Parrillo, M.D.

Reference

1. Kette F, et al: *Circulation* 81:1660, 1990.

Myocardial Acidosis Associated With CO_2 Production During Cardiac Arrest and Resuscitation
von Planta M, Weil MH, Gazmuri RJ, Bisera J, Rackow EC (Univ of Health Sciences/Chicago Med School, North Chicago, Ill)
Circulation 80:684–692, 1989   2–4

Significant hypercarbic acidosis is found in pulmonary arterial blood during cardiac arrest and cardiopulmonary resuscitation (CPR) in both patients and animals. The acid-base state of the myocardium was investigated during cardiac arrest, which was induced electrically in 11 anesthetized, mechanically ventilated domestic pigs. Precordial compression was begun 3 minutes after onset of ventricular fibrillation and continued for 8 minutes.

Intramyocardial hydrogenion concentration $[H^+]$ increased significantly during ventricular fibrillation and promptly fell when spontaneous circulation returned. Cardiac venous P_{CO_2}, $[H^+]$, and lactate peaked in the fourth minute of fibrillation, 1 minute after the start of external chest compression. Marked myocardial production of CO_2 accompanied CPR, but the cardiac venous HCO_3^- was only modestly reduced. Coronary perfusion pressure correlated closely with the end-tidal P_{CO_2}.

Myocardial acidosis during cardiac arrest is associated with intramyocardial production of CO_2 and lactate but no marked change in extracellular bicarbonate. Bicarbonate therapy may be counterproductive if it increases production of CO_2.

▶ The P_{CO_2} of cardiac vein blood was significantly greater than that of mixed venous blood, indicating that the myocardial production of CO_2 during CPR is disproportionately increased. Evidence is presented suggesting that this precipitous rise in myocardial CO_2 production accounts for the profound intramyocardial acidosis that was observed. The authors argue that administration of bicarbonate buffer during CPR may actually increase myocardial CO_2 levels. When administered HCO_3^- combines with $H+$, carbonic acid is formed, generating CO_2. This excess CO_2 readily diffuses across cell membranes, and the diffusion of HCO_3^- is delayed. Theoretically, this should result in worsening intracellular acidosis. However, in a subsequent study, the authors failed to demonstrate such an adverse effect on intramyocardial pH (1). It is our opinion that the imprimatur against the use of bicarbonate in arrest situations needs more experimental support before it is applied generally.—J.T. Barron, M.D., Ph.D., and J.E. Parrillo, M.D.

Reference

1. Kette F, et al: *Circulation* 81:1660, 1990.

Early Predictors of Mortality for Hospitalized Patients Suffering Cardiopulmonary Arrest
Roberts D, Landolfo K, Light RB, Dobson K (Univ of Manitoba, Winnipeg)
Chest 97:413–419, 1990   2–5

Factors predicting mortality were sought in 310 consecutive patients who required advanced cardiac life support. Whereas 37% of the patients were successfully resuscitated, only 10% survived to be discharged from the hospital. Compliance with advanced cardiac life support standards was good.

Age did not correlate with survival. Patients with chronic renal failure and those with cardiogenic shock or left ventricular failure in association with acute myocardial infarction had very poor outcomes, but increased age was not predictive of mortality. In addition, survivors were among those with sepsis, pneumonia, or malignancy. Unwitnessed events and the need for epinephrine both correlated closely with in-hospital mortality, as did identification of electromechanical dissociation or asystole as the initial rhythm. A cardiac, rather than a respiratory, mechanism of arrest also was closely associated with hospital mortality. The duration of resuscitative effort did not distinguish survivors from patients who died in the hospital. Patients who were resuscitated but then died in hospital took up more time in intensive care after cardiopulmonary resuscitation than did those who were discharged.

Prearrest variables are generally not useful in predicting survival. In many patients, it is possible to make decisions on proceeding with or extending resuscitative efforts only after resuscitation is in progress.

▶ Identification of variables associated with a fatal outcome after cardiopulmonary resuscitation (CPR) has the potential to reduce resource expenditure on ultimately futile medical support and to avoid inappropriate prolongation of the lives of dying patients. Unlike previous studies (1,2), this report suggests that advanced age is *not* associated with significantly poorer outcome. Further, in contrast to Bedell et al. (1), malignancy and sepsis were not uniformly associated with fatal outcome, suggesting that the decision to offer CPR in those settings should be individualized.

The uniform association of electromechanical dissociation and prolonged asystole with fatal outcome suggests that intra-arrest variables may be of more use than prearrest variables in clinical decision making with reference to ultimate outcome. In particular, based on this study, the utility of resuscitation of asystolic, electromechanical dissociative and unwitnessed in-hospital arrests should be reassessed.—A. Kumar, M.D., and J.E. Parrillo, M.D.

References

1. Bedell SE, et al: *N Engl J Med* 309:569, 1990.
2. George AL, et al: *Am J Med* 87:28, 1989.

New and Old Paradoxes: Acidosis and Cardiopulmonary Resuscitation
Jaffe AS (Washington Univ)
Circulation 80:1079–1083, 1989   2–6

Some time ago, metabolic acidosis was considered to be frequent during cardiopulmonary resuscitation (CPR) and to compromise cellular metabolism and promote ventricular fibrillation. The physiology on which these assumptions were based has proved to be quite complex. Studies by von Planta et al. demonstrated that intramyocardial acidosis caused by anaerobic metabolism was greater than expected from measurements in mixed venous blood or coronary effluent. Acidosis in arterial blood, however, was less frequent and severe than formerly thought, for reasons that are not clear.

Sodium bicarbonate, once thought to be a benign and obvious intervention during CPR, has since been shown to induce hyperosmolarity, hypernatremia, and transient alkalosis, with induction of arrhythmias. In addition, the ventricular de fibrillation threshold in animals has been shown to be independent of arterial pH, and attentuation of vasopressor effects of high-dose exogenous catecholamines as a result of a low pH has not been proven. Adverse effects of intravenous bicarbonate administration attributable to accentuation of intracellular acidosis have been proposed by a number of authorities.

Early definitive care is the best means of optimizing resuscitation and avoiding the problems of acidosis and low perfusion. An aggressive approach to defibrillation will reduce the number of cardiac arrests in any setting. The American Heart Association is promoting the use of automated and semiautomated defibrillators in advanced cardiac life support programs. The widespread presence of such devices in public places may minimize the sequelae of intramyocardial acidosis and save lives.

▶ The use of bicarbonate during CPR remains controversial. Evidence has accumulated that the effects of sodium bicarbonate, once a mainstay of CPR, are useless at best and potentially detrimental. Recent animal studies have not shown a benefit of bicarbonate administration in models of CPR (1). Unfortunately, viable alternative buffering strategies have not been proven. Currently, the routine administration of sodium bicarbonate is no longer recommended in advanced cardiac life support protocols. The use of sodium bicarbonate based on arterial blood gas analysis is still recommended, however.

The controversy regarding the use of buffering agents such as sodium bicarbonate reflects other current concerns about improvements in the delivery of CPR, such as the use of α-adrenergic agents in place of epinephrine and improvements in techniques and understanding of compression-ventilation. Such techniques, as well as automation of defibrillation devices to allow their use by paramedical personnel, may dramatically alter the delivery of CPR in the future.—A. Kumar, M.D., and J.E. Parrillo, M.D.

Reference

1. Guerci AD, et al: *Circulation* 74:IV75, 1986.

Four Case Studies: High-Dose Epinephrine in Cardiac Arrest
Martin D, Werman HA, Brown CG (Ohio State Univ)
Ann Emerg Med 19:322–326, 1990   2–7

Results of hemodynamic studies in animals and human beings suggest that epinephrine at doses higher than currently recommended may improve resuscitation rates after prolonged cardiac arrest. Data were reviewed on 4 patients who failed to respond to a standard protocol for cardiac arrest and were given larger doses of epinephrine.

The 4 cardiac arrest victims failed to respond after 20–45 minutes of cardiopulmonary resuscitation (CPR) and standard 1-mg doses of epinephrine. Thereafter, larger doses of epinephrine, .12–.22 mg/kg, were administered by peripheral intravenous bolus injection. Within 5 minutes perfusing rhythms developed in all 4 patients, with maximum systolic blood pressures ranging from 134 mm Hg to 222 mm Hg. Cardiac dysrhythmias and metabolic alterations did not occur after these high doses.

Cardiac enzymes were increased in all patients, but only 1 had pathologic evidence of acute myocardial infarction, which, historically, appeared before the administration of high-dose epinephrine. All patients sustained severe brain injury and died. This was probably because of prolonged cardiopulmonary arrest and global brain ischemia. Clinical trials are warranted to establish the role of high-dose epinephrine as the initial pharmacologic intervention in selected patients during prehospital CPR.

▶ High dosages of epinephrine are commonly used in arrest situations as a "last ditch" effort after prolonged CPR when no or an insufficient response is obtained with a conventional regimen using low dosages of epinephrine. However, by the time the high-dose regimen is employed, there probably is significant compromise of blood flow to critical organs, very commonly resulting in irreversible organ injury. Therefore, the use of high dosages in the early stages of CPR has been advocated. Against this approach, however, is the potentially deleterious effect of high dosages of epinephrine on the cardiovascular system, which could negate the salutary effects. The deleterious effects include induction of malignant ventricular arrhythmias, elevation of blood pressure to dangerous levels, adverse metabolic effects, and direct myocardial cell toxicity. In these 4 cases, high-dose epinephrine was indeed of benefit in reestablishing the circulation, but all 4 patients subsequently died nevertheless. Had these patients received high dosages of epinephrine earlier, would the outcome have been more favorable? We agree that clinical trials comparing the low-dose and high-dose regimens are desperately needed.—J.T. Barron, M.D., Ph.D., and J.E. Parrillo, M.D.

Time-Dependent Risk of and Predictors for Cardiac Arrest Recurrence in Survivors of Out-of-Hospital Cardiac Arrest With Chronic Coronary Artery Disease
Furukawa T, Rozanski JJ, Nogami A, Moroe K, Gosselin AJ, Lister JW (Miami Heart Inst, Miami Beach)
Circulation 80:599–608, 1989   2–8

Survivors of out-of-hospital cardiac arrest unassociated with acute myocardial infarction have an increased risk of subsequent life-threatening ventricular tachyarrhythmias. To assess the risk of cardiac arrest recurrence with time and the influence of various clinical, angiographic, and electrophysiologic parameters on subsequent cardiac arrest recurrence with time, 101 patients with chronic coronary artery disease but without acute myocardial infarction who had survived out-of-hospital cardiac arrest were followed prospectively for a mean period of 27 months (range, 6 days to 63 months).

In the control state, 76 patients (75%) had inducible ventricular tachyarrhythmias that could be suppressed by antiarrhythmic drugs or surgery in 32. During follow-up, cardiac arrest recurred in 21 patients, including 2 of 25 patients without inducible ventricular tachyarrhythmias in the control state, 3 of 32 patients with inducible ventricular tachyarrhythmias in the control state that was suppressed after treatment, and 16 of 44 patients with inducible ventricular tachyarrhythmias in the control state that could not be suppressed after treatment (Fig 2–1). Cumulative cardiac arrest recurrence at 4 years was significantly higher

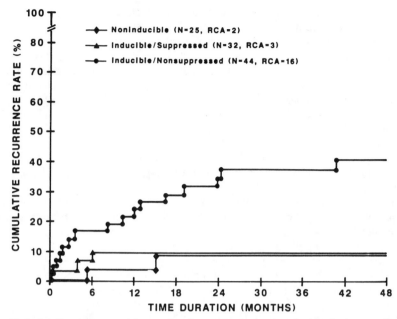

Fig 2–1.—Cumulative actuarial curve of cardiac arrest recurrence in each of the 3 subgroups of ventricular tachyarrhythmia inducibility. Patients who had nonsuppressible tachyarrhythmia had a significantly higher recurrence rate than those with no inducible tachyarrhythmia ($P = .0154$) or those with an inducible tachyarrhythmia that was suppressible by treatment ($P = .0191$). *Abbreviation: RCA,* recurrence of cardiac arrest. (Courtesy of Furukawa T, Rozanski JJ, Nogami A, et al: *Circulation* 80:599–608, 1989.)

among patients with inducible ventricular tachyarrhythmias in the control state that could not be suppressed by treatment.

The actuarial rate of cardiac arrest recurrence was 11.2% during the first 6 months of follow-up (high-risk early phase) and then decreased to less than 4% for each subsequent 6-month period. Multivariate Cox proportional hazards analysis showed that an ejection fraction of less than 35% was the only significant predictor for early phase (≤6 months) recurrence, whereas persistent inducibility of ventricular tachyarrhythmia was the strongest predictor for late phase (>6 months) recurrence. Although clinical congestive heart failure was also predictive, an ejection fraction of less than 35% had only marginal predictive value of late-phase recurrence. Time-dependent risk factor analysis allows ongoing assessment of risk on an individual basis.

► This study of survivors of out-of-hospital cardiac arrest with coronary artery disease but without evidence of acute myocardial infarction suggests that the incidence of subsequent cardiac mortality varies with the duration of survival after the initial cardiac arrest. Specifically, early mortality is dependent on cardiac function, whereas late mortality is most strongly associated with persistent inducibility of ventricular tachyarrhythmias on electrophysiologic studies. Such studies of the changing time dependence of various predictors of cardiac arrest recurrence will help to develop ongoing protocols to assess individual risk and tailor therapy.

In addition, this study clearly demonstrates that patients with a history of cardiopulmonary arrest, congestive heart failure (or ejection fraction less than 35%), and inducible ventricular tachyarrhythmias in the control state that are not suppressed after treatment have an impressively higher cumulative mortality rate than other groups. This group, in particular, must have early assessment for placement of an implantable defibrillator.—A. Kumar, M.D., and J.E. Parrillo, M.D.

Biogenic Amine Metabolites in Human CSF After Hypoxia Due to Cardiac Arrest

Odink J, Kärkelä J, Thissen JTNM, Marnela K-M (TNO-CIVO Toxicology and Nutrition Inst, Zeist; TNO Inst of Applied Computer Science, Wageningen, The Netherlands; Univ Central Hosp, Tampere; Univ of Tampere, Finland)
Acta Neurol Scand 80:6–11, 1989   2–9

Changes in the metabolism of biogenic amines in the CNS caused by hypoxia resulting from cardiac arrest have been reported, but the significance of these changes is unclear. To determine whether the concentrations of monoamine metabolites in the CSF may be predictive of the outcome of hypoxic brain damage, concentrations of 3-methoxy-4-hydroxyphenylglycol (MHPG), 5-hydroxyindole-3-acetic acid (5-HIAA), and homovanillic acid (HVA) were measured in the CSF of 20 resuscitated patients with hypoxia attributable to circulatory arrest and 10 controls who had spinal anesthesia. Among the resuscitated subjects, 8 recovered neurologically and 12 recovered with neurologic deficits. Of the latter, 5 lived longer than 76 hours after resuscitation and 12 died within 76 hours.

Among the neurologically disabled patients, initial CSF concentrations of MHPG, 5-HIAA, and HVA were significantly higher in the subgroup who died within 76 hours. In comparison with values in controls, the MHPG concentration showed a linear increase with time in neurologically disabled patients but decreased with time in the recovered patients. Similarly, 5-HIAA concentrations increased with time in the neurologically disabled patients but declined in the recovered patients after an initial rise. There were no significant changes with time in HVA concentrations. Concentrations of monoamine metabolites in the CSF may be prognostic for hypoxic brain injury after cardiac arrest, with high concentrations of MHPG, 5-HIAA, and HVA suggesting a poor prognosis.

▶ These authors have investigated the correlation of CSF levels of biogenic amine metabolites in humans after transient ischemia produced by cardiac arrest. Patients who had the highest CSF levels of biogenic amine metabolites 4 hours after onset of spontaneous circulation had the worst overall outcome. Although these results may lead one to mechanistic questions, it is impossible to determine from this study whether elevated CSF concentrations of biogenic amine metabolites indicate that catecholamines are important mediators in ischemic brain injury, or whether elevated amine metabolites are simply non-specific indicators of brain injury.

It is of concern that CSF is obtained from patients via the lumbar subarachnoid space because the amine concentration of fluid in this space may not accurately represent the concentrations of fluid around the cerebral hemispheres and the lateral ventricles. In addition, taking fluid from this space may lead to herniation of brain from the intracranial vault if intracranial pressure is elevated from diffuse brain edema. Additional studies will be needed before results from this study can be used clinically. For example, it would be interesting to know whether changes in the concentration of CSF biogenic amine metabolites predicted outcome independent of other predictors (i.e., CC-CPK, duration of arrest, serum glucose, concurrent diseases).—J.R. Kirsch, M.D.

Epinephrine and Norepinephrine in Cardiopulmonary Resuscitation: Effects on Myocardial Oxygen Delivery and Consumption

Lindner KH, Ahnefeld FW, Schuermann W, Bowdler IM (Universitaet Ulm, Germany)
Chest 97:1458–1462, 1990   2–10

Myocardial blood flow appears to be increased after administration of epinephrine during cardiopulmonary resuscitation (CPR), although cardiac output is unchanged or even diminished. Epinephrine, the accepted drug of choice in all forms of cardiac arrest, may fail to improve the balance between myocardial oxygen delivery and myocardial oxygen consumption. Norepinephrine was evaluated as an alternative to epinephrine in such cases.

The comparison between epinephrine and norepinephrine was carried out in 21 pigs with induced cardiac arrest. The animals received 7 minutes of open-chest cardiac massage after a period of 5 minutes of cardiopulmonary arrest. Seven animals each received placebo, epinephrine (45 μg/kg), or norepinephrine (45 μg/kg).

The 2 treatment groups each had significantly higher mean arterial blood pressure at 90 seconds than the control group. During CPR but before drug treatment, myocardial blood flow increased from 71 mL/min/100 g to 126 mL/min/100 g in the epinephrine-treated group and from 74 mL/min/100 g to 107 mL/min 100 g in the norepinephrine-treated group. Myocardial oxygen consumption increased from 4 mL/min/100 g to 9.4 mL/min/100 g after epinephrine, but from only 4.2 mL/min/100 g to 5.1 mL/min/100 g after norepinephrine. The greater increase in myocardial oxygen consumption with epinephrine resulted in an unchanged oxygen extraction ratio. But norepinephrine led to improvement in the ratio of myocardial oxygen delivery and myocardial oxygen consumption.

All of the animals in the norepinephrine group survived the 15-minute period of observation. In contrast, only 3 animals in each of the other groups survived. In this animal model, norepinephrine was superior to epinephrine in easing restoration of spontaneous circulation.

▶ The major determinant of survival after cardiopulmonary arrest is the time interval that precedes institution of effective CPR and restoration of cardiac function. Recently, considerable attention has been devoted to modifying resuscitation techniques in order to improve efficacy. The most important goals of any technique are to deliver adequate blood flow to the brain and heart. Epinephrine is a potent vasoconstrictor that increases central blood pressure during CPR. This presumably improves vital organ blood flow and accounts for its efficacy. The current paper indicates that norepinephrine results in similar increases in blood pressure and coronary blood flow. However, norepinephrine produces a smaller increase in myocardial oxygen consumption, suggesting that it may improve the oxygen supply:demand relationships in the heart. Consistent with this, more animals receiving norepinephrine were able to be successfully resuscitated. This is not the first paper to suggest a role for norepinephrine during CPR. I look forward to human trials.—M.J. Breslow, M.D.

3 Shock

Transformation of Neutrophils as Indicator of Irreversibility in Hemorrhagic Shock
Barroso-Aranda J, Schmid-Schönbein GW (Univ of California, San Diego)
Am J Physiol 257:H846–H852, 1989   3–1

Recent studies have shown that the presence of circulating polymorphonuclear neutrophils (PMNs) is prognostic of a lethal outcome after hemorrhagic shock. Polymorphonuclear neutrophils are thought to plug the microvasculature under low flow states of hypotension, leading to multiple organ failure.

The relationship between levels of activated circulating PMNs and survival was investigated in 30 rats that were subjected to a modified Wiggers hemorrhagic shock protocol. Hypotension was induced by a graded withdrawal of blood via a femoral artery catheter to an arterial pressure

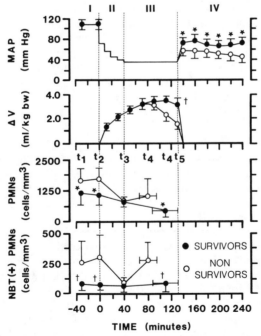

Fig 3–1.—Time course of hemorrhagic shock protocol (no. = 30) with 50% survival. *MAP*, mean arterial pressure; Δ V, volume removed; *PMNs*, total circulating neutrophil count; *NBT(+) PMNs*, nitro blue tetrazolium-positive PMNs. Each point represents mean ± 1 SD. In nonsurvivors, maximum shed volume was reached (t_4) on average 30 minutes earlier than in survivors. *$P < .01$, † $P < .005$. (Courtesy of Barroso-Aranda J, Schmid-Schönbein GW: *Am J Physiol* 257:H846–H852, 1989).

of 35 mm Hg. Hypotension was maintained at this pressure for 90 minutes. At the end of the hypotensive period, Plasma-lyte with albumin was infused at a volume equal to that of the shed blood. The animals were then observed for 24 hours for survival. Because activated PMNs have an increased capacity for reducing nitro blue tetrazolium (NBT) dye, NBT staining was used to count the number of circulating NBT-positive PMNs. Concentrations of circulating PMNs were recorded at baseline, just before bleeding, at the onset of hypotension, at the time of maximum shed volume, and at the end of the 90-minute hypotensive period.

Fifteen animals (50%) did not survive the 24-hour observation period. Four animals died abruptly during the hypotensive period, and the other 11 died later in the postshock period. None of the animals with circulating NBT-positive PMN counts of more than 225 cells per mm^3 before hemorrhage survived (Fig 3–1). All animals with circulating NBT-positive PMN counts of up to 135 cells per mm^3 before bleeding that maintained those low counts during the hypotensive period survived. Animals with low NBT-positive PMN counts before hemorrhage that had significantly elevated counts during the hypotensive period had a low probability for survival. Thus PMN activation is an index for survival after hemorrhagic shock.

▶ Polymorphonuclear neutrophils have been implicated in playing a role in the cascade from shock to endothelial injury and subsequent multisystem organ failure. These authors have demonstrated that in a rat model of hemorrhagic shock, PMN activation is associated with a poor prognosis. Presumably, reactive oxygen species generated by activated PMNs may be responsible for the end organ damage. In hemorrhagic as well as other forms of shock, pharmacologic maneuvers that limit or alter PMN activation may have a therapeutic application.— F.P. Ognibene, M.D., and J.E. Parrillo, M.D.

Emergency Percutaneous Cardiopulmonary Bypass Support in Cardiogenic Shock From Acute Myocardial Infarction
Shawl FA, Domanski MJ, Hernandez TJ, Punja S (Washington Adventist Hosp, Takoma Park, Md; Natl Heart, Lung, and Blood Inst, Bethesda, Md)
Am J Cardiol 64:967–970, 1989   3–2

In 8 consecutive patients with acute myocardial infarction in whom cardiogenic shock developed, cardiopulmonary bypass was established percutaneously to gain hemodynamic stability before coronary angioplasty. The systolic pressure was 80 mm Hg or below despite inotropic or in 1 patient intra-aortic balloon pump support. Signs of hypoperfusion was present. All patients had been in shock for less than 4 hours. Five patients were hospitalized at the time cardiogenic shock developed.

Bypass was instituted within 10 minutes in all cases. In most patients, bypass cannulas were placed in the right femoral system. Hemodynamic stability was achieved consistently, and the mixed venous saturation was at least 70%. Angioplasty was done in all but 1 of the patients. The average time on bypass was 66 minutes. Urine output improved during bypass in all instances. Six patients required transfusion.

Cardiopulmonary bypass can safely be established percutaneously to hemodynamically stabilize patients in cardiogenic shock. The procedure facilitates emergency coronary angioplasty. It remains to be learned whether this approach is superior to intra-aortic balloon counterpulsation.

▶ Despite a variety of therapeutic interventions, the mortality rate associated with cardiogenic shock complicating acute myocardial infarction exceeds 80%. Revascularization of the infarct-related artery using coronary angioplasty in the acute setting may improve survival. However, these patients are frequently too unstable hemodynamically to tolerate the angioplasty procedure. Shawl and co-investigators have demonstrated that emergency percutaneous cardiopulmonary bypass can be rapidly and safely performed with resultant cardiovascular stability so that angioplasty and attempts at revascularization can be undertaken. The large size of the catheters necessary for bypass (20 Fr) affords significant risk to patients with iliofemoral disease and complicates their use in these patients. Local hemorrhage is also a problem. In addition, there have been no data generated that this technique offers a greater advantage than intra-aortic balloon counterpulsation in most patients with cardiogenic shock. Intra-aortic balloon counterpulsation should be attempted initially and bypass used only if this fails. These authors suggest that in cases of cardiac arrest or profound cardiac failure this technique seems to provide the only modality possible to stabilize the patient in order to undergo coronary angioplasty. Pending more definitive data, it seems that this temporizing technique should be reserved only for the patient with either cardiac arrest or severe pump failure in whom angioplasty and coronary revascularization will be attempted, and it should be performed only by operators adequately skilled in the technique of percutaneous bypass.—F.P. Ognibene, M.D., and J.E. Parrillo, M.D.

O_2 Uptake in Bled Dogs After Resuscitation With Hypertonic Saline or Hydroxyethylstarch

Reinhart K, Rudolph T, Bredle DL, Cain SM (Univ of Alabama, Birmingham)
Am J Physiol 257:H238–H243, 1989   3–3

It is not clear how relatively small volumes of hypertonic saline are of clinical benefit. To detect a local effect of hypertonic saline on tissue oxygen extraction, and to determine whether improved peripheral oxygen utilization might help to explain the usefulness of hypertonic saline in resuscitation from shock, studies were performed on both the whole body and isolated hindlimb of anesthetized dogs during resuscitation from hemorrhagic shock. A mean arterial pressure of 40 mm Hg was maintained for 30 minutes before resuscitation with either hypertonic saline, 5 mL/kg (about 16% of the shed blood volume), or hydroxyethylstarch in fourfold greater volume.

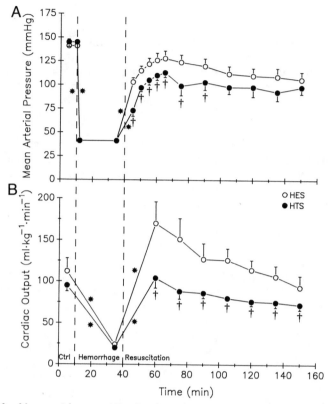

Fig 3–2.—Mean arterial pressure *(A)* and cardiac output *(B)* across all experimental conditions, control *(ctrl)*, hemorrhage, and resuscitation. All values are means ± SE. *HTS* indicates hypertonic saline group; *HES*, hydroxyethylstarch group. *Dagger* indicates significant difference *(P < .05)* between adjacent values within group. (Courtesy of Reinhart K, Rudolph T, Bredle DL, et al: *Am J Physiol* 257:H238–H243, 1989.)

Cardiac output, but not oxygen delivery, returned to baseline with hypertonic saline administration. After administration of hydroxyethylstarch, the cardiac output was greater than baseline and oxygen delivery was near baseline. Only with hydroxyethylstarch was excess oxygen uptake in recovery greater than the oxygen deficit during bleeding. Changes in vascular resistance in the isolated hindlimb were comparable with both regimens. As blood flow declined, the ability of limb muscle to extract oxygen was the same in both groups (Figs 3–2 and 3–3).

When acellular fluid is used for resuscitation from hemorrhagic shock, oxygen delivery may not be adequate even if the cardiac output and arterial pressure are restored to baseline. Overall resuscitation was better with larger amounts of hydroxyethylstarch than with small volumes of hypertonic saline in the present study.

▶ Resuscitation from hemorrhagic shock requires aggressive volume replacement. Whether to give colloid or crystalloid remains controversial, as does the quantity of volume replacement. The goals of this acute volume resuscitation

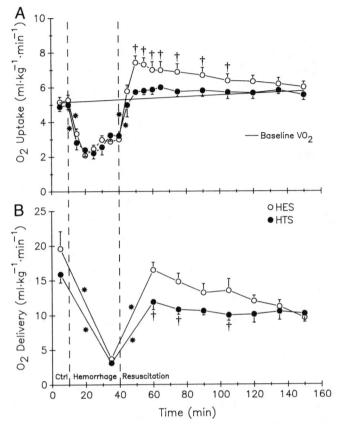

Fig 3–3.—Oxygen *(O₂)* uptake *(VO₂; A)* and *O₂* delivery *(B)* across all conditions. Definitions and symbols are as in Figure (Courtesy of Reinhart K, Rudolph T, Bredle DL, et al: *Am J Physiol* 257:H238–H243, 1989.)

remain restoration of blood pressure and maintenance of organ blood flow with end-organ vitality. These authors have demonstrated that restoration of blood pressure and cardiac output with an acellular fluid (hypertonic saline) in a hemorrhagic shock model may not deliver enough oxygen to a variety of vital tissues. Extrapolating to the clinical scenario, one must be aware that volume resuscitation measures in humans must be developed that restore blood pressure as well as provide optimal oxygen delivery and oxygen uptake. The ideal fluid for acute human volume resuscitation, as well as the quantities required for adequate organ function, will have to be determined in human clinical trials.—F.P. Ognibene, M.D., and J.E. Parrillo, M.D.

Effect of Lactic Acidosis on Canine Hemodynamics and Left Ventricular Function

Teplinsky K, O'Toole M, Olman M, Walley KR, Wood LDH (Univ of Chicago)
Am J Physiol 258 H1193–H1199, 1990   3–4

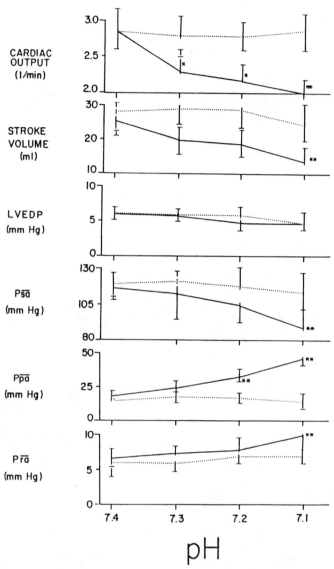

Fig 3-4.—Hemodynamic variables during progressive acidosis. Four stages of progressive acidosis (*solid lines*) are shown on *x*-axis along with time controls (*dotted lines*). P_{sa}, mean systemic arterial pressure; P_{pa}, mean pulmonary artery pressure; P_{ra}, mean right atrial pressure. Error bars are ± SD. *$P <$ .05 and $P <$ .01 compared with baseline stage. (Courtesy of Teplinsky K, O'Toole M, Olman M, et al: *Am J Physiol* 258:H1193–H1199, 1990).

Hypoperfusion states produce lactic acidosis. The acidemia further decreases the inadequate cardiac output. The adverse effect of lactic acidemia on cardiac output may be caused by depressed contractility shown in isolated myocardium. Alternatively, the factors that govern venous return may cause a relative hypovolemic state and/or acidemic pulmonary vasoconstriction-induced right ventricular dysfunction. It was hypothesized that examination of left ventricular (LV) pressure-volume relationships at end systole and end diastole would determine which of these possible mechanisms accounts for decreased cardiac output during progressive lactic acidosis in anesthetized, mechanically ventilated, dogs.

Nine mongrel dogs were studied. Left ventricular volume was estimated from 2 pairs of epicardial ultrasonic crystals in the anteroposterior and longitudinal planes. Left ventricular pressure was determined from a catheter-tipped transducer. Progressive acidemia was induced by a continuous intravenous infusion of .5N lactic acid.

During acidemia, cardiac output, stroke volume, and mean systemic arterial pressure dropped significantly, whereas mean pulmonary artery pressure and right atrial pressure significantly increased. Lactic acidemia produced a 40% decrease in stroke volume, which was attributable to depressed LV contractility, characterized by a reduction in maximum dP/d*t* and a drop in slope with no change in volume intercept of the LV pressure-volume relationship at end systole. Neither the measured LV end-diastolic pressure nor the estimated LV end-diastolic volume dropped with acidemia, which suggests that the reduced venous return did not result from relative hypovolemia. Acidemic pulmonary hypertension may have interfered with the expected response to myocardial depression, however (Fig 3–4).

Lactic acidosis results in a reduction in cardiac output as a consequence of decreasing stroke volume. This occurs primarily through a depression of myocardial contractility, possibly because of an inability to increase end-diastolic volume as a result of acute pulmonary hypertension.

▶ Progressive metabolic acidosis is typically characterized hemodynamically by a fall in cardiac output and hypotension that is difficult to reverse. In anesthetized dogs administered exogenous lactic acid, the authors document a reduction in ventricular performance evidenced by a decrease in the slope of the LV pressure/volume relationship at end systole and a reduction in stroke volume. The data also indicated that the fall in stroke volume did not result solely from absolute hypovolemia but, rather, may have been caused by the effects of acute pulmonary hypertension on LV filling. Because hypoperfusion itself leads to a lactic acidosis, it is clear that a vicious cycle develops unless both the acidosis and hypotension are resolved. In clinical practice, alkaline therapy alone is probably not effective in treating progressive lactic acidosis. Efforts to determine the cause of the lactic acidosis and to treat it aggressively are essential to reversing the hypotensive and hypocontractile clinical state characterized by progressive acidemia.—F.P. Ognibene, M.D., and J.E. Parrillo, M.D.

Hemodynamic and Oxygen Transport Variables in Cardiogenic Shock Secondary to Acute Myocardial Infarction, and Response to Treatment

Creamer JE, Edwards JD, Nightingale P (Univ Hosp of South Manchester, Manchester, England)
Am J Cardiol 65:1297–1300, 1990   3–5

Little is known about oxygen transport in cardiogenic shock after acute myocardial infarction. Oxygen transport variables in 19 such patients were examined and their responses to treatment assessed when possible.

Femoral and pulmonary arterial catheters were inserted before any treatment except for correction of hypoxemia in 8 patients, defibrillation in 3, or pacing in 5. Three patients had mean arterial pressures greater than 80 mm Hg and cardiac indices greater than 2.1 L/min/m^2, with normal mixed venous oxygen saturation despite simultaneous clinical shock. These patients recovered with no further intervention. Sixteen patients received varying combinations of intravenous fluids and dobutamine. Fourteen survived long enough for a second set of measurements to be taken. Mean heart rates rose from 83 beats per minute (bpm) to 101 bpm and mean cardiac indices from 1.4 L/min/m^2 to 2.5 L/min/m^2. Oxygen consumption was maintained even when oxygen delivery was less than 330 mL/min/m^2. Oxygen delivery rose from 230 mL/min/m^2 to 397 mL/min/m^2 and oxygen consumption from 103 mL/min/m^2 to 124 mL/min/m^2 after treatment. Mean mixed venous oxygen saturation rose from 54% to 69%, and the mean oxygen extraction ratio dropped from 48% to 31%. Cuff systolic blood pressure was not related to mean arterial pressure before or after resuscitation. Thirteen patients lived to be discharged from the hospital.

It may be relevant to measure oxygen transport variables during resuscitation from cardiogenic shock and to titrate treatment against increases in mixed venous saturation. When this approaches 60%, oxygen availability is such that survival may be possible.

▶ Oxygen transport variables have been measured in patients with many types of shock, and attempts have been made to associate improved survival with critical levels of oxygen delivery and oxygen consumption in these disease states. Creamer and co-authors have assessed these variables in a small group of patients with cardiogenic shock caused by myocardial infarction before and after resuscitative treatment with fluids and dobutamine. Survival data suggest that early increments in cardiac indices as well as secondary improvements in oxygen transport variables were associated with improvements in survival. However, the optimal pharmacologic agent and its optimal dose have not necessarily been identified, because therapy was limited only to fluids and dobutamine. As a result, it is difficult to determine what is the optimal mode of therapy, as well as the optimal goal of therapy, in patients with cardiogenic shock and impaired oxygen transport. Further study is necessary to confirm these preliminary data.—F.P. Ognibene, M.D., and J.E. Parrillo, M.D.

Effects of Coenzyme Q$_{10}$ in Hemorrhagic Shock
Yamada M (Showa Univ, Tokyo)
Crit Care Med 18:509–514, 1990   3–6

The extent of pulmonary injury caused by hemorrhagic shock and subsequent resuscitation is debated. Ubiquinone (coenzyme Q$_{10}$) (CoQ$_{10}$)

was recently reported to have salutary effects in various forms of shock and membrane-stabilizing effects. Cardiovascular and pulmonary functions and the mode of action of chemical mediators after CoQ_{10} pretreatment in hemorrhagic shock were investigated in a canine model of hemorrhagic shock.

One group of animals received CoQ_{10}, 10 mg/kg, before hemorrhage. The percent change from baseline of peak airway pressure, total lung compliance of the lung and chest wall, and blood lactate levels seemed to be significantly smaller in dogs pretreated with CoQ_{10} than in control dogs. Coenzyme Q_{10} was also found to maintain blood histamine levels and to attenuate the rise in leukotriene C_4.

Coenzyme Q_{10} significantly improved respiratory and metabolic functions during hemorrhagic shock in this animal study. It also had beneficial effects on chemical mediators. Further study of the pharmacology of CoQ_{10} is needed.

▶ Alterations in a variety of hemodynamic and pulmonary parameters in hemorrhagic as well as other types of shock are produced by a variety of known and as yet unknown mediators. Coenzyme Q, an important component of the electron transport chain of cell membranes, may limit some of the deleterious effects of these mediators in a canine model of hemorrhagic shock. However, much additional data will be required before its consideration for use in human clinical trials.—F.P. Ognibene, M.D., and J.E. Parrillo, M.D.

4 Septic Shock

Pentoxifylline Increases Survival in Murine Endotoxin Shock and Decreases Formation of Tumor Necrosis Factor
Schade UF (Forschungsinstitut Borstel, Borstel, Germany)
Circ Shock 31:171–181, 1990   4–1

Lipopolysaccharide (LPS), the active component in endotoxin-generated gram-negative bacterial infection, acts via endogenous mediators, particularly tumor necrosis factor (TNF). Previous studies have shown that treatment with pentoxifylline (POF), a xanthine derivative, improves survival in experimental lethal endotoxemia. To determine whether pretreatment with POF can protect against endotoxin shock after an LPS challenge, LPS was isolated from *Salmonella abortus equi* and administered to mice given POF usually 1 hour before challenge. The experiments were carried out under different conditions of endotoxin susceptibility, including normal, LPS tolerant, LPS hyperreactive, and D-galactosamine sensitized.

Pretreatment with POF in normal and LPS-tolerant mice significantly increased survival compared to that in nonpretreated controls challenged with LPS. Overall survival increased from 50% in controls to 90% in POF-pretreated normal and LPS-tolerant mice. The protective effect of POF in LPS-hypersensitized and D-galactosamine-sensitized animals against the LPS challenge was even more pronounced. Survival increased from 20% in non–pretreated controls to 90% in POF-pretreated animals. Pentoxifylline did not interfere with the development of tolerance to endotoxin. The protective effects of POF were dose dependent. A pretreatment dose of POF, 2 mg/kg, resulted in 40% survival, compared with 35% survival in untreated controls and 90% survival in mice pretreated with POF, 50 mg/kg. The protective effects were observed even when POF was administered up to 4 hours after the LPS challenge. Pentoxifylline effectively inhibited the appearance of TNF in the serum of D-galactosamine-sensitized animals on LPS challenge. In this series, POF prevented LPS lethal toxicity in mice under various conditions of endotoxin susceptibility.

▶ Several studies using models of septic shock have demonstrated some therapeutic benefit of POF. In particular, this study in rodents supports a widely held hypothesis that POF alters endotoxin-induced tissue injury by inhibiting TNF release from macrophages. No data from large animal models of sepsis are available to demonstrate that POF has an effect on survival. Thus further studies of POF in large animals are warranted to confirm its potential therapeutic role in human septic shock.—C. Natanson, M.D., and J.E. Parrillo, M.D.

Renal Effects of Norepinephrine Used to Treat Septic Shock Patients
Martin C, Eon B, Saux P, Aknin P, Gouin F (Hôp Sainte Marguerite, Marseille, France)
Crit Care Med 18:282–285, 1990   4–2

Several studies have demonstrated that norepinephrine (NE) is effective in the treatment of patients with hyperdynamic septic shock. However, in normotensive and hypertensive patients NE can have deleterious effects on the renal circulation that may lead to acute renal failure. A study in normotensive dogs showed that the addition of low-dose dopamine to NE enhances renal blood flow. Thus the concomitant administration of low-dose dopamine and NE in patients with hyperdynamic septic shock may prevent renal ischemia and renal failure.

To assess renal function in patients with septic shock treated with NE infusion, with or without the addition of dobutamine and/or dopamine, a review was made of the records of 19 men and 5 women (mean age, 55 years) admitted to the intensive care unit with septic shock. All required mechanical ventilation because of concomitant acute respiratory failure. After fluid resuscitation 8 patients were treated with NE alone, 8 were given NE plus dobutamine, and 8 received NE plus dobutamine and low-dose dopamine.

Infusion of NE resulted in either an increase in blood pressure, no change, or an increase in the cardiac index; it restored the systemic vascular resistance index to the normal range. In 20 of the 24 patients normalization of systemic hemodynamic variables was followed by reestablishment of urinary flow, a decrease in the serum concentration of creatinine, and an increase in creatinine clearance. None of the 20 had received low-dose dopamine. The other 4 patients remained oliguric despite normalization of systemic hemodynamic variables. All had received low-dose dopamine. Two of these patients died and acute renal failure developed in the other 2.

It appears that NE can be used safely to increase vascular resistance in patients with hyperdynamic septic shock. It may improve renal blood flow and renal vascular resistance.

▶ Martin and co-workers have shown in a small, retrospective study that the early use of NE to support the blood pressure in patients with septic shock is frequently associated with improvement in renal function. The use of low-dose dopamine with NE could not be properly addressed in this retrospective study. Nonetheless, this study confirms the clinical findings of several other investigators that NE is useful to stabilize the hemodynamic status of patients with septic shock who remain hypotensive despite adequate fluid resuscitation. Whether concomitant low-dose dopamine administration will provide any additional benefit must be addressed in a larger, prospective study. There is at least a theoretical rationale for this regimen supported by data from animal studies. Until further studies in humans are reported, the clinician must use his/her own judgment in choosing vasopressor support based on knowledge of the usual cardiovascular and multisystem abnormalities typical of septic shock.—M.M. Parker, M.D.

Endotoxin-Induced Shock in the Rat: A Role for C5a
Smedegård G, Cui L, Hugli TE (Pharmacia A, Uppsala, Sweden; Chinese Academy of Med Sciences, Beijing; Scripps Clinic, LaJolla, Calif)
Am J Pathol 135:489–497, 1989   4–3

Gram-negative sepsis, a prominent cause of circulatory failure, is believed to be an underlying cause of adult respiratory distress syndrome. Results of previous studies have implicated activation of the complement system and the subsequent formation of anaphylatoxins such as C3a and C5a. A rat model of sepsis was developed to assess the role of C5a in the changes induced by lipopolysaccharide (LPS) injection.

Results of in vitro studies indicated that both the IgG fraction and $F(ab')_2$ fragments of rabbit antirat C5a antibody neutralized purified C5a or C5a in serum. In vivo studies used only the $F(ab')_2$ fragments. Injection of $C5a_{des\ Arg}$ into rats led to an immediate fall in arterial pressure followed by rapid recovery. Polymorphonuclear cell counts decreased markedly at the same time and circulating platelets decreased. Injection of LPS produced increased plasma levels of both C3a and C5a. Levels of C5a were significantly reduced in animals given $F(ab')_2$ fragments, and the LPS-induced decrease in arterial pressure was attenuated. The decrease in polymorphonuclear cells induced by LPS was not influenced by administration of $F(ab')_2$ fragments of antirat C5a. Lung edema also was unaffected.

These findings confirm a role for complement activation in mediating the changes produced by LPS. Antianaphylatoxin antibodies are helpful in studying the role of complement whenever activation of the complement system is implicated pathophysiologically.

▶ Like many other mediators, C3a and C5a have been implicated as having a role in the pathophysiology of septic shock. This study used antibodies to C5a to provide further support for this role. Specific neutralizing antibodies are valuable tools for studying the place of various mediators in septic shock, as well as in other disorders. Whether the use of neutralizing antibodies will provide clinical benefit in humans with septic shock will require extensive investigation, but the first step is defining the role of each mediator and its interaction with other mediators.—M.M. Parker, M.D.

Survival of Primates in LD_{100} Septic Shock Following Therapy With Antibody to Tumor Necrosis Factor (TNF-α)
Hinshaw LB, Tekamp-Olson P, Chang ACK, Lee PA, Taylor FB Jr, Murray CK, Peer GT, Emerson TE Jr, Passey RB, Kuo GC (Oklahoma Med Research Found, Oklahoma City; Univ of Oklahoma; Chiron Corp, Emeryville, Calif; Miles Inc, Berkeley)
Circ Shock 30:279–292, 1990   4–4

In previous studies, pretreatment of baboons with fragments of monoclonal antibody (MoAB) to tumor necrosis factor (anti-TNF) before *Es-*

Dosages of *Escherichia coli* Administered to Baboons, and Survival Times

Baboon No. and expt.*	Wt (kg)	Sex	Dose	Survival time
3 C	7.7	M	6.6×10^{10}	12 hr
4 C	7.3	M	6.0×10^{10}	13 hr
5 C (+ isotype)	6.4	FM	6.5×10^{10}	21 hr
6 C (+ isotype)	6.5	FM	4.1×10^{10}	34 hr
8 C	6.4	FM	5.6×10^{10}	15 hr
11 C (+ isotype)	6.8	FM	6.3×10^{10}	18 hr
Mean	6.9		5.9×10^{10}	19 hr
7 E	6.0	M	4.8×10^{10}	> 7 days
8B E	7.3	M	5.0×10^{10}	> 7 days
9 E	6.8	FM	3.5×10^{10}	> 7 days
10 E	6.1	FM	6.0×10^{10}	> 7 days
12 E	6.8	FM	5.3×10^{10}	> 7 days
13 E	6.4	FM	5.8×10^{10}	> 7 days
Mean	6.6		5.1×10^{10}	> 7 days

*C, *control* (*E. coli* only); E, experimental (*E. coli* and antibody to TNF).
(Courtesy of Hinshaw LB, Tekamp-Olson P, Chang ACK, et al: *Circ Shock* 30:279–292, 1990.)

cherichia coli infusion prevented septic shock. Whether early posttreatment with anti-TNF MoAB would prevent death in baboons subjected to lethal *E. coli*-induced shock was determined.

Twelve baboons were given 2-hour infusions of a lethal dose of *E. coli*. Thirty minutes after the infusion was begun, 6 animals received a bolus of anti-TNF MoAB at a dose of 15 mg/kg. The 6 control animals were left untreated. The animals were monitored for 10 hours, observed continuously for another 36 hours, and observed daily thereafter for a maximum of 7 days. After all *E. coli* organisms had been delivered, all animals were treated with gentamicin for up to 3 days. Surviving animals were killed after the seventh day of observation for gross and histologic evaluations.

The mean survival time in the control group was 19 hours; survival ranged from 12 to 34 hours (table). All 6 animals treated with anti-TNF MoAB survived for the 7-day study period. The quality of life of the MoAB-treated animals was significantly improved compared with that of the controls. The MoAB-treated baboons were active, alert, and drinking on the day after the *E. coli* challenge, whereas the control animals were either moribund or already dead by the next day. Near-normal arterial pressures were maintained in the MoAB-treated animals during the monitoring period, and serum urea nitrogen and creatinine levels also remained normal. The severe histopathologic changes seen in the lungs, liver, adrenals, kidneys, and spleen of control animals were absent in the treated animals.

▶ This paper by Hinshaw et al. confirms the results of Tracey et al. (1), showing that MoABs directed at TNF improve survival in baboons injected with a lethal dose of bacteria. In addition, Hinshaw et al. demonstrate that MoABs to TNF are therapeutic even when given 30 minutes after the start of a bacterial infusion. In the previous study by Tracey et al., MoABs to TNF were beneficial only when administered more than 30 minutes before the bacterial challenge. This investigation supports results from other studies indicating that TNF is an important mediator in septic shock. The findings further suggest that therapies directed against TNF may be efficacious in treatment of the disease.—C. Natanson, M.D., and J.E. Parrillo, M.D.

Reference

1. Tracey KJ, et al: *Nature* 330:662, 1987.

Cardiopulmonary Dysfunction in a Feline Septic Shock Model: Possible Role of Leukotrienes
Schützer K-M, Haglund U, Falk A (Renström's Hosp, Göteborg; Univ Hosp, Uppsala; Östra Hosp, Göteborg, Sweden)
Circ Shock 29:13–25, 1989   4–5

The arachidonic acid cascade, when activated in septic shock, produces different eicosanoids. The effects of eicosanoids derived from the cyclooxygenase pathway have been well studied, but less is known about the products derived from the lipooxygenase pathway. Previous studies demonstrated that leukotriene can reduce myocardial contractility and pulmonary compliance, and increase pulmonary airflow resistance.

Whether the LTs are involved in the development of cardiopulmonary dysfunction of septic shock was investigated in a feline septic shock model. Live *Escherichia coli* bacteria infusion was used to induce sepsis in anesthetized cats. Six cats had been pretreated with the 5-lipooxygenase inhibitor diethylcarbamazine (DEC), 7 cats had been pretreated with the LT antagonist FPL 55712, and 8 cats served as septic controls.

After 2 hours of bacteremia, there were no differences in cardiac function in any of the groups. However, after the heart was subjected to volume load by rapid intravenous dextran infusion, DEC-pretreated cats had significantly better preserved left ventricular function than cats in the other 2 groups. Pretreatment with either DEC or FPL 55712 did not affect early pulmonary vascular reactions, although the tracheal pressure response in pretreated animals was less pronounced than that in the controls. The increase in calculated airway resistance and the decrease in pulmonary compliance were also smaller in pretreated animals than in untreated controls. Furthermore, pretreatment prevented arterial hypoxia.

Leukotrienes may be involved in the development of myocardial insufficiency of experimental bacteremic septic shock. They are associated with compromise of pulmonary gas exchange, in part by their effects on the smaller airways.

▶ Recently, inhibitors of arachidonic acid metabolism such as ibuprofen (1) have been demonstrated to have beneficial hemodynamic effects in animal models of endotoxic shock. Most emphasis in such studies has centered on products (such as prostacyclin and thromboxane A2) and inhibition of the cyclo-oxygenase pathway.

This study expands on the mechanisms by which activation of the arachidonic cascade may cause cardiopulmonary dysfunction in septic shock. Leukotrienes, arachidonic acid metabolites derived from the 5-lipo-oxygenase pathway, are shown to be potential mediators of both the myocardial depression and the compromised pulmonary gas exchange seen in clinical sepsis.

Although the immediate potential of the leukotriene antagonists/inhibitors is limited by the fact that only pretreatment studies were performed, this and other studies (2,3) strongly argue that specific leukotriene inhibitors and antagonists should continue to be assessed as potential therapy in septic shock. If beneficial effects can be demonstrated with posttreatment protocols, human trials could follow. At this time, however, there is insufficient evidence to recommend the clinical use of any arachidonic acid cascade inhibitor.—A. Kumar, M.D., and J.E. Parrillo, M.D.

References

1. Balk RA, et al: *Crit Care Med* 16:1128, 1988.
2. Toth PD, et al: *Circ Shock* 15:89, 1985.
3. Hall-Angeras M, et al: *Circ Shock* 20:231, 1986.

Calcium Administration Increases the Mortality of Endotoxic Shock in Rats

Malcolm DS, Zaloga GP, Holaday JW (Uniformed Services Univ of Health Sciences, Bethesda, Md; Wake Forest Univ, Winston-Salem, NC; Walter Reed Army Inst of Research, Washington, DC)

Crit Care Med 17:900–903, 1989   4–6

Calcium chloride is often given to improve cardiac output and blood pressure in patients with septic shock. Recent studies have implicated calcium as a cause of shock and ischemic cell injury. To test the hypothesis that calcium may be deleterious to shock outcome, the effect of hypercalcemia and hypocalcemia on the hemodynamic responses to endotoxin and on short-term survival was studied in rats.

Hypercalcemia was induced in Sprague-Dawley rats by infusion of calcium chloride, and hypocalcemia was induced by infusion of ethylenebis (oxyethylenenitrilo) tetraacetic acid (EGTA). All boluses were given in a volume of 1 mL/kg and all infusions at a rate of 1 mL/hr. Two different calcium chloride doses were used. Controls received saline solution only. Blood samples were obtained after 30 minutes of infusion, after which the animals were given either *Escherichia coli* endotoxin or saline injection. The second blood sample was taken 60 minutes after endotoxin or saline injection. Mortality was assessed at 24 hours.

Infusion of EGTA lowered the ionized calcium level by 12%. The lower dose of calcium chloride increased the ionized calcium level by 20% and the higher dose by 107%. Endotoxin-induced mortality at 24 hours was 20%. Increasing the circulating ionized calcium concentration

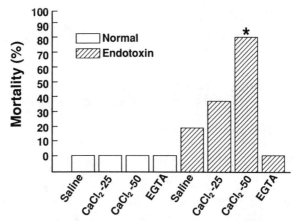

Fig 4–1.—Twenty-four-hour mortality in animals infused with saline, EGTA (30 mg/mL/hr), and calcium chloride (25 and 50 mg/mL/hr) in the presence *(striped bars)* and absence *(open bars)* of endotoxin (5 mg/kg intravenously to 10 animals per treatment group). *$P \leq .05$ compared with saline-treated animals for the endotoxin-treated groups only. (Courtesy of Malcolm DS, Zaloga GP, Holaday JW:*Crit Care Med* 17:900–903, 1989.)

progressively increased endotoxin lethality to 37% in the low-dose group and to 80% in the high-dose group, even though the mean arterial pressure (MAP) was slightly improved after calcium chloride administration (Fig 4–1). Administration of EGTA lowered endotoxin lethality to 0 without having any significant effect on the MAP. Calcium chloride, EGTA, and saline infusions given without endotoxin were not associated with any mortality.

High levels of circulating ionized calcium increase endotoxin lethality despite some improvement in MAP, whereas lowering the concentration of circulating ionized calcium decreases endotoxin lethality without affecting MAP. Caution should thus be used when administering calcium chloride to patients with septic shock.

▶ The study by Malcom et al. calls into question the benefit of using calcium in the management of hypotension from septic shock. Calcium infusions are not routinely part of the management of septic shock, but many clinicians occasionally use calcium either as a bolus or as an infusion in patients with refractory hypotension. This study suggests that calcium should be used with caution, if at all. Furthermore, if one extrapolates data from an animal model to humans, one might conclude that if calcium is used in the treatment of septic shock, care must be taken not to produce hypercalcemia. It would be very premature to suggest the use of calcium antagonists in humans, a point the authors emphasize in their discussion.—M.M. Parker, M.D.

Naloxone in Septic Shock
Hackshaw KV, Parker GA, Roberts JW (Columbia Univ; Harlem Hosp, New York)
Crit Care Med 18:47–51, 1990

Fluid replacement and antibiotic therapy are accepted treatments for septic shock, but the use of such agents as corticosteroids and naloxone remains controversial. Data on 13 consecutive patients in whom naloxone therapy was part of the routine management for septic shock were reviewed.

If blood pressure returned to near baseline values after a 1-L fluid challenge, naloxone was withheld while other forms of support were instituted. Patients resisting the challenge were given naloxone in an initial bolus of .03 mg/kg followed by infusion at a rate of .2 mg/kg.hr for 1 hour. After the infusion, continued supportive measures were maintained.

The mean arterial pressure (MAP) was significantly increased over baseline after the initial naloxone bolus. There was also a marked increase in systemic arterial blood pressure. All patients had at least a partial response to naloxone, defined as an increase in systolic blood pressure of 15 mm Hg and/or an increase of MAP of 13 mm Hg. Cardiac index, pulmonary capillary wedge pressure, and systemic vascular resistance were moderately, although not significantly, increased. There were no adverse reactions to the infusion. Only 1 patient survived. The remaining 12 patients died within an average of 69.4 hours after naloxone administration. Blood cultures were positive for bacterial organisms in 12 patients. The dosage of naloxone used in these patients was considerably higher than that previously reported. Its beneficial effect on MAP in early septic shock makes the drug useful as a temporizing agent while more appropriate antibiotic therapy is readied.

▶ Many studies, both in animals and in humans, have reported that naloxone can produce a temporary increase in blood pressure in patients with septic shock. No human study, however, has demonstrated any effect on outcome. This study by Hackshaw and co-workers also reports a transient (1 hour) increase in blood pressure after the administration of naloxone to a small number of patients with septic shock. Other than the increase in blood pressure, no effects were seen, including no other hemodynamic effects and no improvement in pH. Twelve of the 13 patients in the study died. Despite the fact that there were no adverse reactions to naloxone, there was clearly no meaningful benefit. To treat only blood pressure in a patient with septic shock is to lose sight of the complexity of the process and the therapeutic goals one is trying to reach. Although naloxone may not be harmful to patients with septic shock, it should be considered an experimental agent and should not be used routinely.— M.M. Parker, M.D.

Renal Hemodynamics and Prostaglandin E₂ Excretion in a Nonhuman Primate Model of Septic Shock

Schaer GL, Fink MP, Chernow B, Ahmed S, Parrillo JE, with the technical assistance of Reusch D, Caneal D (Natl Insts of Health, Bethesda, Md; Naval Med Research Inst, Bethesda, Md; Georgetown Univ)
Crit Care Med 18:52−59, 1990   4−8

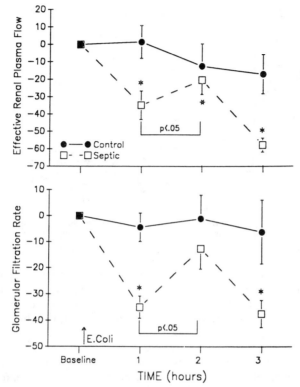

Fig 4–2.—Effect of SS on effective renal plasma flow and glomerular filtration rate. Data expressed as mean percent change from baseline values ± SEM; *asterisk* indicates *P* < .05 vs. baseline. (Courtesy of Schaer GL, Fink MP, Chernow B, et al: *Crit Care Med* 18:52–59, 1990.)

Renal dysfunction is a serious complication of septic shock, although the mechanisms responsible for renal insufficiency in human septic shock are not fully understood. A nonhuman primate model that closely simulates human septic shock was studied to examine the renal excretion of prostaglandin E_2 (PGE_2). In septic shock the kidney may produce PGE_2, a potent endogenous vasodilator, to increase renal blood flow.

Escherichia coli was used to induce septic shock in 18 cynomolgus monkeys; 5 saline-treated animals served as controls. Systemic and renal hemodynamic measurements and urine concentrations of PGE_2 were obtained every 30 minutes during the 3 hours after the infusions.

The *E. coli* infusion was lethal in 80% of the animals within 24 hours. Both mean arterial pressure and systemic vascular resistance were significantly depressed in the septic group. Compared with controls, septic animals also had significantly lower effective renal plasma flow and glomerular filtration rate (Fig 4–2). Urine flow, which was significantly reduced in the septic animals throughout the experiment, remained stable in the control group. Renal excretion of PGE_2 was dramatically increased by the induction of septic shock (Fig 4–3).

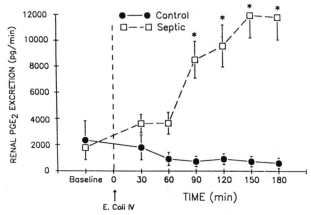

Fig 4–3.—Effect of SS on the renal excretion of PGE_2. Data expressed as mean $\pm$ SEM; *asterisk* indicates $P < .05$ vs. baseline. (Courtesy of Schaer GL, Fink MP, Chernow B, et al: *Crit Care Med* 18:52–59, 1990.)

The renal hemodynamic response to septic shock was biphasic. In the second hour post sepsis, significant increases in effective renal plasma flow and glomerular filtration rate occurred despite the continued severe systemic hypotension. These values decreased during the third postseptic hour.

In this animal model of low systemic vascular resistance septic shock, the renal excretion of PGE_2 was associated with a transient recovery in renal hemodynamics during the second postseptic hour. Treatment with agents that are inhibitors of prostaglandin synthesis may interfere with renal autoregulation in patients with septic shock, dramatically worsening renal function.

▶ Human septic shock is characterized by hypotension with low systemic vascular resistance (SVR) and increased cardiac index. In this study, anesthetized cynomolgus monkeys given a lethal intravenous dose of *E. coli* were used to determine the effects of severe septic shock on renal hemodynamics and on renal excretion of PGE_2. Although this model resulted in hypotension and a low SVR, the cardiac index was not increased. Excretion of PGE_2 was found to increase in the second hour post sepsis and was associated with improvement in effective renal plasma flow and glomerular filtration rate (GFR). However, despite continued significant PGE_2 excretion the improvement in effective renal plasma flow and GFR could not be maintained beyond the second hour post sepsis. Further, in the septic shock model employed, the cardiac index became significantly depressed compared to baseline values at 15 minutes and 165 minutes post *E. coli* challenge. Fluctuations in renal hemodynamics over the course of the study may have been caused in part by changes in the cardiac index. The authors correctly point out that a lethal infusion of *E. coli* does not simulate accurately an infectious process. In addition, normal cardiovascular responses to septic shock could have been blunted by anesthesia. This study would have been more interesting if the effects of a prostaglandin synthesis inhibitor on renal hemodynamics were observed. Despite these limitations, PGE_2 may have an important role in regulating renal hemodynamics in septic shock. These findings may have important implications for clinical trials using ibuprofen in septic shock.—A.L. VanDervort, M.D., and R.L. Danner, M.D.

Detoxification of Plasma Containing Lipopolysaccharide by Adsorption
Bysani GK, Shenep JL, Hildner WK, Stidham GL, Roberson PK (St Jude's Children's Research Hosp, Memphis; Univ of Tennessee, Memphis; LeBonheur Children's Med Ctr, Memphis)
Crit Care Med 18:67–71, 1990   4–9

Increased plasma levels of lipopolysaccharides (LPS) can induce coagulopathy, hypotension, and shock. Patients with gram-negative bacillary septic shock may have levels of LPS as high as 400 µg/mL of plasma. It has been hypothesized that circulating LPS is responsible for many of the features of gram-negative bacterial sepsis. The ability of 13 materials with known affinity for LPS to detoxify plasma containing LPS by adsorption was compared.

Each material was used to adsorb water and pooled normal human plasma to which *Escherichia coli* 0111:B4 LPS was added. In addition, each substance was used to adsorb plasma obtained by plasmapheresis of a patient with fatal *Klebsiella pneumoniae* sepsis. To determine whether the patient's plasma could be detoxified by adsorption, LPS-sensitized mice were treated with 3 of the experimental materials.

Although LPS was most readily removed from water and least readily removed from plasma obtained from the patient with sepsis, some of the materials did remove substantial amounts of LPS from the patient's plasma. The most effective adsorbent was activated charcoal, which removed 100% of the LPS from water and plasma containing added LPS and 98% of *K. pneumoniae* LPS from plasma obtained from a patient with sepsis. Bentonite and Kaopectate, which contains bentonite, were almost as effective as activated charcoal. All mice in a control group were dead within 12 hours. In contrast, all mice in the group treated with activated charcoal and 85% of mice in the Kaopectate-treated group were alive at 36 hours.

These findings suggest that selective removal of LPS from plasma might be beneficial for patients with gram-negative septic shock. The effective adsorbents may have also removed bacterial toxins other than LPS from the patient's plasma.

▶ The removal of endotoxin or other mediators from the blood of patients with septic shock has been suggested to have potential therapeutic benefit. To this end, Bysani and colleagues have demonstrated that a variety of adsorbents, most notably activated charcoal and bentonite, can in fact remove endotoxin from human plasma. These adsorbents, however, are not specific for endotoxin and may remove essential substances from the blood. In a canine model of septic shock, Natanson and co-workers (1) have demonstrated that plasmapheresis increases mortality. The ability to remove specific harmful mediators while leaving intact the beneficial proteins in the blood must be convincingly demonstrated in animal models before this technique can be applied to humans.— M.M. Parker, M.D.

Reference

1. Natanson C, et al: *Clin Res* 37:346, 1989.

Beneficial Effect of a Platelet-Activating Factor Antagonist, WEB 2086, on Endotoxin-Induced Lung Injury

Chang S-W, Fernyak S, Voelkel NF (Univ of Colorado; Denver VA Med Ctr)
Am J Physiol 258:H153–H158, 1990   4–10

Platelet-activating factor (PAF), a potent vasoactive lipid that may be an important mediator of endotoxic shock, appears to have a particular potential to cause lung injury. To define the role of PAF in acute lung vascular injury, the effect of WEB 2086 on lung vascular leak in endotox-in-treated rats was studied. A synthetic derivative of triazolodiazepine, WEB 2086 is a potent and specific antagonist of PAF action.

Lung vascular leak was assessed by means of ^{125}I-labeled bovine serum albumin. Intraperitoneal injections of *Salmonella enteritidis* endotoxin increased the extravascular leakage of ^{125}I-labeled albumin in the perfused lungs of the animals at 30 minutes, 2 hours, 6 hours, and 48 hours.

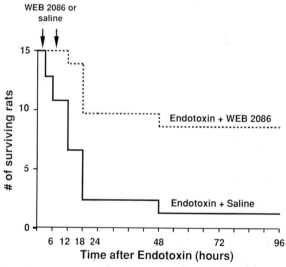

Fig 4–4.—Effect of WEB 2086 posttreatment on endotoxin-induced lethality. Shown are number of surviving rats at various time points after intraperitoneal injection of endotoxin, 20 mg/kg. WEB 2086, 10 mg/kg, or saline was injected at 2 hours (intravenously) and 6 hours (intraperitoneally) after endotoxin. All deaths occurred during the first 48 hours after endotoxin injection. The 2 survival curves are significantly different (P < .005) by the method of Mantel and Haenszel. (Courtesy of Chang S-W, Fernyak S, Voelkel NF: *Am J Physiol* 258:H153–H158, 1990.)

Lung injury was significantly reduced at 2 hours after endotoxin injection when the animals were treated with intraperitoneally administered WEB 2086, 10 mg/kg, either 20 minutes before or 30 minutes after the endotoxin injection. Post treatment with WEB 2086 starting at 90 minutes after endotoxin resulted in a marked reduction in lung leak at 6 hours. Some animals received a lethal dose of intraperitoneally administered endotoxin, 20 mg/kg. In this group, post treatment with WEB 2086, starting at 2 hours, significantly improved survival compared with vehicle-treated rats (Fig 4–4).

The protective effect of WEB 2086 did not result from a reduction of endotoxin-induced oxidative stress. The release of thromboxane B_2 by endotoxin-treated lungs was not affected by WEB 2086. In addition, neither pretreatment nor post treatment with WEB 2086 brought about a significant reduction in the endotoxin-induced increase in plasma glutathione disulfide, a marker of in vivo oxidative stress. During the early periods of endotoxemia, the lung injury process is perpetuated by persistent activation of PAF. Thus PAF receptor antagonists may have a potential role in the treatment of sepsis-associated lung injury.

▶ Several previous studies in small animal models of sepsis by these authors and others have shown WEB 2086 and other PAF antagonists to have a therapeutic effect. This study in rodents attempts to explain the beneficial effect of PAF in septic shock; however, the findings are essentially negative in identifying a pathophysiologic mechanism for the beneficial response. The authors do not show that PAF reduced endotoxin-induced oxidative stress or eicosanoid metabolites. Studies using large animal models and humans are needed to confirm a pathophysiologic and therapeutic role for PAF and PAF antagonists in septic shock.—C. Natanson, M.D., and J.E. Parrillo, M.D.

Prognostic Values of Tumor Necrosis Factor/Cachectin, Interleukin-1, Interferon-α, and Interferon-γ in the Serum of Patients With Septic Shock
Calandra T, Baumgartner J-D, Grau GE, Wu M-M, Lambert P-H, Schellekens J, Verhoef J, Glauser MP, and the Swiss-Dutch J5 Immunoglobulin Study Group (Ctr Hosp Univ Vaudois, Lausanne, Switzerland; Univ of Geneva; State Univ of Utrecht, The Netherlands)
J Infect Dis 161:982–987, 1990   4–11

Results of experimental studies have shown tumor necrosis factor/cachectin (TNF) to be a primary mediator of the adverse effects of endotoxin. To determine the evolution of serum levels of TNF during the course of septic shock and the association between these levels and patient outcome, serum concentrations of immunoreactive TNF were measured in 70 patients. Serum concentrations of immunoreactive interleukin-1β (IL-1β), interferon-α (IFNα), and interferon-γ (IFNγ) were also measured to examine the interplay of these cytokines and TNF.

Gram-negative bacteria were the cause of septic shock in 77% of the

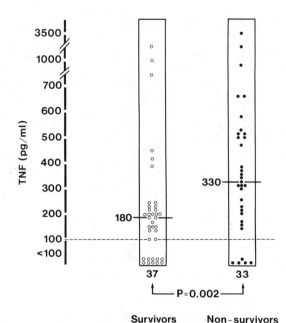

Fig 4–5.—Serum levels of immunoreactive TNF measured at study entry (before infusion of immunoglobulins) in survivors and nonsurvivors. *Horizontal bars* represent median concentrations of TNF in each group of patients. *Broken line* shows limit of detection of radioimmunoassay (<100 pg/mL). (Courtesy of Calandra T, Baumgartner J-D, Grau GE, et al: *J Infect Dis* 161:982–987, 1990.)

patients. Immunoreactive TNF was detected in 55 patients (79%); 37 patients survived and 33 died.

The median serum levels of TNF at study entry were greater in the nonsurvivors than in the survivors (Fig 4–5). In survivors the median concentration of TNF decreased from 180 pg/mL at study entry to 150 pg/mL at day 1 and to less than 100 pg/mL at day 10. In nonsurvivors the median concentration of TNF remained high: 330 pg/mL at study entry, 250 pg/mL at day 1, and 305 pg/mL at day 10.

Although median concentrations of IL-1β at study entry were significantly greater in nonsurvivors than in survivors, this difference did not persist at day 1. Serum concentrations of IFNα and IFNγ remained unchanged during the course of septic shock and did not correlate with patient outcome or with serum levels of TNF. Stepwise logistic regression analysis revealed that levels of TNF had a negligible impact on prediction of outcome. In contrast, 5 simple clinical and laboratory variables were of prognostic significance: severity of the underlying disease, patient age, documentation of infection, urine output, and arterial pH (table).

▶ This study examines the role of TNF in septic shock by investigating the time course and relationship to outcome of serum TNF elevations during human

Results of Logistic Regression Analysis

Variables	Coefficient (C)	Standard error (SE)	C:SE ratio	P
Severity of underlying disease	−2.05	0.81	−2.52	.01
Age	0.06	0.03	2.41	.02
Documentation of infection				
Nonbacteremic infections vs. bacteremias	1.93	0.86	2.24	.03
Bacteremias vs. no organism isolated	−1.37	1.55	−0.89	.38
Urine output	−0.02	0.01	−2.12	.04
Arterial pH	−0.09	0.04	−2.03	.05
TNF	2.08	1.14	1.82	.07
Temperature	−0.06	0.03	−1.68	.10
Constant	90.63	34.65	2.62	

Note: The ratio of coefficient to SE *(C:SE)* can be read roughly as *t* statistics. Absolute value less than 2 indicates variable of minor effect in presence of other variables.
(Courtesy of Calandra T, Baumgartner J-D, Grau GE, et al: *J Infect Dis* 161:982–987, 1990.)

septic shock. The analysis is sound, and the conclusions are clear.— C. Natanson, M.D., and J.E. Parrillo, M.D.

Comparison of Halothane, Isoflurane, Alfentanil, and Ketamine in Experimental Septic Shock

Van der Linden P, Gilbart E, Engelman E, Schmartz D, de Rood M, Vincent J-L (Erasme Univ Hosp, Brussels)
Anesth Analg 70:608–617, 1990   4–12

The anesthetic agents used when patients with septic shock require surgery can adversely affect cardiovascular function and oxygen balance. Because few data are available on the effects of anesthesia in septic shock, 2 commonly used inhalation anesthetics, halothane and isoflurane, and 2 intravenous agents, ketamine and alfentanil, were studied in a canine septic shock model.

A total of 45 dogs were randomized in 5 groups of 9 dogs each. All received intravenous injections of *Escherichia coli* endotoxin (3 mg/kg). A control group was given a bolus dose of phenobarbital to maintain controlled ventilation. The remaining groups each received 1 of the 4 study agents.

Endotoxin administration resulted in severe decreases in arterial pressure and cardiac index in all groups, together with a significant increase in blood lactate. Initial fluid resuscitation restored the cardiac index to baseline levels. Heart rate and arterial pressure increased slightly in the control animals; the cardiac index increased significantly. The cardiac index remained unchanged in the halothane group, whereas heart rate, arterial pressure, and systemic vascular resistance decreased significantly. Heart rate and arterial pressure were not significantly altered in the isoflurane group. With alfentanil, the cardiac index increased despite a reduction in heart rate. Arterial pressure and systemic vascular resistance decreased in this group. Arterial pressure, cardiac index, and systemic vascular resistance showed no significant changes with ketamine, although the heart rate decreased. Blood lactate increased significantly with halothane and isoflurane, was unchanged with alfentanil, and tended to decrease with ketamine.

Overall, halothane had the fewest desirable effects. Ketamine appeared to result in the least harm to hypoxic tissues and best preserved cardiac function. Ketamine may be the anesthetic agent of choice in septic shock.

▶ The authors clearly state in the Discussion the problems with this study: (1) different anesthetic agents are compared and no analgesic equivalents are determined (except for the inhalation agents) to compare hemodynamic data; (2) the effects of anesthetics are mostly dose dependent and only single doses of each anesthetic are used; (3) only physiologic variables (and not survival) are measured. The manuscript defines an area of great clinical importance—an area with little available data. The problems described above limit the conclusions of the study and its usefulness for clinical practice. Additional studies using various models of septic shock are necessary to compare different anesthetic agents (over a range of doses) at equivalent analgesic doses.—C. Natanson, M.D., and J.E. Parrillo, M.D.

Detection of Renal Blood Flow Abnormalities in Septic and Critically Ill Patients Using a Newly Designed Indwelling Thermodilution Renal Vein Catheter
Brenner M, Schaer GL, Mallory DL, Suffredini AF, Parrillo JE (Natl Insts of Health, Bethesda, Md)
Chest 98:170–1179, 1990   4–13

Mortality from septic shock is increased in patients with renal dysfunction. Although knowledge of the mechanisms leading to renal failure in septic shock could lead to methods of preserving renal function in these critically ill patients, the measurement of alterations in renal blood flow (RBF), a major mechanism of acute renal failure in animal models, is difficult. A catheter was designed to evaluate alterations in RBF accurately.

The specially shaped catheter is placed percutaneously under fluoroscopic guidance into the renal vein, allowing direct sampling of renal venous blood and reliable calculations of para-aminohippurate clearance (C_{PAH}). The study group included 8 critically ill patients, 7 with septic shock.

The catheter can determine RBF by 2 techniques: C_{PAH} levels (with extraction coefficient determination) and thermodilution-derived RBF. The 2 techniques showed a strong correlation, confirming reliability of the thermodilution method. A decrease was noted in PAH extraction, supporting the need for renal vein sampling to determine C_{PAH} in sepsis. Extractions of PAH ranged from 28% to 90% in these patients, whereas normal values exceed 90%. Significant errors in the estimation of RBF would result if such decreases were not taken into account.

Renal vascular resistance did not change significantly throughout the study. During recovery from sepsis the fraction of total body arterial blood flow going to the kidneys increased significantly. In 4 of 7 septic patients a reduced glomerular filtration rate correlated with the fraction of total blood flow going to the kidneys.

Renal vein catheterization can be performed safely and provide measurements over a period of several days. Renal vein catheters may be helpful in defining the pathophysiology of renal dysfunction in septic patients and in evaluating the effects of various interventions on RBF.

▶ This interesting study describes the use of a newly designed renal vein catheter for the purpose of directly determining RBF. At present, data on the perfusion of specific organs during septic shock are sparse and in need of further investigation. This new method has the advantage of directly measuring RBF by thermodilution and determining the true PAH clearance by sampling from the renal vein. Disadvantages of this method include the need for fluoroscopy during insertion and frequent catheter migration into the inferior vena cava. The results demonstrate that PAH extraction is decreased in critically ill patients, and that sepsis-induced renal dysfunction may occur despite normal total RBF. This investigational technique could provide useful information on the effects of various interventions on RBF and renal function in critically ill patients.—A.L. VanDervort, M.D., and R.L. Danner, M.D.

Plasma Tumor Necrosis Factor in Patients With Septic Shock: Mortality Rate, Incidence of Adult Respiratory Distress Syndrome, and Effects of Methylprednisolone Administration
Marks JD, Marks CB, Luce JM, Montgomery AB, Turner J, Metz CA, Murray JF (Univ of California, San Francisco; San Francisco Gen Hosp; Upjohn Company, Kalamazoo, Mich)
Am Rev Respir Dis 141:94–97, 1990   4–14

Previous studies have suggested that the cytokine tumor necrosis factor (TNF) may be an important mediator of the pathophysiology of septic shock. If this is the case, then TNF should be detectable in the plasma of patients with gram-positive or gram-negative septic shock. The plasma of patients with suspected septic shock was studied to determine the presence of TNF and characterize the time course of its release.

The 86 patients were enrolled in a trial to determine the value of methylprednisolone (MPSS) in preventing the development of adult respiratory distress syndrome (ARDS) in septic shock. The TNF was measured by an enzyme-linked immunosorbent assay. The effects of MPSS were as-

Presence of TNF in Patients With Septic and Nonseptic Shock

	Total Patients (n)	Patients with Measurable TNF		Peak TNF Level* (pg/ml)
		(n)	(%)	
Nonseptic shock	12	1	8	323
Septic shock	74	27	37†	181 ± 35
Bacteremic	48	18	38	168 ± 30
Nonbacteremic	26	9	35	206 ± 89
Gram-positive	32	12	38	196 ± 67
Gram-negative	25	9	36	167 ± 53
Mixed infection	17	6	35	172 ± 44

*Mean peak TNF level ± SEM for patients with measurable TNF.
†P < .05 compared with nonseptic shock; Fisher's exact test.
(Courtesy of Marks JD, Marks CB, Luce JM, et al: *Am Rev Respir Dis* 141:94–97, 1990.)

sessed by comparing initial and posttreatment plasma levels in patients who received the active drug and those given placebo.

Septic shock occurred in 74 patients; TNF was more common in patients with shock from sepsis than in those with shock from other causes (table). In 25 of 27 patients with septic shock and measurable TNF levels, TNF was present in the initial blood sample. Levels of TNF decreased significantly during the 24 hours after study enrollment, whether MPSS or placebo was given (Fig 4–6). The 12-hour parenchymal lung injury scores were higher in patients with detectable TNF (Fig 4–7). Measur-

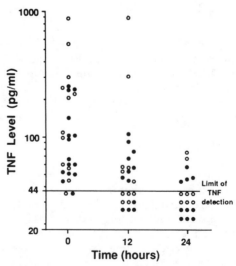

Fig 4–6.—Effect of time on TNF levels during the first 24 hours after admission to the study in patients with septic shock who received *(open circles)* or did not receive *(filled circles)* methylprednisolone. There are fewer data points and 12 and 24 hours because some patients died. (Courtesy of Marks JD, Marks CB, Luce JM, et al: *Am Rev Respir Dis* 141:94–97, 1990.)

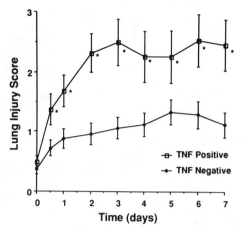

Fig 4–7.—Lung injury scores in patients with septic shock with and without detectable TNF. Asterisks indicate $P < .05$ compared with patients without detectable TNF. (Courtesy of Marks JD, Marks CB, Luce JM, et al: *Am Rev Respir Dis* 141:94–97, 1990.)

able levels of TNF were associated with a higher rate of mortality (81% vs. 43%) and a greater risk of ARDS (55% vs. 26%).

Tumor necrosis factor is present early in the course of septic shock, regardless of bacterial type. The administration of MPSS does not affect the tendency of TNF levels to decrease. Because TNF release appears to occur before the clinical appearance of septic shock, anti-TNF therapies would have to be administered prophylactically to patients at risk.

▶ Understanding the pathophysiology of septic shock is essential to the development of new, more effective therapeutic interventions. Marks et al. present data in this study that implicate TNF as a factor in ARDS and in higher mortality from septic shock. Because TNF is found very early in the course of septic shock and decreases within 24 hours, it is unlikely that therapeutic interventions aimed at blocking TNF will be effective unless they can be instituted prophylactically, before the onset of septic shock. It is likely that by the time the syndrome of septic shock has been recognized clinically, the pathophysiologic events, of which TNF is probably a part, are already well established, and that blocking the early mediators (such as TNF) may not be effective.—M.M. Parker, M.D.

Right Ventricular Dysfunction and Dilatation, Similar to Left Ventricular Changes, Characterize the Cardiac Depression of Septic Shock in Humans
Parker MM, McCarthy KE, Ognibene FP, Parrillo JE (Clinical Ctr, NIH, Bethesda, Md)
Chest 97:126–131, 1990   4–15

Left ventricular dysfunction is characteristic of septic shock, but the relationship of left to right ventricular function is not well understood. This

Initial to Final Ejection Fraction and End Diastolic Volume
Index in Survivors and Nonsurvivors of Septic Shock

Parameters	Survivors (n = 22)			Nonsurvivors (n = 17)		
	Initial	Final	p*	Initial	Final	p
Left ventricular ejection fraction	.31	.47	.001	.40	.43	NS†
Left ventricular end diastolic volume index, ml/m²	145	106	.012	124	102	NS
Right ventricular ejection fraction	.35	.51	.001	.41	.39	NS
Right ventricular end diastolic volume index, ml/m²	124	88	.03	120	114	NS

*Paired sample t test.
†NS indicates not statistically significant.
(Courtesy of Parker MM, McCarthy KE, Ognibene FP, et al: *Chest* 97:126–131, 1990.)

relationship was examined by serial hemodynamic and nuclide angiographic studies in 39 patients with septic shock, 22 of whom survived. The right ventricular ejection fraction was calculated by the 2-regions-of-interest method.

Hemodynamic findings generally returned toward normal in surviving patients, whereas nonsurvivors had no significant hemodynamic changes except for a rise in heart rate. The initial ejection fraction was substantially depressed but rose significantly with recovery (table). Left and right ventricular end-diastolic volume fell toward normal during recovery. Nonsurvivors had no significant change in left ventricular or right ventricular ejection fraction. Pulmonary vascular resistance correlated negatively with the right ventricular end-diastolic volume only in surviving patients.

Myocardial depression affects both ventricles simultaneously in human septic shock. It is hoped that a more complete understanding of the effects of septic shock on the myocardium will allow more effective treatment.

▶ This study conclusively demonstrates the biventricular nature of the myocardial depression observed in septic shock. The fact that this dysfunction is a biventricular phenomenon lends credence to the idea of a circulating myocardial depressant substance(s) that is thought to be involved pathophysiologically in ventricular dilatation. Coronary flow limitations, which had once been thought to be responsible for the fall in myocardial performance, would not be as likely to affect the right ventricle as severely as the left.

Also of particular interest in this study, as in previous studies regarding the responses of the left ventricle to sepsis, is the failure of ventricular dilatation to develop in nonsurvivors. This would suggest that biventricular dilatation is an important physiologic response to the events that occur in septic shock. Why the ventricles of nonsurvivors do not dilate is unknown. Also, whether this failure of ventricular dilatation plays a causal role in their subsequent death also remains unclear.

Optimal management of patients with septic shock requires an understanding of the cardiovascular performance changes occurring in most of these patients. The clinician must realize that, despite a high cardiac output, most septic shock patients have significant dysfunction of both left and right ventricular performance.—A.C. Dixon, M.D., and J.E. Parrillo, M.D.

Skeletal Muscle Blood Flow and Venous Capacitance in Patients With Severe Sepsis and Systemic Hypoperfusion
Astiz ME, Rackow EC, Haydon P, Karras G, Weil MH (Chicago Med School, North Chicago, Ill)
Chest 96:363–366, 1989   4–16

An altered peripheral vascular tone is thought to be a factor in septic circulatory failure. Lowered venous tone with pooling may decrease the effective circulating blood volume, and decreased arterial tone can compromise nutrient flow to the tissues. Forearm vascular tone and blood flow were quantified in 10 severely septic patients and 10 control patients without sepsis who were admitted for elective surgery. Venous tone and flow were determined by plethysmography.

Thirty percent of septic patients were discharged from the hospital. Mean arterial pressure, central venous pressure, and cardiac index did not differ significantly in the septic and nonseptic groups. Peak forearm venous capacitance was reduced in the septic group. Forearm venous tone was nearly twice as great in the septic subjects. There were no significant differences in forearm blood flow or forearm arteriolar resistance. Increased venous capacitance and a redistribution of skeletal muscle blood flow are not characteristic of severe sepsis.

▶ The response of the peripheral vasculature to the mediators implicated in the pathophysiology of sepsis is very important to the overall syndrome produced in the patient. Regional blood flow has been difficult to study, and different species may have different responses to the same mediators. This study reports regional blood flow to skeletal muscle in humans with sepsis. The absence of the expected decreased forearm venous tone or increased venous capacitance may be a result of the method used, or may imply that skeletal muscle blood flow is not altered in sepsis, although blood flow to other organ systems may be. Regional blood flow in human sepsis remains poorly understood and yet is crucial to the understanding of the pathophysiology of septic shock.—M.M. Parker, M.D.

The Effects of Aminophylline and Pentoxifylline on Multiple Organ Damage After *Escherichia coli* Sepsis

Harada H, Ishizaka A, Yonemaru M, Mallick AA, Hatherill JR, Zheng H, Lilly CM, O'Hanley PT, Raffin TA (Stanford Univ)
Am Rev Respir Dis 140:974–980, 1989   4–17

Aminophylline can lessen the increase in pulmonary vascular permeability occurring in various models of acute lung injury. The effects of aminophylline and pentoxifylline, another methylxanthine, on organ damage were compared in guinea pigs subjected to *Escherichia coli* sepsis. Organ damage was assessed using measurements of ^{125}I-albumin accumulation in bronchoalveolar lavage fluid and in the lungs, kidneys, liver, heart, adrenals, and spleen.

Albumin indices in all organs and in lavage fluid increased significantly in septic control animals compared with those given saline, aminophylline, or pentoxifylline. Similarly, lung wet-to-dry weight ratios increased in the septic control animals but not in the methylxanthine-treated groups. The mean arterial pressure did not fall significantly in pentoxifylline-treated septic animals, but it did decline in septic animals given aminophylline.

Both aminophylline and pentoxifylline attenuate organ albumin leak in septic guinea pigs, the latter with no apparent effect on mean arterial pressure. Pentoxifylline may be preferable for use in clinical trials of treatment for adult respiratory distress syndrome and multiple organ damage in sepsis.

▶ It is of great interest that methylxanthines may ameliorate at least one measure of organ damage caused by sepsis. It must be remembered, however, that in this study the animals were pretreated with the study drug. Humans with sepsis are always treated after the onset of sepsis. It is important to study drugs that have shown some benefit in animal models, but drugs that are beneficial before the onset of sepsis may not prove to be helpful after sepsis is established. Furthermore, this study looked only at organ damage as assessed by albumin leak. A beneficial effect on outcome was not an end point in this study but, obviously, is of prime importance in humans.—M.M. Parker, M.D.

Fig 4–8.—Change (mean ± SEM) in the core temperature (**A**) and the percentage change from baseline in pulmonary wedge pressure (*PCW*, **B**) and mean pulmonary-artery pressure (*PAP*, **C**) measured over 8 hours in the endotoxin and control groups. Volume loading (represented here and in Figures 2 and 3 by an *arrow*) was initiated at 3 hours and completed by 5 hours. The values at 2 end points (3 hours and 5 hours) were evaluated statistically. Temperature increased significantly at 3 and 5 hours after injection in the endotoxin group. The PWP and the PAP did not vary significantly at either end point. (Courtesy of Suffredini AF, Fromm RE, Parker MM, et al: *N Engl J Med* 321:280–287, 1989.)

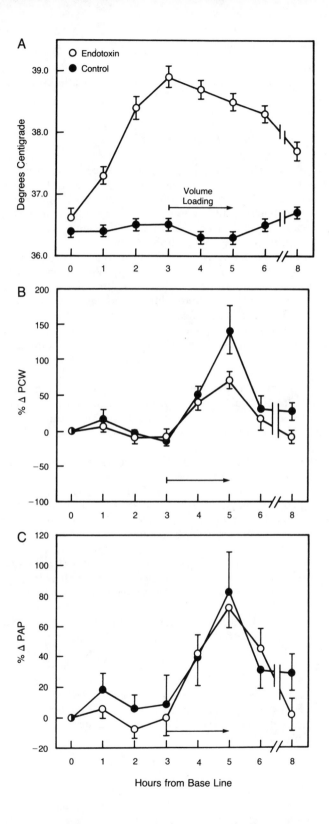

The Cardiovascular Response of Normal Humans to the Administration of Endotoxin

Suffredini AF, Fromm RE, Parker MM, Brenner M, Kovacs JA, Wesley RA, Parrillo JE (Clinical Ctr, Natl Insts of Health, Bethesda, Md)

N Engl J Med 321:280–287, 1989   4–18

Endotoxin is considered to be an important mediator of cardiovascular dysfunction in septic shock. Hemodynamics were studied in 9 normal persons aged 23–38 years who were administered a bolus of *Escherichia coli* endotoxin, 4 ng/kg intravenously; 6 other persons were administered saline instead. All underwent volume loading with normal saline 4–5 hours after endotoxin or saline administration.

The expected flulike symptoms and an increased core temperature followed endotoxin administration (Fig 4–8). Pulmonary vascular resistance indices were similar in the endotoxin and saline recipients. The cardiac index rose much less after volume loading in endotoxin recipients (Fig 4–9). Ejection fraction decreased in the endotoxin group but increased in controls after volume infusion (Fig 4–10). Ventricular performance is compared in Figure 4–11). No hemodynamic differences from baseline were present 24 hours after endotoxin administration.

Endotoxin produces a hyperdynamic cardiovascular state in normal human beings. Depressed left ventricular function is independent of changes in left ventricular volume or vascular resistance. The changes are similar to those seen in septic shock, suggesting that endotoxin is a major factor in cardiovascular dysfunction in this state.

▶ This study has significantly advanced our understanding of myocardial performance in gram-negative septic shock in several respects. First, the study demonstrated that exogenously administered endotoxin causes a reversible reduction in myocardial performance similar to that seen in clinical septic shock. This provides strong evidence that endotoxin plays a major role in the pathogenesis of the cardiovascular abnormalities of human septic shock.

Secondly, the simultaneous evaluation of ejection fraction and a load independent measure of ventricular performance, the ratio of peak systolic pressure to end-systolic volume index, demonstrates that left ventricular dysfunction is intrinsically abnormal, rather than simply altered by changes in preload and afterload.

Lastly, the concomitant measurement of serum tumor necrosis factor activity suggests that this substance either exerts a delayed effect on the myocardium or, alternatively, may not be directly involved in the observed myocardial depression.

Ongoing studies using animal models, or the administration to humans of monoclonal antibodies against endotoxin or tumor necrosis factor, should help resolve many of the remaining questions regarding the mechanisms of the observed fall in ventricular performance in endotoxic shock.—A.C. Dixon, M.D., and J.E. Parrillo, M.D.

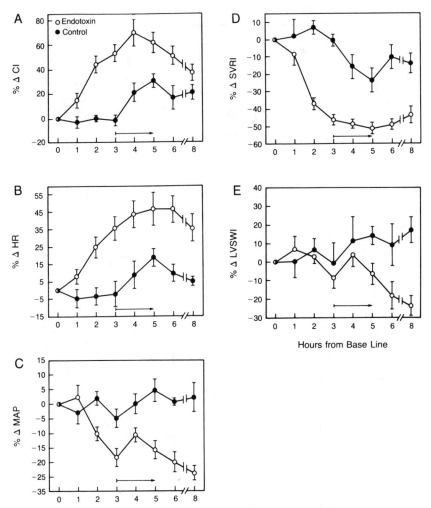

Fig 4–9.—Percentage change (mean ± SEM) from baseline in the cardiac index (*CI*, **A**), heart rate (*HR*, **B**), mean systemic arterial pressure (*MAP*, **C**), systemic vascular-resistance index (*SVRI*, **D**), and left ventricular stroke-work index (*LVSWI*, **E**). The CI and HR increased, and the SVRI decreased significantly at 3 hours after endotoxin administration. At 5 hours, the CI, SVRI, and MAP in the endotoxin group were significantly different from values in the control group. (Courtesy of Suffredini AF, Fromm RE, Parker MM, et al: *N Engl J Med* 321:280–287, 1989.)

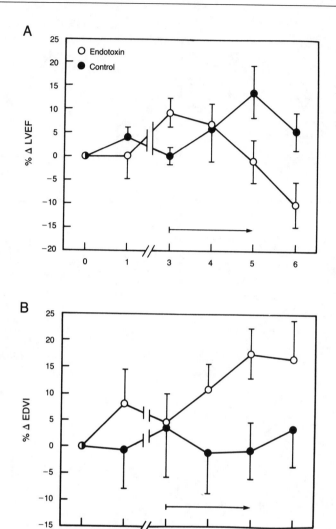

Fig 4–10.—Percentage change (mean ± SEM) from baseline in the left ventricular ejection fraction (*LVEF,* **A**) and ventricular end-diastolic volume index (*EDVI,* **B**) over a 6-hour period. The LVEF increased significantly at 3 hours and then decreased significantly at 5 hours in the endotoxin group compared with the control group. The EDVI increased at 5 hours to a value that was slightly, but not significantly, greater than that in the control group. (Courtesy of Suffredini AF, Fromm RE, Parker MM, et al: *N Engl J Med* 321:280–287, 1989.)

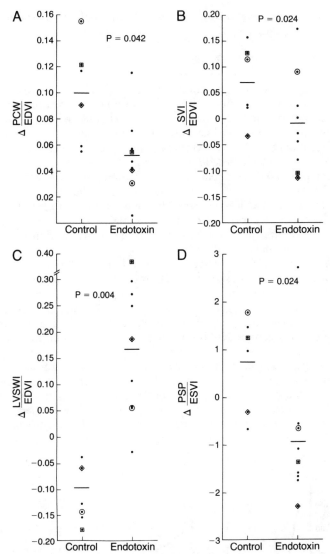

Fig 4–11.—Change from baseline to the point of maximal volume load in ratios reflecting ventricular performance. *PCW/EDVI* denotes the ratio of pulmonary capillary wedge pressure to left ventricular end-diastolic volume index; *SVI/EDVI,* the ratio of stroke-volume index to left ventricular end-diastolic volume index; *LVSWI/EDVI,* the ratio of left ventricular stroke-work index to left ventricular end diastolic volume index, and *PSP/ESVI,* the ratio of peak systolic pressure to left ventricular end-systolic volume index. Each *symbol* within a *circle, square,* or *diamond* represents a value of each of 3 individuals who participated in both the control and endotoxin parts of the study at 3-month intervals. The *other symbols* represent values in individuals who participated in only 1 of the parts of the study. The *horizontal lines* indicate the calculated means for each group; they are shown for descriptive purposes only and not for statistical comparisons. (Courtesy of Suffredini AF, Fromm RE, Parker MM, et al: *N Engl J Med* 321:280–287, 1989.)

Effect of Cocarboxylase in Dogs Subjected to Experimental Septic Shock

Lindenbaum GA, Larrieu AJ, Carroll SF, Kapusnick RA (Albert Einstein Med Ctr, Philadelphia)
Crit Care Med 17:1036–1040, 1989   4–19

Cocarboxylase (CC), or thiamine pyrophosphate, is a coenzyme acting to degrade pyruvate in the Krebs cycle. An analogue has protected cyanide-poisoned rats and also has protected ischemic myocardium in animals subjected to coronary ligation. The hemodynamic and metabolic effects of treatment with CC were examined in dogs in endotoxic shock, produced with *Escherichia coli* endotoxin.

Arterial pressure recovered earlier and better in CC-treated animals (Fig 4–12), and the same was the case for the cardiac index (Fig 4–13). Administration of CC lessened the effects of endotoxin on pH and base excess. Sustained recovery of oxygen pressure was seen only in treated animals. No significant deterioration in oxygen consumption was evident in the treated animals (Fig 4–14).

Administration of CC lessens the metabolic and hemodynamic sequelae of endotoxin shock in dogs. It may act at the mitochondrial level to improve the function of pyruvate dehydrogenase, with consequent improved utilization of oxygen and glucose as well as better production of adenosine triphosphate. Future studies should include a direct assay of pyruvate dehydrogenase activity in the presence of endotoxin and CC.

▶ The possibility of treating septic shock with agents that act at the cellular level is an exciting one. Cellular metabolism in septic shock is not well understood. Cocarboxylase may well provide one method to study the pathophysiology of septic shock at the cellular level. The results reported by Lindenbaum et al. suggest that cocarboxylase may have a beneficial effect on cellular metabolism in endotoxin shock, at least for a few hours. Whether the beneficial ef-

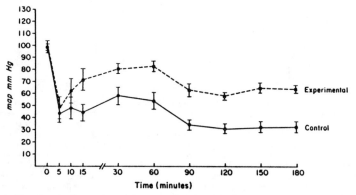

Fig 4–12.—Changes in mean arterial pressure *(map)* preinjection (time = 0 minutes) and postinjection on endotoxin. Cocarboxylase administered at time = 2 minutes. There were significant ($P < .5$) differences between the control and the experimental (cocarboxylase) groups at all times after 15 minutes (mean ± SEM). (Courtesy of Lindenbaum GA, Larrieu AJ, Carroll SF, et al: *Crit Care Med* 17:1036–1040, 1989.)

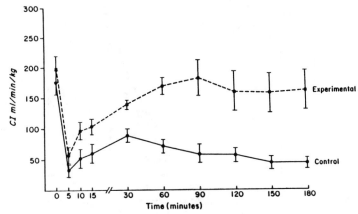

Fig 4–13.—Changes in cardiac index *(CI)* preinjection (time = 0 minutes) and postinjection of endotoxin. Cocarboxylase administration at time = 2 minutes. There were significant (*P* < .05) differences between the control and experimental (cocarboxylase) groups at all times after 15 minutes (mean ± SEM). (Courtesy of Lindenbaum GA, Larrieu AJ, Carroll SF, et al: *Crit Care Med* 17:1036–1040, 1989.)

fects will be long lasting or will result in an improvement in outcome are issues that must be addressed in further studies.—M.M. Parker, M.D.

Sepsis-Induced Diastolic Dysfunction in Chronic Canine Peritonitis
Stahl TJ, Alden PB, Ring WS, Madoff RC, Cerra FB (Univ of Minnesota)
Am J Physiol 258:H625–H633, 1990   4–20

There is increasing evidence that sepsis compromises myocardial function when volume support is used, but its effects on diastolic function remain uncertain. These effects were examined in a chronic dog model of

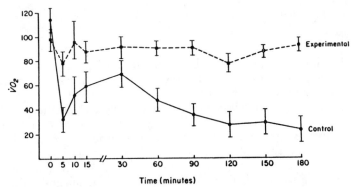

Fig 4–14.—Oxygen consumption ($\dot{V}O_2$) preinjection (time = 0 minutes) and postinjection of endotoxin. With the exception of the 30-minute time point, there were significant (*P* < .05) differences between the control and experimental (cocarboxylase) groups at all times after injection. Cocarboxylase administered 2 minutes after endotoxin (mean ± SEM). (Courtesy of Lindenbaum GA, Larrieu AJ, Carroll SF, et al: *Crit Care Med* 17:1036–1040, 1989.)

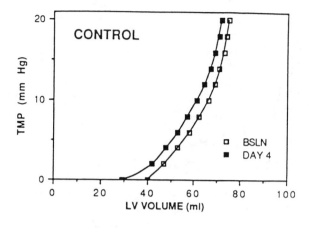

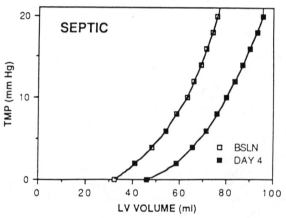

Fig 4–15.—Mean computed-fitted transmural pressure *(TMP)* vs. left ventricular *(LV)* volume curves for control and septic groups. Curves are generated from all individual curves in each group at baseline *(BSLN)* and day 4. (Courtesy of Stahl TJ, Alden PB, Ring WS, et al: *Am J Physiol* 258:H625–H633, 1990.)

hyperdynamic sepsis, produced by cecal ligation and puncture combined with ongoing high-volume fluid resuscitation. Cardiac function was assessed ultrasonically and by pressure measurements.

The animals became febrile and leukocytic and had positive blood cultures for enteric organisms. They also were hyperdynamic, but systolic blood pressure, stroke volume, and ejection fraction remained stable. Pressure-volume curves (Figs 4–15 and 4–16) showed significantly reduced intrinsic contractility during systole and markedly abnormal diastolic function. Myocardial compliance decreased significantly. Results of ultrastructural studies showed more marked myofibrillar and mitochondrial edema and myofibrillar disruption in study than in control biopsy specimens.

Early, progressive ventricular dysfunction characterizes this model of

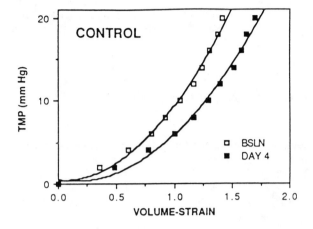

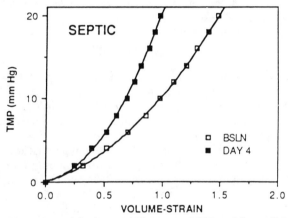

Fig 4–16.—Mean computed-fitted transmural pressure *(TMP)* vs. left ventricular volume-strain curves for control and septic groups. Curves are generated from all individual curves in each group at baseline *(BSLN)* and day 4. (Courtesy of Stahl TJ, Alden PB, Ring WS, et al: *Am J Physiol* 258:H625–H633, 1990.)

systemic hyperdynamic sepsis. Reduced myocardial contractility may be primary effect of sepsis. Ventricular dilation associated with reduced compliance may reflect a compensatory mechanism preserving global ventricular function in the hyperdynamic state.

▶ In this elegant study, Stahl and co-workers use ultrasonic cardiac crystals to measure ventricular volume and intraventricular catheters to measure pressure. Using sophisticated measures of cardiac performance, they confirm the decrease in cardiac contractility and increase in ventricular volume reported using conventional techniques in human studies and another dog model of septic shock. Unlike Natanson's dog model, this study reports a decrease in diastolic compliance, which may explain the findings of Ognibene et al. in humans (1).

Ventricular dysfunction in septic shock has been well documented. The effects of sepsis on diastolic function require further investigation to be fully understood.— M.M. Parker, M.D.

Reference

1. Ognibene FP, et al: *Chest* 93:903, 1988.

Effect of Leukotriene Inhibitor LY-171883 on the Pulmonary Response to *Escherichia coli* Endotoxemia
Gross D, Ben Dahan J, Landau EH, Krausz MM (Hadassah Univ Hosp, Jerusalem)
Crit Care Med 18:190–197, 1990   4–21

Despite the highly developed technology for ventilatory support, respiratory failure is a major cause of increased morbidity and mortality in sepsis. Inhibition of the lipoxygenase system in endotoxemia could change the ventilatory response that results in respiratory insufficiency. The effect of the leukotriene D_4 receptor antagonist, LY-171883, on the respiratory and hemodynamic response to endotoxemia in sheep was determined.

Twenty awake sheep were used. In 2 sheep (group 1) LY-171883, 4 mg/kg, was injected intravenously; in 12 other animals (group 2) *Escherichia coli* endotoxin was infused intravenously; and in 6 animals (group 3), LY-171883, 4 mg/kg was given 15 minutes before and 30 minutes after the same dose of endotoxin.

Infusion of LY-171883 in group 1 did not change baseline ventilatory and cardiovascular measures. In group 2, a 2-phase pulmonary response was seen: an early pulmonary hypertension in which pulmonary artery pressure (PAP) rose from 18.7 to 51.2 mm Hg, with a drop in cardiac index (CI) from 171 mL/min·kg to 114 mL/min·kg. The ratio of peak inspiratory/expiratory flow rate (PIF/PEF) rose from 1.08 to 1.35. The respiratory rate rose from 50 to 70 breaths per minute 30 minutes after the endotoxin was given. The flow rate measured at midexpiration time dropped from 81% to 25% of its peak expiration. The airway resistance increased from 3.8 cm H_2O/L·sec to 32.7 cm H_2O/L·sec.

In the second permeability phase, there was an increase in pulmonary lymph flow from 8.5 mL/hr to 35.2 mL/hr, a drop in PaO_2 from 76 torr to 61 torr, and a rise in the pulmonary shunt ratio from 16% to 31%. In group 3, LY-171883 administration was followed by a rise in CI to 202 mL/min·kg and in PAP only to 35.1 mm Hg. Such treatment prevented the increase in PIF/PEF and oxygen consumption and delivery. It also prevented the drop in $\dot{V}_{50}$ and the rise in pulmonary resistance after endotoxin. Changes in pulmonary lymph flow, lymph protein clearance, Hgb, white blood cell count, PaO_2, pulmonary shunt ratio, and oxygen consumption were comparable to those in group 2.

In endotoxemia, LY-171883 attenuates pulmonary hypertension and changes in airway resistance. The reduction in $\dot{V}_{50}$ was prevented, and the CI response to endotoxemia was reversed. However, this lipoxygenase product did not affect hypoxemia and the late permeability response to endotoxin.

▶ The authors have used a well-characterized sheep model of lung injury to evaluate a specific arm of the pulmonary inflammatory response to endotoxin. Sheep have a characteristic 2-phase response to the infusion of endotoxin, including an early phase of pulmonary hypertension, with reduced cardiac output and hypoxemia, and a later phase of increased microvascular permeability. Additionally, responses of airways and the pulmonary circulation to constrictor stimuli are altered (1). The LD4 receptor antagonist resulted in partial improvement of the lung response to endotoxin, diminishing the increase in pulmonary artery pressure and airway resistance, but did not alter the increased in lung permeability. The data suggest that in sheep, LD4 is a potent vasoconstrictor and bronchoconstrictor and mediates an early portion of the pulmonary response to endotoxin administration. Other mediators including cytokines, nonarachidonate metabolites, and free oxygen radicals presumably contribute to the accompanying development of lung inflammation, noncardiogenic pulmonary edema, and respiratory failure (1).—A.F. Suffredini, M.D., and J.E. Parrillo, M.D.

Reference

1. Brigham KL, Meyrick B: *Am Rev Respir Dis* 133:913, 1986.

Endotoxin-Induced Myocardial Depression in Rats: Effect of Ibuprofen and SDZ 64-688, a Platelet Activating Factor Receptor Antagonist
Baum TD, Heard SO, Feldman HS, Latka CA, Fink MP (Univ of Massachusetts, Worcester)
H Surg Res 48:629–634, 1990   4–22

Myocardial dysfunction is known to occur in sepsis and endotoxicosis; however, the mechanisms underlying this phenomenon are not well understood. The hypothesis that lipopolysaccharide (LPS)-induced myocardial dysfunction is mediated by cyclooxygenase-derived metabolites of arachidonic acid or platelet-activating factor (PAF) was tested.

Ether-anesthetized rats were given intravenous injections of normal saline, ibuprofen, or SDZ 64-688 (a PAF receptor antagonist). Thirty minutes later, normal saline (NS) or *Escherichia coli* 0111:B4 LPS was injected. Atria was harvested 2 hours later, connected to an isometric force transducer-amplifier-recorder apparatus, and maintained in vitro in oxygenated 37.5° C Krebs-Henseleit buffer.

The force of contraction indexed to body weight was significantly lower in the 7 animals in the NS/LPS group than in the 7 in the NS/NS group. Ibuprofen pretreatment did not affect the adverse influence of LPS on the atrial force of contraction indexed to body weight. Pretreatment with SDZ 64-688 did ameliorate the deleterious effect of LPS on contractility. The PAF antagonist did not manifest intrinsic positive inotropic activity in 8 animals.

Lipopolysaccharide induces myocardial contractile dysfunction in rats. This phenomenon appears to be ameliorated by pretreatment with a PAF receptor antagonist. Studies using other animal species are needed before the findings can be generalized.

▶ A wide variety of mediators have been implicated in the development myocardial depression that results from septic shock. The authors evaluated cardiac performance in isolated strips of atrial muscle by evaluating contractile indices as a function of preload, rate, and isoproterenol infusion. A PAF receptor antagonist, but not a cyclooxygenase inhibitor, blocked the atrial contractile dysfunction induced by endotoxin. These results are intriguing because of the beneficial hemodynamic effects that occur with ibuprofen, a cyclooxygenase inhibitor in several animal models of septic shock (1). The current study demonstrates that, although cyclooxygenase inhibitors improve systemic hemodynamics in models of septic shock, they have little effect on myocardial contractile dysfunction. Platelet-activating factor has potent negative inotropic effects in isolated animal hearts (rat, guinea pig, rabbit, dog) that are not blocked by leukotriene or cyclooxygenase inhibitors (2). The PAF released by endotoxin may act directly or through other inflammatory mediators to cause myocardial contractile dysfunction.—A.F. Suffredini, M.D., and J.E. Parrillo, M.D.

References

1. Metz CA, Sheagren JN: *J Crit Care* 5:206, 1990.
2. Pinckard RN, et al., in Gallin JI, et al (eds): *Platelet Activating Factors in Inflammation: Basic and Clinical Correlates*. New York, Raven Press, 1988, p 139.

Activation of Coagulation After Administration of Tumor Necrosis Factor to Normal Subjects
van der Poll T, Büller HR, ten Cate H, Wortel CH, Bauer KA, van Deventer SJH, Hack CE, Sauerwein HP, Rosenberg RD, ten Cate JW (Univ of Amsterdam; Beth Israel Hosp, Boston; Netherlands Red Cross Blood Transfusion Service, Amsterdam)
N Engl J Med 322:1622–1627, 1990   4–23

Tumor necrosis factor (TNF) is an important mediator of the activation of coagulation in septicemia. A controlled study was undertaken to investigate the early dynamics and route of coagulation activation after administration of recombinant TNF. Indices of activation of the common and intrinsic pathways of coagulation were measured sequentially in 6 healthy men who received an intravenous bolus injection of recombinant TNF, 50 $\mu g/m^2$, of or saline during 2 study periods.

Compared with saline, recombinant TNF induced a rapid but transient activation of the common pathway of coagulation. There was a brief increase in plasma levels of factor X activation peptide that reached maximal values after 30–45 minutes. This was followed by a gradual increase in plasma levels of the prothrombin fragment F_{1+2} that peaked after 4–5 hours and remained elevated for 6–12 hours. The circulating levels of factor XIIa–C1 inhibitor complexes, kallikrein–C1 inhibitor complexes, factor XII, and prekallikrein remained within normal range after injection of TNF, indicating that the intrinsic pathway of coagulation was not stimulated. This was further supported by the observation that plasma levels of factor IX activation peptide, a measure of in vivo activation of factor IX, were not affected by TNF. The delay between the maximal activation of factor X and that of prothrombin amounted to several hours and indicated that neutralization of factor Xa was slow.

Low-dose TNF induces rapid, sustained activation of the common pathway of coagulation system in healthy subjects, probably through the extrinsic route. Tumor necrosis factor could play an important role in the early activation of the hemostatic mechanism in septicemia.

▶ In this study, Van der Poll et al. show that TNF injections in normal volunteers activates the coagulation system. These results suggest that release of endogenous mediators in response to bacterial toxins is a potential pathway for sepsis-induced coagulation disorders. Studies such as this using safe, low-dose challenges of exogenous and endogenous toxins in normal volunteers in combination with various agonists and antagonists can be used to examine the pathophysiologic mechanisms of septic shock and define potential therapies for the disease.— C. Natanson, M.D., and J.E. Parrillo, M.D.

Circulating Interleukin-1 and Tumor Necrosis Factor in Septic Shock and Experimental Endotoxin Fever

Cannon JG, Tompkins RG, Gelfand JA, Michie HR, Stanford GG, van der Meer JWM, Endres S, Lonnemann G, Corsetti J, Chernow B, Wilmore DW, Wolff SM, Burke JF, Dinarello CA (New Engl Med Ctr; Tufts Univ; Massachusetts Gen Hosp; Brigham and Women's Hosp; Harvard Med School, Boston)
J Infect Dis 161:79–84, 1990   4–24

Several endogenous factors have been implicated in the mediation of host responses to infection and injury. To assess their relative roles in vivo, plasma concentrations of interleukin-1 (IL-1), IL-1α and IL-1β, and tumor necrosis factor or cachectin (TNF-α) were measured by radioimmunoassay in 44 healthy subjects, 15 patients in septic shock, and 6 volunteers infused with *Escherichia coli* endotoxin.

Plasma IL-1α levels were low (40 pg/mL) or undetectable in all plasma samples. Plasma IL-1β levels were <70 pg/mL in 67% of healthy subjects but were significantly higher in septic patients (mean, 120 pg/mL). Plasma IL-1β levels did not correlate with the severity of illness but were in fact significantly higher among patients who survived than those who died. Plasma TNF-α levels in septic patients were significantly higher than in healthy subjects (mean, 119 pg/mL vs. 73 pg/mL). Plasma TNF-α

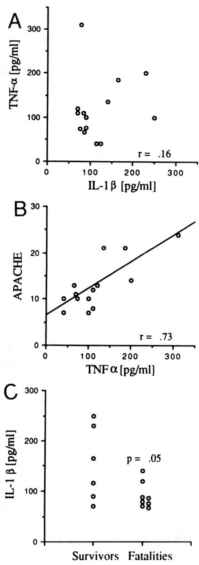

Fig 4–17.—A, lack of association between interleukin (IL)-1β and tumor necrosis factor (TNF)-α concentrations in initial plasma samples obtained from patients in septic shock (*P* = .58). **B,** positive association of TNF-α with severity of illness (*P* = .003). **C,** plasma IL-1β levels of surviving patients, compared with those of patients who died. Significance determined by Student's t test. (Courtesy of Cannon JG, Tompkins RG, Gelfand JA, et al: *J Infect Dis* 161:79–84, 1990.)

concentrations in septic patients correlated with severity of illness but not with plasma IL-1β levels (Fig 4–17). After infusion of endotoxin, plasma IL-1β levels increased by twofold within 180 minutes. In contrast, peak TNF-α levels were 15 times higher and were reached more rapidly (90 minutes) than IL-1β levels.

Plasma IL-1β and TNF-α concentrations are regulated independently and are associated with different outcomes. Plasma Il-1β and TNF-α responses are dissociated in both time course and magnitude with respect to acute responses to infection.

▶ Defining patterns of inflammatory mediator release is an important step in developing therapeutic approaches for the organ damage that results from severe infections. The authors evaluated patients who had preexisting infections with gram-negative, gram-positive, or fungal infections for a mean duration of 4.4 days (18 hours to 21 days) and obtained blood within 20 minutes to 4 hours from onset of septic shock. The acute cytokine response evaluated was thus well after onset of septicemia and very close to the time of progression to septic shock.

Interleukin-1α was essentially undetectable in the patients with septic shock as well as in the normal reference population, consistent with its role as a cell-associated mediator, which may be important in inflammatory events in the local cell environment (1). Interleukin-1β was difficult to measure in plasma without extensive modifications to the radioimmunoassay system, including eliminating background interference from rabbit serum used as a carrier protein in the assay and extracting the plasma with chloroform to remove lipids and lipoproteins, which are elevated during the acute-phase response and may interfere with the assay. The IL-1β levels were higher in the survivors, although this has not been found uniformly in other studies of the IL-1β response to acute infection (2, 3). When natural Il-1β or TNF-α was added to the plasma of healthy persons, less was recovered in patients with septic shock (83% TNF-α and 71% IL-1β recovered in healthy subjects vs. 61% TNF-α and 54%-1β recovered from patients with septic shock). This suggests that the cytokines measured may underestimate the amount of endogenous cytokine, and that acute-phase proteins and cytokine inhibitory proteins bind these cytokines and may play a role in the control of their effects in vivo (4). This study illustrates the difficulties in performing liquid-phase immunoassays for cytokines in critically ill patients and emphasizes the independent regulation of TNF and IL-1β during acute inflammatory responses and during septic shock.—A.F. Suffredini M.D., and J.E. Parrillo, M.D.

Refrences

1. Endres S, et al: *Eur J Immunol* 19:2327, 1989.
2. Giardin E, et al: *N Engl J Med* 319:397, 1988.
3. Calandra T, et al: *J Infect Dis* 161:982, 1990.
4. Arend WP, Dayer JM: *Arthritis Rheum* 33:305, 1990.

Platelet Activating Factor Receptor Antagonist Improves Survival and Attenuates Eicosanoid Release in Severe Endotoxemia
Fletcher JR, DiSimone AG, Earnest MA (Vanderbilt Univ, Nashville; Univ of South Alabama, Mobile)
Ann Surg 211:312–316, 1990   4–25

Exogenous platelet activating factor (PAF) can result in hypotension, plasma extravasation, metabolic acidosis, and death. These effects are like those of endotoxin and the eicosanoids. The effects of BN52021, a specific PAF receptor antagonist, on the hemodynamic events and survival in rat endotoxemia were determined, and the effects of this antagonist on eicosanoid production in endotoxemia were assessed.

Male Sprague-Dawley rats were used. Endotoxin alone significantly caused hypotension, prostaglandin release, and death. In contrast, pretreatment with BN52021 significantly changed the hypotension, significantly attenuated the eicosanoid release, and improved survival rates, which suggests that PAF receptor activation is an early event in endotoxemia.

The results support the hypothesis that there may be an intimate relationship between PAF and the eicosanoids. Some of the effects of PAF in endotoxemia may be mediated through the cyclooxygenase pathway. Eicosanoid release in endotoxemia might be associated with PAF synthesis and PAF receptor activation.

▶ This well-controlled study adds support to a role of PAF in the pathogenesis and mortality of septic shock. Platelet-activating factor is part of the family of lipid autocoids, including eicosanoids that orchestrate a wide variety of inflammatory processes through primary and secondary mediators (1). These agents are generated rapidly after a stimulus and are intimately involved in a wide variety of normal and abnormal processes that regulate cardiovascular, pulmonary, renal, liver, neurologic, and reproductive function. Platelet-activating factor is formed by a variety of inflammatory cells, including neutrophils, macrophages-monocytes, endothelial cells, mast cells, eosinophils, and natural killer cells as well as platelets, and has myriad effects through its ability to contract smooth muscle and endothelial cells (1). The role of a PAF antagonist in increasing the survival of rats challenged with endotoxin and limiting the increase in thromboxane and PGE_2 is notable in the face of previous data that shows a role for improvement in survival and hemodynamic responses in animals given cyclooxygenase inhibitors (2). Through direct and indirect pathways (i.e., arachidonate metabolites), PAF plays a significant role in this lethal animal model of shock caused by endotoxin.—A.F. Suffredini, M.D., and J.E. Parrillo, M.D.

References

1. Pinckard RN, et al. in Gallin JI, et al (eds): *Platelet Activating Factors in Inflammation: Basic and Clinical Correlates.* New York, Raven Press, 1988, p 139.
2. Metz CA, Sheagren JN: *J Crit Care* 5:206, 1990.

Plasma Tumor Necrosis Factor Levels in Patients With Presumed Sepsis: Results in Those Treated With Antilipid A Antibody Vs Placebo
de Groote MA, Martin MA, Densen P, Pfaller MA, Wenzel RP (Univ of Iowa; VA Med Ctr, Iowa City)
JAMA 262:249–251, 1989

Cachectin, tumor necrosis factor (TNF), is presumed to play a major role in mediating the physiologic effects of endotoxin in gram-negative bacterial infection. However, in 1 study detectable levels of TNF were found only at the onset of the clinical responses and in another there was only a transient response of TNF to infusion of endotoxin.

In the present study an enzyme-linked immunosorbent assay was used to detect TNF in the plasma of patients with gram-negative sepsis. This double-blind, placebo-controlled study was designed to evaluate the efficacy of an IgM-neutralizing monoclonal antibody to endotoxin, J-5, in reducing the morbidity and mortality of patients with presumed gram-negative sepsis.

Thirty-eight patients were randomized to receive either antilipid A antibody (19 patients) or placebo for presumed gram-negative bacteremia. Blood samples for TNF analysis were drawn immediately before infusion of the antibody-placebo and again at 3, 6, 12, 18, 24, 36, and 48 hours after infusion. All patients received appropriate antibiotics; 84% had already begun treatment when the first blood sample was drawn.

Sixteen of the 38 patients had positive blood cultures. Fourteen had gram-negative rods, and 2 had *Streptococcus pneumoniae*. One of 20 plasma samples from healthy volunteers showed detectable TNF. Six of the 38 patients had detectable levels of TNF, including 4 of 14 with positive cultures for gram-negative rods but only 2 of 22 patients with negative blood cultures. Of the 6 patients with detectable TNF, 4 had received placebo and 2 had received the antibody. The level of TNF did not predict shock, adult respiratory distress syndrome, disseminated intravascular coagulation, renal failure, or mortality.

The highest levels of TNF were found in 2 patients with *Entobacter cloacae* bacteremia, 1 of whom had received placebo. The other 2 patients with bacteremia and detectable levels of TNF had positive blood cultures for *Hemophilus influenzae* and *Bacteroides fragilis*. The 2 patients with detectable levels of TNF and negative findings on blood cultures had clinical findings consistent with gram-negative sepsis.

It is difficult to study the levels of TNF in human beings, as evidenced by elevated levels of TNF in healthy subjects and undetectable levels in clinically septic patients. Large prospective studies are needed to determine the pattern of release, of TNF in patients with gram-negative sepsis.

▶ Tumor necrosis factor appears transiently in normal humans who are given intravenous endotoxin, peaking at 90 minutes and then rapidly disappearing from the circulation within 3 hours (1). The authors obtained blood samples 2–72 hours after onset of the clinical signs of sepsis. Only 6 of 38 (16%) had detectable TNF, and these levels did not predict the development of organ failure (adult respiratory distress syndrome, renal failure), shock, or death. Of interest was the detection of TNF immunoreactivity (1,600 pg/mL) in a normal subject who represented part of the reference population. On further examination with a cytotoxicity assay that measures actual bioactivity, no TNF was found. This emphasizes that false positives may occur in a small percentage of samples tested with immunoassays, as noted in other studies (1).

This report is in contrast to several large studies that found detectable immunoreactive TNF in a larger percentage of patients with sepsis and septic shock. Presumably, this represents differences in patient selection, time of blood sampling, and TNF assay sensitivity. Calandra et al. (2) found that of 70 patients with septic shock, 55 (79%) had detectable levels of immunoreactive TNF at study entry and levels were associated with outcome. Offner et al. (3) found detectable TNF in 23 of 34 patients (68%) with sepsis and noted a persistent elevation, rather than a precipitous increase, at the onset of septic shock. Marks et al. (4) found elevated TNF in 27 of 74 patients (37%) with septic shock and observed a significant association with an increased incidence and severity of ARDS in these patients. Although the authors of the original study conclude that further investigations are required to evaluate the role of TNF in gram-negative sepsis, it is apparent that a rise in TNF occurs in infections with gram-negative, gram-positive, and fungal infections (2–4), and that elevation of TNF represents a common pathway of host response to infection.—A.F. Suffredini M.D., and J.E. Parrillo, M.D.

References

1. Michie HR, et al: *N Engl J Med* 318:1481, 1988.
2. Calandra T, et al: *J Infect Dis* 161:982, 1990.
3. Offner F, et al: *J Lab Clin Med* 116:100, 1990.
4. Marks JD, et al: *Am Rev Respir Dis* 141:94, 1990.

Tumor Necrosis Factor's Effects on Lung Mechanics, Gas Exchange, and Airway Reactivity in Sheep
Wheeler AP, Jesmok G, Brigham KL (Vanderbilt Univ; Cetus Corp, Emeryville, Calif)
J Appl Physiol 68:2542–2549, 1990   4–27

The most common cause of adult respiratory distress syndrome (ARDS) is gram-negative bacterial sepsis. When endotoxin is infused into awake sheep, a lung injury similar to human ARDS can be produced. Recent studies have proposed tumor necrosis factor-α (TNF-α) as a major mediator of the endotoxin reaction, and animal studies have shown that high doses of TNF-α can cause shock and death. Because of the similarities in biologic effect of TNF-α and endotoxin, the results of sublethal infusions of TNF-α in awake sheep were examined to test the hypothesis that TNF-α would bring about the lung changes seen with endotoxemia.

Five sheep received intravenous doses of human recombinant TNF-α, 10 μg/kg, on 2 occasions. Within 15 minutes of the infusion, rigors, mild agitation, and tachypnea developed in all animals. They were assessed for changes in lung mechanics, pulmonary and systemic hemodynamics, gas exchange, and number and type of peripheral blood leukocytes. Airway reactivity was determined by use of aerosolized histamine before and after TNF-α infusion.

The administration of TNF-α caused rapid onset of systemic and pulmonary arterial hypertension, hypoxemia, and neutropenia. There were prompt, profound, and sustained reductions in dynamic lung compliance and increases in resistance to airflow across the lung. As with endotoxin, there was a profound decrease in total peripheral blood leukocytes after TNF-α. The dose of aerosolized histamine needed to alter lung compliance was acutely reduced with TNF-α.

The findings support the hypothesis that TNF-α is a key mediator in the endotoxin response. Changes in airway activity were more pronounced with TNF-α than with endotoxemia, but changes in lung mechanics, hemodynamics, gas exchange, and leukocyte counts were less severe. Thus TNF-α may not be the sole mediator of endotoxin-induced injury.

▶ It is widely appreciated that most of the systemic disturbances associated with gram-negative bacteria are the result of the host's response to the lipopolysaccharide cell wall component, endotoxin. Endotoxin is a potent cellular activator that results in elaboration of many macrophage products. Recently, TNF has been identified as an endogenous compound that appears to be an important intermediary in many endotoxin-induced disturbances. This study by Wheeler et al. demonstrates a variety of pulmonary alterations induced by TNF, and these are qualitatively similar to those seen with endotoxin. The obvious hope is that therapeutic intervention can be developed that will prevent either TNF production or TNF-induced responses, and these will prevent many of the sequelae of gram-negative bacteremia. Several laboratories are involved in investigations using monoclonal antibodies to clear TNF. The results of these immunotherapy trials are eagerly awaited.—M.J. Breslow, M.D.

Extracorporeal Membrane Oxygenation Therapy in Neonates With Septic Shock

McCune S, Short BL, Miller MK, Lotze A, Anderson KD (George Washington Univ; Children's Natl Med Ctr, Washington, DC; Inst of Child Health, and Development, NIH, Bethesda, Md)
J Pediatr Surg 25:479–482, 1990   4–28

Extracorporeal membrane oxygenation (ECMO) therapy has been used successfully in infants with cardiorespiratory decompensation who did not respond to conventional intensive medical management. However, many centers remain reluctant to use ECMO in neonates with septic shock because of the risk of bleeding complications and the history of poor survival.

Among 100 infants who qualified for ECMO therapy, as defined by a greater than 80% mortality when conventional medical management is used, 10 had a documented diagnosis of septic shock. In these septic infants, heparin management and weaning techniques were altered, with ECMO flows being maintained at full (60% to 70%) bypass, allowing activated clotting times to be kept as low as 190–210 seconds. Weaning was accomplished by decreasing the percent of oxygen to the membrane via the blender, rather than by decreasing the ECMO blood flow rates.

All 10 infants with septic shock who received ECMO therapy survived. Compared with other infants treated with ECMO, these septic infants required significantly more ventilatory support after ECMO and had a higher incidence of chronic lung disease, which suggests that this condition may be associated with additional parenchymal or vascular damage that is not seen with meconium aspiration syndrome or respiratory distress syndrome. Intracranial hemorrhage was noted in 40% of septic infants, compared to 20% of other infants.

Extracorporeal membrane oxygenation therapy appears to be a viable alternative for neonates with septic shock that is unresponsive to conventional medical management. Reduced heparin dose and maintenance of high ECMO flows can help to decrease the risk of bleeding diathesis in these septic infants.

▶ The authors have shown that ECMO can be applied successfully to neonates with septic shock. The associated bleeding complications are controlled with maintenance of high ECMO blood flow rates and reduced heparin administration. With the ever-expanding indications for ECMO, it remains important to confirm such retrospective observations with controlled, prospective trials.— D.G. Nichols, M.D.

Hyperdynamic Sepsis Modifies a PEEP-Mediated Redistribution in Organ Blood Flows
Bersten AD, Gnidec AA, Rutledge FS, Sibbald WJ (Univ of Western Ontario, London)
Am Rev Respir Dis 141:1198–1208, 1990   4–29

The use of positive end-expiratory pressure (PEEP) to treat arterial oxygen desaturation during acute hypoxemic respiratory failure can compromise tissue oxygen delivery. Although redistribution of blood flow (Q) to the organs with greatest need should compensate for the decrease in tissue oxygen delivery to organ systems, septic multiple system organ failure may interfere with this process. To examine this issue, the effects of PEEP on organ Q was studied in an awake sheep model before and during hyperdynamic sepsis.

During the nonseptic study, PEEP was associated with a 9% decrease in thermodilution-measured systemic Q, although arterial perfusing pressures were not affected. Microsphere-derived Q was maintained to the brain and heart, but fell in the liver, spleen, pancreas, and other organs. Positive end-expiratory pressure depressed systemic Q by 17% in the septic animals. However, Q fell only in the pancreas, liver, and spleen. Infusion of Ringer's lactate did not restore Q to pre-PEEP levels in the septic animals.

Differences in the distribution of post-PEEP organ Q between the nonseptic and septic animals were probably caused by the vasculopathy of sepsis and/or an alteration in the function of specific organ microcirculations. The inability to restore PEEP-mediated changes in organ Q suggests the need for alternative methods of support for organ Q in acute respiratory failure secondary to sepsis.

▶ Positive end-expiratory pressure (PEEP) is utilized in a variety of pathophysiologic conditions to improve oxygenation. However, PEEP-induced decreases in cardiac output can offset increases in oxygen content, leading to a reduction in oxygen delivery. In this study, Bersten et al. provided detailed information on how PEEP affects individual organ blood flow in a conscious hyperdynamic sepsis model in sheep. Overall, the response to PEEP was similar in septic and control animals. Of note, although fluid administration increased cardiac output, it did not reduce PEEP-induced decreases in organ blood flow. Whether similar decreases in organ blood flow exist in human sepsis during PEEP is unknown. It goes without saying, however, that PEEP is not without adverse effects and should be used only to achieve clear-cut therapeutic objectives.—M.J. Breslow, M.D.

Atypical Staphylococcal Toxic Shock Syndrome: Two Fatal Pediatric Cases
Tyson W, Wensley DF, Anderson JD, Fraser GC, Wilson EM (British Columbia Children's Hosp, Vancouver)
Pediatr Infect Dis 8:642–645, 1989   4–30

Strict criteria for the diagnosis of toxic shock syndrome (TSS) may be essential for epidemiologic studies, but it may be difficult to make a diagnosis in mild disease or atypical presentations. Two fatal pediatric cases that involved toxin-producing strains of *Staphylococcus aureus* did not entirely meet the standard criteria for TSS.

The first patient had surgery for appendicitis. The appendectomy specimen, as well as the second and third laparotomies, failed to reveal the etiology. At autopsy *S. aureus* was cultured from the cecal contents, and there was diffuse hemorrhagic necrosis of the ileocecal region. The second patient was neutropenic from chemotherapy for neuroblastoma and presented with *S. aureus* septicemia and diffuse peritonitis.

The clinical course in both children was characterized predominantly by an uncontrollable "capillary leak syndrome," with massive third-space fluid loss and failure to maintain intravascular volume. Erythroderma was absent in the first patient and delayed in the second. The *S. aureus* strain from both patients produced TSS toxin-1 and enterotoxins. The second patient did not respond to therapy although antistaphylococcal treatment was begun well before death.

These 2 cases illustrate that adoption of the term "atypical toxic shock syndrome" may aid in the recognition and treatment of disease in cases that do not entirely satisfy current criteria for TSS at the time of presentation. The diagnosis should be considered in the differential diagnosis of children with acute onset of massive ascites and generalized anasarca of unknown cause, particularly in those who remain unresponsive to conventional therapy.

▶ This interesting case report describes 2 patients who had uncontrollable "capillary leak syndrome" with massive third-space fluid loss. This occurred despite the lack of typical rash in the first patient and before its development in the second. This lack of rash was extremely important in that it made the diagnosis of TSS very difficult. As a result, intensivists should be aware that this sequence of events can occur.—M.C. Rogers, M.D.

Control of Endotoxemia in Burn Patients by Use of Polymyxin B
Munster AM, Xiao G-X, Guo Y, Wong LA, Winchurch RA (Johns Hopkins Univ; Francis Scott Key Med Ctr, Baltimore)
J Burn Care Rehabil 327–330, 1989   4–31

The reduction of endotoxin load in patients with major burns is a desirable clinical objective. In 2 sequential prospective experiments, 62 patients with burns of at least 20% of the total body surface area were randomly assigned to an experimental polymyxin B (PB) or control group.

In the first study, consisting of the "early treatment" group, patients received PB intravenously during the first week after burn injury in a bell-shaped dosage form that resembled the level of endotoxemia after burn injury as previously documented. There was a highly significant reduction in endotoxin levels, as measured by the chromogenic limulus lysate assay, in the PB group as compared with the control group. In addition, there was a trend for a reduction in wound infection and mortality in the PB group, but the difference was not statisically significant.

In the second study, patients received intravenous PB perioperatively during excisional surgery of the burn wound. Although endotoxin levels were markedly reduced postoperatively in the PB-treated group, there was no significant reduction in clinical complication rate and mortality.

Despite the lack of statistically significant clinical results, the reduction in endotoxemia with the intravenous administration of PB in both the early treatment and perioperative groups is quite impressive. Treatment with PB remains a promising technique for reducing endotoxemia.

▶ This was a prospective randomized trial designed to reduce endotoxemia. The agent tested was intravenous PB and the results were encouraging. Nevertheless, there was a lack of statistically significant clinical results despite the reduction of endotoxemia. As a result, I conclude with the authors that the drug is promising, but that more trials are needed.—M.C. Rogers, M.D.

Septic Shock in Children: Bacterial Etiologies and Temporal Relationships

Jacobs RF, Sowell MK, Moss MM, Fiser DH (Univ of Arkanasas; Arkansas Children's Hosp, Little Rock)

Pediatr Infect Dis J 9:196–200, 1990   4–32

Septic shock occurs in 5% to 30% of children with bacterial sepsis, with a case fatality rate ranging from 45% to 98%. A retrospective analysis of 2,110 admissions to the pediatric intensive care unit was undertaken to determine the incidence of septic shock in children, ascertain the relationship between septic shock and common bacterial pathogens, and evaluate the temporal relationship between onset of septic shock and admission to the hospital. Septic shock was defined as the presence of clinical evidence of sepsis, fever (>38.3° C) or hypothermia (<35.6° C), tachycardia, tachypnea, and inadequate organ perfusion.

There were 564 patients who met the criteria for septic shock. Of these, 143 (25%) had confirmed bacterial sepsis or meningococcemia, the majority of the cases being attributable to *Hemophilus influenzae* type b (41%), *Neisseria meningitidis* (18%), and *Streptococcus pneumoniae* (11%). Meningitis was the most frequent localized infection, occurring in 50% of cases with septic shock. The overall mortality rate in patients with septic shock caused by bacterial infections was almost 10%. In 8 children who had no evidence of hypotension or hypoperfusion on initial evaluation, septic shock developed within a mean 4.6 hours after admission.

Septic shock is relatively common among children with clinical sepsis and/or meningitis and may develop after the patient's admission to the hospital. Infants and children with bacterial meningitis or sepsis should be monitored closely for at least the first 24 hours of admission and until stable perfusion is achieved.

▶ This review of 564 cases of septic shock in children concludes that this condition occurs more frequently in children than has been previously appreciated. In only 25% of these patients, however, was septic shock confirmed by bacterial infection. When it was confirmed, organisms implicated most frequently were *H. influenzae* type b (41%), *N. meningitidis* (18%), and *S. pneumoniae* (11%).—M.C. Rogers, M.D.

5 Cardiovascular

Acute Myocardial Ischemia

Prognostic Significance of Mitral Regurgitation in Acute Myocardial Infarction

Barzilai B, Davis VG, Stone PH, Jaffe A, and the MILIS Study Group (Washington Univ)

Am J Cardiol 65:1169–1175, 1990   5–1

The occurrence of mitral regurgitation (MR) after myocardial infarction (MI) is associated with decreased long-term survival. However, it is not known whether MR is an independent contributor to mortality in this setting. To clarify the relationship between clinically detected MR and survival after MI, data obtained from the Multicenter Investigation of the Limitation of Infarct Size (MILIS) trial were analyzed.

The diagnosis of MI was confirmed by measurement of the creatine kinase-MB concentration in 849 of the 985 patients enrolled in the MILIS trial. A murmur suggestive of MR was heard in 169 patients (20%), 76 of whom had a murmur at admission. In the other 93 patients a murmur was first detected during days 1 through 11 of hospitalization. Murmurs not suggestive of MR were excluded.

Patients with MR at the time of admission were older, more commonly women, more likely to be nonwhite, had a significantly greater frequency of previous infarction, and had a greater frequency of signs and symptoms of congestive heart failure than those without MR at admission. The in-hospital mortality was 15% in patients with MR at admission, 10% in patients with MR during hospitalization, and 8% in those without MR. The 12-month mortality rate was 36% for patients with initial MR, 16% in those with a later MR, and 15% in those without MR. This increased mortality persisted at 48 months, with a mortality of 47% in patients with MR at admission, 26% in those with MR detected during hospitalization, and 24% in those without MR. The differences were statistically significant.

Correction for differences in baseline variables showed that the presence of MR on admission did not contribute independently to mortality. Rather, patients with MR on admission had a significantly decreased wall motion score in the anterior segments, and both systolic and diastolic volumes were significantly enlarged. Thus the murmur of MR derives its prognostic significance from a combination of clinical, radiographic, and ECG variables.

▶ The use of careful auscultation was the basis for diagnosis. Auscultation alone without more objective documentation, by Doppler for example, may be a relatively weak objective criterion as a basis for evaluation of prognostic end points. Indeed, Doppler echocardiography appears to demonstrate evidence for mitral regurgitation in 40% to 50% of patients with acute MI.[1,2] No effort was made to quantify the degree of mitral regurgitation, which may be difficult using auscultation alone. This study points out the importance of multivariate analysis in determination of significant prognostic risk factors. Clearly, it is not necessarily the mitral regurgitation per se but, rather, the underlying conditions, e.g., extensive myocardial infarction, previous infarction, left ventricular (LV) size, female sex, age, and systolic performance, that are significant variables. The most important clinical prognostic variables for long-term survival after acute MI remain LV systolic performance and degree and complexity of ventricular arrhythmias.—P.R. Liebson, M.D., and J.E. Parrillo, M.D.

References

1. Barzilai B, et al: *Am J Cardiol* 61:220, 1988.
2. Loperfido F, et al: *Am J Cardiol* 58:692, 1986.

Diagnostic Efficiency of Lactate Dehydrogenase Isoenzymes in Serum After Acute Myocardial Infarction

Jensen AE, Reikvam Å, Åsberg A (Central Hosp of Sogn og Fjordane, Førde, Norway)
Scand J Clin Lab Invest 50:285–289, 1990   5–2

Measurement of serum lactate dehydrogenase (LD) isoenzymes provides useful information in the diagnosis of acute myocardial infarction (MI). When MI is present, the activity of serum LD isoenzyme-1 (LD-1) peaks between 24 and 48 hours after the onset of chest pain. Thus levels of LD-1 are particularly informative when patients are admitted more than 24 hours after onset of symptoms because levels of total creatine kinase (CK) and CK-MB isoenzymes may have returned to normal by that time. A serum LD-1–LD-2 ratio of more than 1 is generally considered diagnostic of MI, but some have found the LD-1-total LD ratio to be more useful.

To assess the diagnostic efficacy of levels of LD isoenzymes in acute MI, serial levels of LD isoenzymes were measured in 117 patients with symptoms suggestive of acute MI. Diagnoses were based on clinical and ECG criteria and on changes in serum levels of aspartate aminotransferase, CK, and total levels of LD measured over a 5-day period from admission. The results of LD isoenzyme tests were not made available to the physicians who made the diagnoses.

Forty-one of the 117 patients were considered to have acute MI, and 5 of them died. Eighteen patients without acute MI were discharged before completion of the study. Complete data sets were available for 41 patients with acute MI and 76 patients without.

By using receiver operating characteristic curves and logistic discriminant analysis, the serum level of LD-1 on day 2 proved to be the most accurate diagnostic parameter. On that day the various ratios between LD-1 and the other LD isoenzymes did not improve discrimination. The LD-1–LD-5 ratio was the least efficient. The LD-1–total LD ratio had the highest diagnostic efficiency on day 3, whereas the LD-1–LD-3 ratio had the highest efficiency on day 5. On the day after onset of symptoms in patients with suspected acute MI, serum LD-1 is a more reliable indicator than the LD-1–total LD ratio.

▶ Measurement of lactate dehydrogenase isoenzymes (LD-1 through LD-5) is generally recommended when patients with suspected MI are seen more than 24 hours from onset of chest pain. This paper convincingly shows that a single isoenzyme, LD-1, has the greatest diagnostic efficiency on the second day after admission, and that simultaneous assessment of LD-2 through LD-5 may not be necessary.—G.L. Schaer, M.D., and J.E. Parrillo, M.D.

Diabetic Patients and Beta-Blockers After Acute Myocardial Infarction
Kjekshus J, Gilpin E, Cali G, Blackey AR, Henning H, Ross J Jr (Univ of California, San Diego; VA Hosp, San Diego; Naval Hosp of San Diego; Univ of British Columbia, Vancouver)
Eur Heart J 11:43–50, 1990   5–3

Although the longterm use of β blockers after myocardial infarction (MI) reduces mortality, there is controversy about their use in diabetic patients, who are at increased risk for early and late mortality after acute MI. In a recent small study it was reported that long-term timolol therapy after an acute MI in diabetic patients reduced mortality. In the present large multicenter study, the benefit of β-blocker therapy after acute MI was examined in 2,024 patients including 281 with diabetes who were discharged from the hospital. Survivors were followed by telephone or mail at 3, 6, and 12 months after hospital discharge. One-year follow-up data were available for 268 diabetic patients and 1,418 who were not diabetic.

At 1 year after hospital discharge the mortality rate in diabetics was 17%, compared with 10% in nondiabetics. The mortality rate in diabetics treated with β blockers was 10.2%, compared with 23.4% in diabetics who did not receive β blockers. The mortality rates in nondiabetics were 6.5% in patients taking β blockers and 12.8% in those not taking β blockers. The differences in mortality could have been attributable to bias in patient selection for β-blocker therapy because patients were not randomized to treatment. After excluding diabetics who had evidence of pulmonary congestion on chest radiographs, the 1-year mortality rate was 7% in those taking β blockers and 17% in those not taking β blockers.

Multivariate analysis confirmed that long-term β-blocker therapy was an independent predictor of 1-year cardiac survival after hospital discharge for all diabetics but not for nondiabetics. However, the efficacy of β blockers in diabetic survivors of acute MI requires further confirmation in randomized trials.

▶ This retrospective study convincingly demonstrates that β blockers reduce mortality in diabetic patients after acute MI. Because diabetics tend to have more extensive coronary artery disease, and therefore a greater amount of myocardium at risk for reinfarction, these patients may have the most to gain by β-blocker therapy. Pending the results of a randomized, prospective trial specifically addressing this question, the benefits of β-blocker therapy in the post-MI diabetic patient may outweigh the potential risks of aggravating metabolic control.—G.L. Schaer, M.D., and J.E. Parrillo, M.D.

Cardiac Event Rate After Non-Q-Wave Acute Myocardial Infarction and the Significance of Its Anterior Location

Kao W, Khaja F, Goldstein S, Gheorghiade M (Henry Ford Hosp, Detroit)
Am J Cardiol 64:1236–1242, 1989   5–4

Non–Q-wave acute myocardial infarction (MI) has a lower in-hospital mortality rate than Q-wave acute MI, but the incidence of recurrent infarction is higher and the long-term mortality is similar. Because patients with non–Q-wave MI tend to represent a heterogeneous group, a study was done to determine whether any particular subgroup might be at increased risk for the development of postinfarction ischemic events.

The study population consisted of 135 patients recovering from enzymatically confirmed non–Q-wave MI who were followed prospectively for a median of 9.9 months. Of the 135 patients, 65 had an anterior non–Q-wave MI and 70 had an inferior or lateral non–Q-wave MI. Recurrent infarction was documented by repeat cardiac enzyme profiles and ECGs.

At baseline, patients with anterior non–Q-wave MI were older and had a higher incidence of previous acute MI than patients with inferolateral non–Q-wave MI. At last follow-up, 31 (48%) of 65 patients with anterior non–Q-wave MI had sustained either reinfarction or had died of cardiac causes compared with 10 (14%) of 70 patients with inferolateral non–Q-wave MI. After adjusting for baseline variables, including age and complication of heart failure, the differences in survival and reinfarction between the 2 groups were statistically significant. When patients with previous acute MI were excluded, the mortality rate still was 44% for patients with anterior non–Q-wave MI and 11% for patients with inferolateral non–Q-wave MI. Anterior location, along with nitrate use before acute MI, was the strongest predictor of reinfarction or death, as patients with anterior location were 7.2 times more likely to have reinfarction or die of cardiac events than those with an inferolateral location.

Patients with anterior non–Q-wave MI are at very high risk for sustaining a major cardiac event very soon after the index acute MI. This high risk may be related to a larger area of residual viable myocardium in the infarct-related artery when compared with inferolateral non–Q-wave MI.

▶ This study shows that the anatomical location of a non–Q-wave MI has a dramatic effect on short-term prognosis. Patients with a non–Q-wave MI in the anterior distribution have much higher reinfarction and mortality rates than those with inferolateral non–Q-wave MI. The key issue, not addressed in this study, is whether a more aggressive revascularization strategy could improve the otherwise poor outcome. Until further studies are performed, it would seem prudent to recommend coronary angiography and revascularization (coronary angioplasty or coronary artery bypass grafting) for most patients with a recent anterior non–Q-wave MI. This strategy is especially recommended for patients in whom postinfarction angina develops and those who have documented exercise-induced myocardial ischemia.—G.L. Schaer, M.D., and J.E. Parrillo, M.D.

The Effects of Oral Isosorbide 5-Mononitrate on Mortality Following Acute Myocardial Infarction: A Multicentre Study
Fitzgerald LJ, Bennett ED (St George's Hosp Med School, London)
Eur Heart J 11:120–126, 1990   5–5

Intravenous nitrates are widely used in the treatment of acute myocardial infarction (MI), but the role of oral nitrates in management has not been well studied. To study the effects of oral isosorbide 5-mononitrate (ISMN) in the management of acute MI, a multicenter, randomized, double-blind, placebo-controlled trial was undertaken in 360 patients with suspected AMI. Of these, 184 were randomly allocated to treatment with ISMN and 176 to placebo. The mean age was 60 years. The initial oral dose of ISMN or placebo was 40 mg if the systolic blood pressure (SBP) was more than 110 mm Hg and 20 mg if it was 110 mm Hg or less. Thereafter, the ISMN dose for all patients was 20 mg, given 4 times daily for 48 hours, 3 times daily for 24 hours, and 2 times daily for 48 hours. Before analysis of the results, patients were grouped according to the presence or absence of heart failure on admission.

The diagnosis of infarction was confirmed in 93% of the ISMN-treated patients and in 93% of the controls. The 5-day overall mortality rate was 4.9% in ISMN-treated patients and 4% in the controls; the overall mortality rate at 6 months was 14.1% in the ISMN-treated patients and 10.5% in controls. There was a nonsignificant reduction in mortality in ISMN-treated patients with heart failure at 5 days compared with a nonsignificant increase in mortality in ISMN-treated patients without heart failure. Lidocaine requirements in ISMN-treated patients were slightly increased over those in the controls. Oral ISMN produced a mean reduction in SBP of 10 mm Hg at 6 hours and 8 mm Hg at 12 hours, with no effect thereafter.

The hemodynamic effects of oral ISMN are similar to those of intravenous nitroglycerin. Oral ISMN can be of benefit in patients with acute

MI and heart failure. However, the use of nitrates in acute MI in the absence of heart failure needs to be further investigated.

▶ Intravenous nitroglycerin is used increasingly in the management of acute MI, particularly in patients receiving thrombolytic therapy. This study investigated the effects of oral ISMN on mortality in patients with acute MI. This nitrate preparation was chosen because it does not undergo first-pass metabolism (unlike isosorbide dinitrate) and therefore produces more stable plasma levels with less variable hemodynamic effects. There are 2 problems with this study. First, although a trend toward reduced mortality was observed in MI patients with heart failure, the study did not enroll a sufficient number of patients to detect a statistical difference. A second problem is that none of the patients received thrombolytic therapy. The coronary vasodilating properties of nitrates may be particularly beneficial in patients successfully reperfused with thrombolytic therapy. Additional studies are clearly needed.—G.L. Schaer, M.D., and J.E. Parrillo, M.D.

Prognostic Significance of Nonfatal Myocardial Reinfarction
Benhorin J, Moss AJ, Oakes D, the Multicenter Diltiazem Postinfarction Trial Research Group (Univ of Rochester, NY)
J Am Coll Cardiol 15:253–258, 1990   5–6

In most risk stratification and intervention postinfarction trials, cardiac mortality is used as the major outcome end point, either alone or in combination with nonfatal reinfarction, to form a single composite end point.

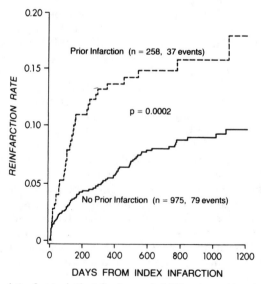

Fig 5–1.—Cumulative first nonfatal reinfarction rate in 1,233 patients with and without earlier (preenrollment) infarction. (Courtesy of Benhorin J, Moss AJ, Oakes D, et al: *J Am Coll Cardiol* 15:253–258, 1990.)

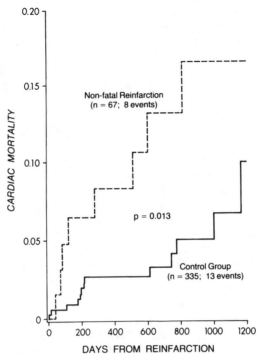

Fig 5–2.—Cumulative cardiac mortality rate in 67 patients after a second nonfatal myocardial infarction and in a 5:1 matched control group (no. = 335). (Courtesy of Benhorin J, Moss AJ, Oakes D, et al: *J Am Coll Cardiol* 15:253–258, 1990.)

This combined end point is based on the assumption that similar pathophysiologic mechanisms contribute to both events. Because the independent risk carried by nonfatal myocardial reinfarction for subsequent cardiac death has not been determined, the prognostic significance of nonfatal reinfarction was assessed, using the data from the previously reported Multicenter Diltiazem Postinfarction Trial. The study population included 1,234 patients, aged 25–75 years, treated with placebo, who were followed for 1–4 years after an acute myocardial infarction (MI).

During an average follow-up of 25 months, 116 patients (9.4%) experienced a first nonfatal reinfarction, of whom 14 (12.1%) subsequently died of cardiac causes and 5 (4.3%) of noncardiac causes (Fig 5–1). Of the remaining 1,118 patients, 110 (9.8%) had a cardiac death and 38 (3.4%) had noncardiac death. Univariate analysis revealed that patients with nonfatal reinfarction were more likely to be women, to have had an MI before their index event, and to have had previous cardiac-related symptoms. Multiple logistic regression analysis revealed that nonfatal reinfarction carried a significant and independent risk for subsequent cardiac mortality greater than that carried by other significant variables. An actuarial comparison of cardiac mortality in patients after a second nonfatal MI with that in a 5:1 matched control group confirmed that cardiac mortality was significantly greater over time in the reinfarction group than in the control population (Fig 5–2).

Nonfatal reinfarction represents a strong, significant, and independent risk for subsequent cardiac death in postinfarction patients. The relative contribution of nonfatal reinfarction to the risk of cardiac death is higher in patients with a first MI than in the total postinfarction population.

▶ It has been amply demonstrated that, in patients leaving the hospital after recovery from an MI, the 1-year mortality rate is higher after non–Q-wave infarction than after Q-wave infarction. Epidemiologic investigations have also demonstrated that mortality in women after MI is generally higher than that in men. Whether posthospitalization mortality in non–Q-wave infarction can be affected beneficially by long-term pharmacologic intervention remains to be demonstrated. The Beta-Blocker Heart Attack Trial demonstrated that β blockers were primarily effective after Q-wave infarction. Meta-analyses of aspirin trials suggest that these agents lower mortality after infarction.

The Diltiazem Reinfarction Trial demonstrated a decrease in reinfarction in patients receiving calcium channel blockers after non–Q-wave infarction. No antiarrhythmic agent has been demonstrated to decrease posthospitalization mortality in infarct patients.

Thus risk stratification currently may be useful for prognosis but not necessarily for decisions on selected medication. It is now prudent to give all postinfarct patients a β blocker and aspirin (usually 160 mg daily) for long-term maintenance after infarction. It is also important, especially with regard to attributable risk for future cardiovascular events after infarction, to lower the low-density lipoprotein cholesterol level to less than 130 mg/dL by diet and, frequently, lipid-lowering agents. Some clinicians would lower this value to below 100 mg/dL in the postinfarction population.—P.R. Liebson, M.D., and J.E. Parrillo, M.D.

Serial Evaluation of Right Ventricular Dysfunction Associated With Acute Inferior Myocardial Infarction
Yasuda T, Okada RD, Leinbach RC, Gold HK, Phillips H, McKusick KA, Glover DK, Boucher CA, Strauss HW (Massachusetts Gen Hosp, Boston; Saint Francis Hosp Med Research Inst, Tulsa; Univ of Oklahoma)
Am Heart J 119:816–822, 1990   5–7

Previous studies have found that 15% to 50% of patients with inferior wall myocardial infarction (MI) have right ventricular (RV) dysfunction. Gated blood pool scans in these patients show an increase in RV size and a decrease in RV ejection fraction (RVEF) when compared with normal controls and patients with anterior MI. Serial evaluation of RV function in patients with acute inferior wall MI and associated RV dysfunction was performed using multigated blood pool imaging.

During a 3-year period, 38 patients were seen with inferior wall MI, in 18 of whom had RV dysfunction was observed on radionuclide ventricu-

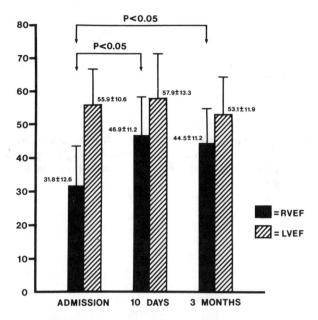

EVOLUTION OF RVEF AND LVEF

Fig 5–3.—Mean right ventricular ejection fraction (RVEF) and left ventricular ejection fraction (LVEF) on admission and at 10 days and 3 months after infarction. (Courtesy of Yasuda T, Okada RD, Leinbach RC, et al: *Am Heart J* 119:816–822, 1990.)

lograms. All patients had ECG evidence of inferior wall MI, but none had clinical evidence of RV dysfunction. Consequently, RV infarction was not clinically suspected initially. All patients underwent multigated blood pool scanning within 18 hours of chest pain and again at 10 days. Fifteen patients also underwent rest and exercise ventriculography at 3 months.

The mean resting RVEF was 31.8% at admission, 46.9% at 10 days, and 44.5% at 3 months; the improvement in RVEF was statistically significant. Left ventricular ejection fraction (LVEF), on the other hand, was 55.9% at admission, 57.9% at 10 days, and 53.1% at 3 months, values that were not different (Fig 5–3). Six of 15 patients undergoing exercise ventriculography at 3 months had a rise in RVEF of greater than a 5% increase with exercise. Eight patients underwent cardiac catheterization. Neither the location, the severity of coronary artery narrowing, nor the presence of collaterals correlated with the RV exercise response. Improvement in RV function over a 10-day interval after acute inferior wall MI suggests the presence of significant reversible RV dysfunction in some patients during the acute phase.

▶ A subpopulation of patients with inferior MI demonstrate RV ischemia and RV dysfunction. It is important to recognize such patients; they may have fluid-responsive hypotension. Of the 18 patients identified here, 3 had a drop in blood pressure in response to nitrates or morphine, and 8 had hypotension requiring rapid volume expansion and pressor agents.

It is not clear, however, that bedside gated blood pool scans are always the best way to identify RV dysfunction in the coronary care unit. A look at the error bars in Figure 5–3 will serve to point up the variability of the technique.— S. Hollenberg, M.D., and J.E. Parrillo, M.D.

The Use of Tissue-Type Plasminogen Activator for Acute Myocardial Infarction in the Elderly: Results From Thrombolysis in Myocardial Infarction Phase I, Open Label Studies and the Thrombolysis in Myocardial Infarction Phase II Pilot Study
Chaitman BR, Thompson B, Wittry MD, Stump D, Hamilton WP, Hillis LD, Dwyer JG, Solomon RE, Knatterud GL, for the TIMI Investigators (Maryland Med Research Inst, Inc, Baltimore)
J Am Coll Cardiol 14:1159–1165, 1989   5–8

Elderly patients with acute myocardial infarction (MI) are at increased risk for in-hospital mortality and morbidity when compared with younger patients. Most clinical trials designed to assess the efficacy of thrombolytic therapy in patients with acute MI exclude patients older than 75 years of age. Consequently, clinical data on elderly patients with acute MI treated with thrombolytic therapy are scarce. Clinical experience with recombinant tissue-type plasminogen activator (rt-PA) for acute MI in patients 65 years of age or older who were enrolled in the Thrombolysis in Myocardial Infarction (TIMI) trials was evaluated. Of 756 patients enrolled in the TIMI study, 577 were 65 years of age or younger, 87 were aged 65–69 years, and 92 were aged 70–76 years.

The in-hospital mortality rates were 3.5% in patients aged 65 years and younger, 11.5% in patients aged 65–69 years, and 12% in patients aged 70–76 years. Thus in-hospital mortality increased significantly with

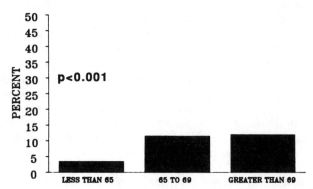

Fig 5–4.—The in-hospital mortality rate was significantly increased in patients >65 years of age ($P < .001$). (Courtesy of Chaitman BR, Thompson B, Wittry MD, et al: *J Am Coll Cardiol* 14:1159–1165, 1989.)

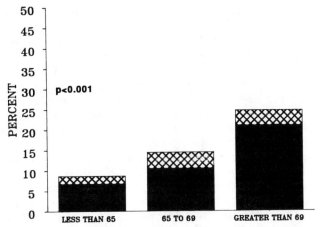

Fig 5–5.—The incidence of major hemorrhagic events among patients not undergoing cardiac surgery significantly increased with age ($p < .001$). The incidence of transfusions among those who had a major hemorrhagic event significantly increased with age. *Filled area*, transfusion; *shaded area*, no transfusion. (Courtesy of Chaitman BR, Thompson B, Wittry MD, et al: *J Am Coll Cardiol* 14:1159–1165, 1989.)

increasing age (Fig 5–4). Female gender, presence of diabetes mellitus or extensive coronary artery disease, history of congestive heart failure, continuing chest pain immediately after rt-PA administration, low systolic blood pressure at the time of admission, and advanced age were variables predictive of in-hospital death.

The incidence of major hemorrhagic events among patients who did not undergo cardiac surgery during hospitalization was 8.7% in patients aged 65 years or younger, 14.5% in patients aged 65–69 years, and 24.7% in patients aged 70–76 years. Thus the incidence of major bleeding events also increased with age (Fig 5–5). Most bleeding events were associated with cardiac catheterization or puncture wounds. Reperfusion status at 90 minutes after rt-PA administration was similar for all 3 age groups and ranged from 60% to 71%.

Early cardiac catheterization in older patients with acute MI who are treated with rt-PA is associated with an increased in-hospital mortality rate and an increased incidence of hemorrhagic events when compared with younger patients. The safety and efficacy of rt-PA therapy in patients older than 76 years of age have not been determined.

▶ With increasing experience with thrombolytics, advanced age is no longer considered an absolute contraindication to such therapy; because mortality is higher, the benefits of reperfusion would be expected to be greater. As this study points out, the risks in the elderly are higher as well (although in these TIMI trials, all patients underwent cardiac catheterization, and some received 150 mg of rt-PA, a dose associated with higher rates of hemorrhage). A randomized trial of rt-PA in patients older than 75 would be of great interest.—S. Hollenberg, M.D., and J.E. Parrillo, M.D.

Patterns of Coronary Artery Disease in Post-Infarction Ventricular Septal Rupture

Skehan JD, Carey C, Norrell MS, de Belder M, Balcon R, Mills PG (London Hosp; London Chest Hosp)
Br Heart J 62:268–272, 1989   5–9

Rupture of the interventricular septum occurs in approximately 1% of survivors of myocardial infarction (MI). A clinical impression that the coronary collateral circulation and the left ventricular anatomy of patients with septal rupture differ from the patterns commonly seen in MI survivors prompted a comparison of the cardiac cineangiograms of 91 patients with septal rupture with those of 123 unselected stable survivors of MI who had a positive submaximal exercise test early after infarction.

Patients with septal rupture were older, had a more even ratio of men to women, and more often had anterior infarctions and total occlusions of the infarct vessel. They had more left ventricular damage, more single-vessel than triple-vessel disease, more aneurysm formation, and minimal collaterals to the infarct territory. The comparison patients had more triple-vessel than single-vessel disease, and two thirds of the patients had well-developed collaterals. Ventricular septal rupture is more likely to occur in patients with coronary occlusion who have little or no collateral support to the infarct territory.

▶ Ventricular septal rupture typically presents within 3–5 days after MI, with rapid onset of biventricular failure and appearance of a new murmur. Doppler echocardiography will establish the diagnosis easily and reliably, but arteriography is usually performed before operating to visualize the coronary anatomy and guide aortocoronary bypass grafting. This report from Skehan et al. summarizes a broad clinical experience and suggests that the absence of coronary collaterals exacerbates regional necrosis, increases the risk of ventricular aneurysmal dilatation, and leads to septal rupture.— R.E. Cunnion, M.D.

Should Thrombolytic Therapy Be Administered in the Mobile Intensive Care Unit in Patients With Evolving Myocardial Infarction? A Pilot Study

Roth A, Barbash GI, Hod H, Miller HI, Rath S, Modan M, Har-Zahav Y, Keren G, Bassan S, Kaplinsky E, Laniado S (Tel-Aviv Med Ctr; Sheba Med Ctr, Tel-Aviv; Sackler School of Medicine, Tel-Aviv)
J Am Coll Cardiol 15:932–936, 1990   5–10

Because timely delivery of thrombolysis is valuable in the successful reperfusion of patients with acute myocardial infarction (MI), it has been suggested that such therapy be started before the patient arrives at the hospital. The feasibility, safety, and effectiveness of prehospital thrombolytic therapy were evaluated in 2 medical centers in Israel, where mobile intensive care units are staffed by physicians or interns as well as by paramedics. The 118 patients eligible for the study received treatment with recombinant tissue-type plasminogen activator (rt-PA), either in the mobile intensive care unit (group A) or in the hospital (group B). A total dose of 120 mg of rt-PA was administered over a 6-hour period.

Intravenous thrombolytic treatment was initiated at a mean of 94 minutes after onset of chest pain in group A (74 patients) and after a mean of 137 minutes in group B (44 patients). The radionuclide left ventricular ejection fraction, measured within 48 hours of arrival at the hospital, did not differ significantly in the 2 groups. A trend toward a lower incidence of congestive heart failure at hospital discharge was noted in group A (7%) compared with group B (16%). The 2 groups did not differ significantly in incidence of recurrent ischemia, bleeding, coronary angioplasty, coronary bypass graft procedures, or death.

The prehospital intravenous administration of rt-PA was safe and shortened the time from onset of chest pain to treatment by an average of 43 minutes. Prehospital thrombolysis did not, however, significantly improve the outcome in this patient group.

▶ Administering thrombolytic agents very early after the onset of chest pain clearly has the potential to maximize their beneficial effects. In this pilot study from Tel-Aviv, the number of patients was too small to demonstrate statistically significant differences in outcomes, i.e., death, heart failure, recurrent ischemia, reinfarction, and stroke. Rather, the principal importance of this study lies in its demonstration that prehospital thrombolysis is feasible. This is true, at least in settings where physicians travel in ambulances, and potentially it may be extrapolated to the much broader patient populations served by paramedics. Additional investigations currently in progress will clarify issues pertaining to patient selection and organization of the mobile health care team.—R.E. Cunnion, M.D.

Selecting the Best Triage Rule for Patients Hospitalized With Chest Pain
Weingarten SR, Ermann B, Riedinger MS, Shah PK, Ellrodt AG (Univ of California, Los Angeles; RAND/UCLA Ctr for Health Policy Study, Santa Monica, Calif)
Am J Med 87:494–500, 1989   5–11

Clinical prediction rules and risk stratification aids have been designed to improve the efficiency of bed utilization by patients hospitalized with chest pain. These rules have dealt both with admission to the coronary care unit (CCU) or intermediate care unit and with subsequent transfer to less intensive care units.

In the present prospective observational study of 498 patients at Cedars-Sinai Medical Center, triage rules were tested both at admission and 24 hours later to determine whether following these rules shortens the stay in the CCU and intermediate care unit without compromising patient care. Admission guidelines were based partially on Brush's classification of the ECG, which was modified to incorporate clinical practices essential for triage. The early transfer guidelines, based on recommendations of Mulley et al., incorporated clinical factors.

Application of an admission triage rule would have increased admissions to the CCU by 3%. Application of the early transfer rule would have reduced bed usage by 860 intermediate care and 82 CCU bed-days, when compared with actual patient triage. This reduction would decrease hospital costs and increase bed availability to incoming patients. Twenty-four patients (9.5%) would have experienced a minor complication after a transfer directed by the triage rule, but their medical care would not have been affected adversely. The use of the admission triage rule did not predict life-threatening complications as well in this population as in that originally reported by Brush and co-workers.

These findings suggest that use of an admission triage rule would have increased bed utilization in the CCU. The use of a triage rule 24 hours after admission appears more promising for improving bed utilization and would do so by shortening the stay in the CU or intermediate care unit.

▶ In many institutions the demand for monitored beds in the CCU and intermediate care unit exceeds the supply, and it becomes necessary on occasion to admit patients with chest pain to unmonitored beds, to send them to other hospitals, or to transfer other patients out of units to create space. The use of formal, explicit triage algorithms potentially could facilitate optimal utilization of monitored beds. Many such triage algorithms have been promoted but relatively few have undergone rigorous prospective evaluation. In this careful study from Cedars-Sinai Medical Center, triage rules failed to reduce unit admissions but did serve at 24 hours to identify low-risk patients for expedited transfer out of units. Although triage algorithms can complement clinical judgment, they cannot substitute for it, and before implementing triage algorithms hospitals must factor into context their own unique resources and capabilities.—R.E. Cunnion, M.D.

Direct Coronary Angioplasty in Acute Myocardial Infarction: Outcome in Patients With Single Vessel Disease
Stone GW, Rutherford BD, McConahay DR, Johnson WL Jr, Giorgi LV, Ligon RW, Hartzler GO (St Luke's Hosp, Kansas City, Mo.)
J Am Coll Cardiol 15:534–543, 1990   5–12

Although recent studies have shown that early reperfusion can limit infarct size and increase survival, the optimal therapy for patients with single-vessel disease who present with acute myocardial infarction (MI) is not known. At the Mid-America Heart Institute patients in the early stages of acute MI are managed by immediate coronary arteriography followed by direct coronary angioplasty, without previous thrombolytic therapy.

The short- and long-term prognosis and clinical and angiographic factors that influence prognosis and myocardial salvage after direct angioplasty were studied in 215 consecutive patients with single-vessel disease who had the procedure between 1981 and 1988. The 161 men and 54 women had a mean age of 56 years. Angioplasty was generally initiated within 1 hour after the patient's arrival in the emergency room.

Coronary angioplasty was successful in 212 patients (99%). One patient required urgent coronary bypass operation. No deaths occurred during the initial angioplasty procedure. In 8 patients (4%) a recurrent ischemic event occurred before discharge. The in-hospital mortality rate was 1%. In 66 of 126 patients in whom predischarge angiography was performed the left ventricular ejection fraction increased. Regional wall motion improved in 60 patients.

After a mean follow-up of 35 months 214 patients had an actuarial 3-year cardiac survival rate of 92%. Nine patients (4%) had a late, nonfatal MI, 11 (5%) underwent late coronary bypass surgery, and 52 (24%) underwent repeat coronary angioplasty procedures. At late follow-up evaluation 149 of 197 patients (77%) were asymptomatic, but 29 (15%) had mild angina.

In patients with single-vessel disease and evolving acute MI, direct coronary angioplasty without previous thrombolytic therapy results in excellent early and late event-free survival. These results are comparable to those achievable with conventional or thrombolytic therapy.

Emergency Angioplasty in Acute Anterior Myocardial Infarction
Flaker GC, Webel RR, Meinhardt S, Anderson S, Santolin C, Artis A, Krol R
(Univ of Missouri Hosps and Clinics; Harry S Truman VA Hosp, Columbia)
Am Heart J 118:1154–1159, 1989   5–13

Because patients with acute occlusion of the left anterior descending (LAD) vessel resulting in anterior infarction have a high rate of in-hospital mortality (10% to 28%), aggressive forms of medical management have been advocated. The outcomes in 93 patients with acute anterior

Predictors of Hospital Mortality in Patients With Anterior Infarction Treated With Emergency PTCA			
	No.	*Hospital mortality*	*p*
Cardiogenic Shock			<0.001
Present	20	10 (50%)	
Absent	73	3 (4%)	
Site of LAD stenosis			<0.002
Proximal	43	11 (26%)	
Mid-distal	50	2 (4%)	
Residual LAD stenosis			<0.0027
Complete success (≤50%)	73	5 (7%)	
Partial success (51-99%)	12	3 (25%)	
Failure	8	5 (63%)	

(Courtesy of Flaker GC, Webel RR, Meinhardt S, et al: *Am Heart J* 118:1154–1159, 1989.)

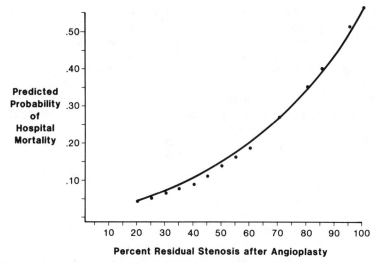

Percent Residual Stenosis after Angioplasty

Fig 5–6.— Predicted probability of hospital mortality as a function of the degree of residual stenosis. The estimated probability of hospital mortality is greated than .50 when the residual stenosis is 95% or greater. (Courtesy of Flaker GC, Webel RR, Meinhardt S, et al: *Am Heart J* 118:1154–1159, 1989.)

myocardial infarction who were treated with percutaneous transluminal coronary angioplasty (PTCA) were reviewed. All had a high-grade obstruction in the LAD vessel or the bypass graft to this vessel; 64 patients had total occlusion and the others had stenosis ranging from 90% to 99%.

In 73 patients (78%) PTCA was considered to be completely successful with a residual lesion of less than 50%. Results in 12 patients were judged partially successful, with a residual lesion of 51% to 99%; PTCA was unsuccessful in 8 patients (9%). Thirteen patients (14%) died in the hospital. Factors independently predictive of hospital mortality were the presence of shock, proximal location of the LAD stenosis, and the degree of residual stenosis of the LAD vessel after PTCA (table). When residual stenosis is 95% or higher, the estimated probability of hospital mortality is greater than .50 (Fig 5–6). Although reocclusion was found in only 11% of the patients, 34% had later evidence of restenosis.

The mortality rate was 9% in the 85 patients in whom PTCA was completely or partially successful. In contrast, the mortality rate was 63% in patients with unsuccessful PTCA. Thus PTCA should be attempted only by cardiologists who are experienced in the procedure, and they should strive for a residual lesion of less than 50%.

▶ The proper role of primary angioplasty in acute myocardial infarction (MI), although widely studied and debated, remains controversial. The report by Stone et al. (Abstract 5–12) presents a retrospective analysis with unbelievably good results. They were able to get most patients to the catheterization laboratory within 1 hour of presentation to the emergency room, and angioplasty was done within 6 hours of symptom onset in more than 75% of cases. In patients with single-vessel disease, they reported a primary success rate of 99% and an in-hospital mortality of 1%. Flaker et al. (Abstract 5–13) retrospectively analyzed patients with disease in the LAD territory (native vessel or bypass graft), with somewhat different results. Their mortality rate was 9% in patients with successful angioplasty, but 63% in the 8% of patients with unsuccessful PTCA. The difference between the 2 studies probably results from the population studied, an unavoidable difficulty with retrospective analyses. The retrospective analysis by Stone et al. also obscures that fact that to find the 43% of patients with single-vessel disease, one must catheterize the 57% of patients who don't have it; the results in the group as a whole were not as impressive (1).

It appears that patients who have successful angioplasty after acute MI do well, whereas patients in whom the procedure is unsuccessful are in big trouble. Predicting beforehand who will do well with PTCA is not easy (and those patients are the ones who are likely to do well with thrombolytic therapy alone). Randomized trials comparing emergent with delayed angioplasty or with conservative therapy have shown no benefit of routine emergency angioplasty (2,3). Thrombolytic therapy (in eligible candidates) decreases mortality (4). The TIMI II-B trial compared routine catheterization and angioplasty with the conservative strategy of "watchful waiting" and found no significant differences (5).

What is a doctor to do? In our opinion, routine coronary angioplasty as primary therapy in acute MI remains unproven. Patients with failed angioplasty do poorly early on, and emergent coronary artery bypass grafting in these patients is generally done using saphenous vein grafts rather than internal mammary arteries, with all the consequent implications for late graft stenosis. Emergent PTCA is a promising therapy for patients who fail to exhibit reperfusion after thrombolytic therapy (these patients can be difficult to identify, but they usually experience ongoing or recurrent chest pain and ST segment elevation) and in those who present early after symptom onset but have contraindications to thrombolysis.—S. Hollenberg, M.D., and J.E. Parrillo, M.D.

References

1. O'Keefe JH Jr, et al: *Am J Cardiol* 64:1221, 1989.
2. TIMI Research Group: *JAMA* 260:2849, 1988.
3. Topol EJ, et al: *N Engl J Med* 317:581, 1987.
4. GISSI: *Lancet* 1:397, 1986.
5. TIMI Research Group: *N Engl J Med* 320:618, 1989.

Percutaneous Cardiopulmonary Bypass Support in High-Risk Patients Undergoing Percutaneous Transluminal Coronary Angioplasty
Shawl FA, Domanski MJ, Punja S, Hernandez TJ (Washington Adventist Hosp, Takoma Park, Md)
Am J Cardiol 64:1258–1263, 1989   5–14

High-risk patients undergoing coronary angioplasty may be supported by the prophylactic use of cardiopulmonary bypass. The outcomes of supported angioplasty in 51 consecutive patients (mean age, 63 years) were reviewed. Most of the patients had a low ejection fraction, a large amount of viable myocardium perfused by the target artery(s), or both.

Of the patients, 23 had Canadian Cardiovascular Society class III and 28 had class IV angina. Most had 3-vessel disease (94%) and impaired left ventricular function (90%). Cardiopulmonary bypass support was instituted using a nonsurgical percutaneous insertion technique, with flows of 2–5 L/min (mean, 3.6 L/min). Support was gradually weaned in approximately 5 minutes after completion of angioplasty. The mean bypass time was 37 minutes.

Angioplasty was successful in 115 of 117 attempted lesions. Most of the complications occurred at bypass cannula insertion sites. Three patients died in the hospital of causes unrelated to bypass. Discharged patients were followed for a mean of 4.9 months. During this period 31 patients remained asymptomatic, 12 were in class I, and 4 in class II; 1 patient died, but the cause was unclear.

In up to 6% of patients, balloon angioplasty results in abrupt closure, an event that can result in hemodynamic collapse or death. Patients with poor left ventricular function at baseline or those in whom the abruptly closed vessel supplies a large amount of myocardium may not survive long enough to undergo emergency bypass surgery. Percutaneous bypass support in such high-risk patients allows systemic perfusion to be maintained and may allow for successful balloon angioplasty.

▶ The concept of supported angioplasty has been gaining increasing acceptance and popularity in recent years. The technique is useful for patients with high-risk lesions who might not be optimal surgical candidates but who would benefit from coronary revascularization. Bypass can be initiated after insertion of percutaneous sheaths by an experienced invasive cardiologist, but it is important to realize that ready availability of qualified pump technicians and surgical backup are essential. The high restenosis rate in this study (9 of 17), and the fact that 40% of the patients required blood transfusions (mean, 2.4 units), argue against the indiscriminate use of this technique. Carefully selected patients, however, may benefit from supported percutaneous transluminal coronary angiography.—S. Hollenberg, M.D., and J.E. Parrillo, M.D.

The Cost:Benefit Ratio of Acute Intervention for Myocardial Infarction: Results of a Prospective, Matched Pair Analysis
Chapekis AT, Burek K, Topol EJ (Univ of Michigan)
Am Heart J 118:878–882, 1989   5–15

Intervention with early reperfusion therapy for acute myocardial infarction (MI) has resulted in decreased mortality, improved left ventricular function, and limitation of infarct size. Nevertheless, declining financial resources necessitate scrutiny of the cost:benefit ratio of such additional procedures. The clinical outcome and costs of intervention and nonintervention strategies were studied prospectively in 78 matched pairs of patients with acute MI who were drawn from a database of 507 patients. The selected patients had a mean age of 61 years; 68% were men, and 43% had an anterior infarct location. In the intervention group, 27 patients had intravenous thrombolysis, 14 had coronary angioplasty, and 34 had thrombolysis followed by angioplasty. No attempt at myocardial reperfusion was made in the nonintervention group, but they were subsequently considered for angiography and revascularization.

Nearly half of the patients undergoing acute intervention had an uncomplicated clinical status at 72 hours, compared with only 19% of those in the nonintervention group. The 10-day mortality rate was 5.3% with intervention and 13% with nonintervention. Diagnostic cardiac catheterization and percutaneous transluminal coronary angioplasty were performed more often in the intervention group than in the nonintervention group (99% vs. 51% and 60% vs. 0%, respectively).

The mean cumulative hospital charges were not statistically different for the 2 groups ($31,684 with intervention and $29,022 with nonintervention). The cost-to-benefit ratio of acute intervention for MI appears to be in the range of other accepted treatments.

▶ Cost:benefit analyses in medicine are extremely difficult to do; this particular analysis compares a group that underwent intervention within the first 6 hours of onset of symptoms with a group not eligible for such therapy (most likely because they presented later or were older than 75). For another thing, such analyses involve assumptions and value judgments that are hard to quantify and that not everyone may share. Still, it is reassuring that thrombolytic therapy, a treatment known to improve mortality in acute MI, is reasonably cost efficient.— S. Hollenberg, M.D., and J.E. Parrillo, M.D.

Angiographic Morphology of Coronary Artery Stenoses in Prolonged Rest Angina: Evidence of Intracoronary Thrombosis
Rehr R, Disciascio G, Vetrovec G, Cowley M (Med College of Virginia, Richmond)
J Am Coll Cardiol 14:1429–1437, 1989   5–16

Angiographic findings of occlusive thrombus, intraluminal filling defects, and complex lesion morphology can indicate the presence of intracoronary thrombosis. To determine whether these findings are also associated with the clinical syndrome of unstable (prolonged rest) angina, a review was made of the coronary angiograms of 92 patients in whom significant coronary artery disease was found.

Coronary angiograms were performed by way of the trancutaneous femoral approach, and each major epicardial vessel was evaluated in all relevant projections by 2 experienced angiographers. Interrater reliability was excellent, with a concordance rate of 87%. Angiograms were defined as "unstable" if they contained at least 1 unstable coronary artery, i.e., an artery exhibiting either evidence of an intraluminal coronary thrombus or the presence of a complex lesion. Angiograms without such findings were classified as "stable."

Group I included 50 patients who were clinically unstable and group II included 42 patients who were clinically stable. Men were significantly underrepresented in the former group (56% vs. 81%). There was no intergroup difference in either aspirin use or overall nonsteroidal anti-inflammatory drug use. The mean severity of significant coronary artery stenoses and the frequency of significant left main coronary artery disease were similar in the 2 groups. Far more patients in the unstable group had evidence of intracoronary thrombus (42% vs. 17%) and complex lesion morphology (44% vs. 14%). This difference was significant by χ^2 analysis.

Overall, acute coronary morphology was found in a significantly higher percentage of patients in group I (70%) than in group II (21%). These findings suggest that there is a strong association between the angiographic descriptors of intraluminal thrombosis and the clinical syndrome of unstable angina. This syndrome and acute transmural myocardial infarction may share a thrombotic mechanism.

▶ The finding of a strong association between intraluminal coronary thrombus or complex lesion morphology and angina at rest suggests that this intracoronary pathology may be important in initiating the syndrome of prolonged rest angina. Although 30% of the patients with unstable symptoms had no evidence of thrombosis, angiography is not completely sensitive in the detection of intracoronary clot; in any case, it provides a view of the coronary anatomy at only a single time point. Other mechanisms such as coronary spasm may play a role in some patients.

This study supports a pathogenic role of intracoronary thrombosis in the initiation of unstable angina and strengthens the theoretical justification for trials of thrombolytic agents in unstable angina. Such trials are underway, and the results are eagerly anticipated.— S. Hollenberg, M.D., and J.E. Parrillo, M.D.

The Predictive Value of Serum Enzymes for Perioperative Myocardial Infarction After Cardiac Operations: An Autopsy Study
Van Lente F, Martin A, Ratliff NB, Kazmierczak SC, Loop FD (Cleveland Clinic Found)
J Thorac Cardiovasc Surg 98:704–710, 1989   5–17

Perioperative myocardial infarction (MI) occurs in 5% to 23% of patients undergoing coronary artery bypass, but the diagnosis is difficult to establish. Cardiac enzymes and isoenzymes were evaluated as predictors of perioperative MI in 79 patients in whom autopsies were performed after coronary artery bypass or valve replacement procedures.

Multiple sections were taken from the myocardium at autopsy and clinical records were reviewed for ECG evidence of perioperative MI. Blood samples for analysis of enzymes had been obtained at admission to the recovery unit.

Histologic examination demonstrated findings consistent with perioperative MI in 37 patients. In the remaining 42 patients there was either no evidence of myocardial injury or the age of the infarct was not consistent with the time between operation and death. Death resulted from cardiac causes in 30 patients (81%) with infarction and in 8 patients (19%) without infarction.

Enzyme activities, including those of creatine kinase, creatine kinase-MB, asparate aminotransferase, and the lactate dehydrogenase-1/lactate dehydrogenase-2 ratio, differed significantly in patients with and without infarction. All enzyme parameters were greater in the infarction group. Creatine kinase-MB levels showed the closest relationship with the presence of perioperative MI.

Myocardium-derived enzymes are released during cardiac operations involving cardiopulmonary bypass. By using a cutoff of 133 units per liter for creatine kinase-MB activity, 15 infarctions would be diagnosed with 96% accuracy at a prevalence of 10%.

▶ The diagnosis of perioperative MI can be very challenging, and changes in cardiac isoenzymes cannot be used to identify all such patients. This was an autopsy study with histologic evidence of MI; one would expect such fatal infarctions to be less subtle than nonfatal MIs. The premortem diagnosis of perioperative MI on the basis of symptoms, ECG changes, or wall motion abnormalities may be very difficult. Nonetheless, the findings of these investigators suggest that measurement of creatine kinase-MB fractions may be useful, provided that the lower threshold value is adjusted to make the test more specific.—S. Hollenberg, M.D., and J.E. Parrillo, M.D.

Multiple Microemboli After Disintegration of Clot During Thrombolysis for Acute Myocardial Infarction
Stafford PJ, Strachan CJL, Vincent R, Chamberlain DA (Royal Sussex County Hosp, Brighton, England)
Br Med J 299:1310–1312, 1989   5–18

Hemorrhage and reperfusion injury are potential complications of thrombolytic therapy; another complication appears to be related to disintegration of clots after treatment with anistreplase or streptokinase. Severe symptoms developed in 7 patients soon after they received thrombolytic agents.

The patients with severe embolic complications represent 1.5% of a group of 475 consecutive patients treated with thrombolysis for acute myocardial infarction. Of the 7 patients, 5 complained of severe leg pain, although only 2 lost a major pulse. In 5 patients, symptoms appeared within 12 hours after thrombolysis.

In all of these patients, complications were thought to have resulted from systemic embolization from disintegration of a preexisting clot. The symptoms were not characteristic of those of vasculitic reaction, an alternative explanation. Five patients died. In several patients, necropsy showed evidence of emboli. The response of 1 patient to iloprost, a stable prostaglandin analogue, suggests that this agent may possibly be beneficial in treating peripheral microemboli. Conditions associated with an intravascular clot may contraindicate thrombolysis.

▶ As the use of thrombolytic therapy in acute myocardial infarction becomes more widespread, more potential complications of such therapy are being recognized. These case reports point up another possible complication worth considering. Known intravascular clots probably represent a relative contraindication to thrombolytic therapy. The authors reported a good result with the use of iloprost in 1 patient. This therapy is difficult to evaluate because most American physicians would heparinize patients with microemboli acutely: Of the 7 patients reported here, 5 were given coumadin and none was given heparin.—S. Hollenberg, M.D., and J.E. Parrillo, M.D.

Increased Neutrophil Elastase Release in Unstable Angina Pectoris and Acute Myocardial Infarction

Dinerman JL, Mehta JL, Saldeen TGP, Emerson S, Wallin R, Davda R, Davidson A (Univ of Florida; Univ of Uppsala, Sweden)

J Am Coll Cardiol 15:1559–1563, 1990   5–19

Neutrophils release oxygen free radicals and proteolytic enzymes, including elastase, which can damage vital tissue. Neutrophils have been implicated as contributing to the continued myocardial injury that occurs after successful reperfusion in the management of acute myocardial infarction (MI). Thus elastase may have a role in reperfusion injury. To characterize neutrophil elastase activity in ischemic heart disease, plasma levels of a neutrophil elastase-derived fibrinopeptide, Bβ 30–43, were measured by a specific radioimmunoassay in 25 patients with stable an-

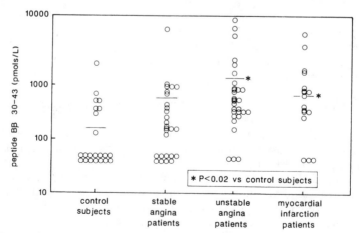

Fig 5–7.—Plasma levels of peptide Bβ 30–43 in myocardial ischemia. Level is increased in patients with unstable angina pectoris and acute myocardial infarction, compared with controls. (Courtesy of Dinerman JL, Mehta JL, Saldeen TGP, et al: *J Am Coll Cardiol* 15:1559–1563, 1990.)

gina pectoris, 29 with unstable angina pectoris, 17 with acute MI, and 22 healthy controls. All study participants were men.

Plasma levels of peptide Bβ 30–43 varied widely in each group. However, the mean plasma level of peptide Bβ 30–43 was 5 times higher in patients with acute MI and 13 times higher in patients with unstable angina pectoris, compared with levels in healthy controls (Fig 5–7). Although the level in patients with stable angina pectoris was higher, compared with that in controls, the difference did not reach statistical significance.

Patients with acute MI or unstable angina pectoris had higher total leukocyte counts and absolute neutrophil counts than patients with stable angina or healthy controls. No significant relationship between plasma levels of peptide Bβ 30–43 and total leukocyte count or absolute neutrophil count could be detected between or within the study groups. The enhanced release of elastase that occurs in patients with acute MI or unstable angina pectoris suggests significant neutrophil activation, which may have a role in the progression and severity of myocardial and coronary endothelial injury following ischemia and reperfusion.

▶ With mounting experimental evidence implicating the neutrophil in the pathogenesis of myocardial reperfusion injury, investigators are questioning whether or not neutrophil-mediated reperfusion injury occurs clinically. Although this study did not investigate the existence of reperfusion injury, it clearly demonstrates that patients with acute MI and unstable angina have higher peripheral blood levels of a neutrophil elastase-derived fibrinopeptide. This indicates that these syndromes are associated with systemic neutrophil activation. Additional studies are required to determine if neutrophil elastase is released within the reperfused myocardium and, more importantly, whether neutrophil elastase (or other neutrophil products) is injurious to reperfused myocardium.—G.L. Schaer, M.D., and J.E. Parrillo, M.D.

Reduction in Reperfusion Injury by Blood-Free Reperfusion After Experimental Myocardial Infarction

Schaer GL, Karas SP, Santoian EC, Gold C, Visner MS, Virmani R (Georgetown Univ; Armed Forces Inst of Pathology, Washington, DC)
J Am Coll Cardiol 15:1385–1393, 1990   5–20

There is increasing evidence that myocardial salvage after acute myocardial infarction (MI) is reduced by adverse events that occur after initially successful reperfusion. Although there is controversy over the pathogenesis of reperfusion injury, recent studies have strongly implicated circulating neutrophils that gradually accumulate in the ischemic myocardium during coronary artery occlusion. The accumulated neutrophils are thought to cause tissue injury by the release of toxic oxygen-derived free radicals and proteolytic enzymes and by plugging the microcirculation.

Whether a transient period of blood-free reperfusion would reduce reperfusion injury was investigated in a closed chest canine model of acute MI. Anesthetized, endotracheally intubated, ventilated dogs were

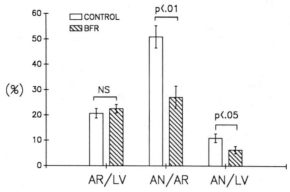

Fig 5–8.—Effect of blood-free reperfusion (BFR) on myocardial infarct size determined by staining with triphenyltetrazolium chloride. (*Abbreviations: AN*, area of necrosis; *AR*, area at risk; *LV*, left ventricle. (Courtesy of Schaer GL, Karas SP, Santoian EC, et al: *J Am Coll Cardiol* 15:1385–1393, 1990.)

subjected for 90 minutes to angioplasty balloon occlusion of the left anterior descending coronary artery. In 13 dogs the balloon was left inflated for an additional 15 minutes while the infarct vessel was perfused with an acellular oxygenated perfluorochemical emulsion (Fluosol). The balloon was then deflated to allow unmodified blood reperfusion. In 13 untreated control dogs the balloon was deflated after 90 minutes of coronary occlusion. One week after infarction the dogs were reanesthetized and the area at risk was defined by injection of monastral blue dye. Left ventricular function was assessed by contrast ventriculography before the dogs were killed.

Despite a comparable area at risk, dogs treated with transient blood-free reperfusion immediately after coronary artery occlusion had a mean 47% reduction in infarct size, compared with untreated dogs (Fig 5–8). Ventriculography performed 1 week after reperfusion demonstrated that the global left ventricular ejection fraction and anterolateral ejection fraction values in treated dogs were superior to values obtained in untreated dogs. Reperfusion injury in a canine model of acute MI can be reduced by a transient period of blood-free reperfusion with an oxygenated cell-free blood substitute.

▶ Various blood components (e.g., neutrophils, platelets, free fatty acids, catecholamines) may be harmful to the newly reperfused myocardium. This study from our laboratory sought to test the benefits of transiently restricting the entry of blood into the previously occluded coronary artery while simultaneously perfusing it with Fluosol (a non-blood oxygen-carrying perfluorochemical emulsion). This approach significantly reduced myocardial infarct size and improved ventricular function. The observed reduction in reperfusion injury probably results from multiple mechanisms, including transient restriction of blood entry, "washout" of metabolites and cellular aggregates within the ischemic microcirculation, and independent effects of Fluosol on inhibiting neutrophil function. A randomized, multicenter clinical trial in progress is evaluating the benefits of intravenous Fluosol during thrombolytic therapy.—G.L. Schaer, M.D., and J.E. Parrillo, M.D.

In Vivo Infusion of Oxygen Free Radical Substrates Causes Myocardial Systolic, But Not Diastolic Dysfunction
Przyklenk K, Whittaker P, Kloner RA (Wayne State Univ; Harper Hosp, Detroit)
Am Heart J 119:807–815, 1990   5–21

Reactive oxygen species are thought to cause contractile dysfunction of previously ischemic "stunned" myocardium. Nevertheless, direct in vivo evidence is lacking. Whether in vivo exposure of canine myocardium to exogenously generated reactive oxygen species produces changes similar to those characteristic of stunned myocardium was investigated in anesthetized open-chest dogs given either saline or a mixture of xanthine oxidase, purine, and iron-saturated transferrin infused into an anterior coronary vein.

Infusion of the free-radical-generating substances did not produce ischemia and was not associated with myocyte injury or death. Nevertheless, marked abnormalities in regional systolic function were seen. Segment shortening in the perfused region averaged 62% of baseline 2 hours after the start of the infusion. The free radical scavengers superoxide dismutase and catalase reversed the systolic dysfunction.

Reactive oxygen species produced systolic but not diastolic dysfunction in this canine model. The systolic and diastolic dysfunction seen in stunned myocardium following transient myocardial ischemia and reperfusion may be caused by different mechanisms.

▶ Myocardial stunning refers to the contractile dysfunction resulting from transient myocardial ischemia and reperfusion. Complete recovery of the systolic and diastolic abnormalities produced by this transient ischemic insult usually takes hours to days. A large body of experimental evidence suggests that toxic oxygen-derived free radicals play a major role in the pathogenesis of this problem. This interesting paper suggests that free radicals are probably responsible for the systolic, but not the diastolic, abnormalities. This suggests that the pathogenesis of stunned myocardium may be even more complex than previously believed. New therapies aimed at reducing stunned myocardium should therefore examine both systolic and diastolic contractile function.—G.L. Schaer, M.D., and J.E. Parrillo, M.D.

Neutrophil Depletion Limited to Reperfusion Reduces Myocardial Infarct Size After 90 Minutes of Ischemia: Evidence for Neutrophil-Mediated Reperfusion Injury
Litt MR, Jeremy RW, Weisman HF, Winkelstein JA, Becker LC (Johns Hopkins Med Insts)
Circulation 80:1816–1827, 1989   5–22

The benefits of early reperfusion of ischemic myocardium may be limited by reperfusion-related necrosis of ischemic myocytes, which is in part ascribed to oxygen free radical formation, causing lipid peroxidation and membrane damage. Because neutrophils are a potential source of oxygen free radicals, the effects of neutrophil depletion during reperfusion were studied in dogs having the proximal circumflex coronary artery occluded for 90 minutes. Either whole blood or blood depleted of neutrophils was used to selectively reperfuse the previously occluded circumflex coronary artery for 2 hours. Infarct size was measured using triphenyltetrazolium chloride.

The ischemic risk region was equally large in neutropenic and control animals, and collateral flow to this region also was the same. When collateral flow was less than .2 mL/min/g, infarct size was about half as great in neutropenic as in control dogs. In neutropenic animals the mean predicted infarct size was 17% of the left ventricle and the mean observed size was 10%. The no-reflow zone was less extensive in neutropenic animals.

Neutropenia limited to the period of reperfusion was associated with significantly smaller infarcts in this canine model. Neutrophils are important mediators of the reperfusion injury seen after prolonged myocardial ischemia. The degree of neutropenia required to prevent necrosis is uncertain. Inhibition of neutrophil function with a monoclonal antibody against a membrane adhesion protein may be a feasible clinical alternative to mechanically filtering neutrophils.

▶ This elegant study lends further support to the hypothesis that neutrophils are a major cause of reperfusion-associated myocardial injury. Recent studies have shown that a prominent inflammatory response develops within the reperfused myocardium, with large numbers of neutrophils rapidly accumulating in the previously ischemic region after reperfusion. These activated neutrophils may then injure endothelial cells and myocytes by releasing toxic oxygen-derived free radicals or proteolytic enzymes, or by mechanically plugging the microcirculation (no-reflow phenomenon). These data raise the possibility that agents capable of inhibiting neutrophil function may reduce reperfusion injury. However, before this strategy is tested clinically, further experimental studies are needed to be certain that neutrophil inhibition does not produce adverse effects on infarct healing or susceptibility to infection.—G.L. Schaer, M.D., and J.E. Parrillo, M.D.

Reperfusion Injury and Its Pharmacologic Modification
Opie LH (Univ of Cape Town, South Africa)
Circulation 80:1049–1062, 1989   5–23

Early thrombolysis has attracted great interest in the treatment of acute myocardial infarction, but reperfusion itself may result in myocardial injury in addition to the preceding ischemic insult. This reperfusion-associated injury may take several forms, including reperfusion arrhythmias, myocardial stunning, and reperfusion-induced myocyte necrosis.

Although it is firmly established that both reperfusion arrhythmias and myocardial stunning occur, it remains unclear whether reperfusion-induced myocyte necrosis reflects an acceleration of damage that would have occurred in any case, or whether a specific added injury occurs. Reperfusion injury is most often ascribed to calcium overload, free radical damage, and adverse effects of neutrophils.

Agents that diminish the extent of ischemic injury (e.g., calcium antagonists and β blockers) should also be effective in reperfusion injury. Much more study is needed under conditions of gradual reperfusion more closely simulating thrombolysis and using agents such as free radical scavengers that are given only at the time of reperfusion.

Reperfusion injury may be limited by minimizing the time from onset of chest pain to reperfusion and by optimizing the metabolic state of the ischemic myocardium, e.g., through early β blockade. In addition, reperfusion should take place slowly. Careful administration of inotropic agents may be indicated in cases of severe mechanical stunning.

▶ This is an informative review of an important but controversial problem: myocardial reperfusion injury. Considerable interest in reperfusion-associated injury has been stimulated by the emergence of thrombolytic therapy as the standard of care for most patients with acute myocardial infarction. Although many animal experiments have indicated that a component of myocardial necrosis is caused by the process of reperfusion, this has not yet been proven clinically. In contrast, myocardial stunning (*reversible* contractile dysfunction following an ischemic event) has been demonstrated both in animals and in clinical studies. Determining an effective pharmacologic strategy to reduce reperfusion-associated myocardial necrosis and myocardial stunning would have great clinical importance. Promising approaches that are currently being investigated include agents that diminish neutrophil-mediated injury to the coronary microcirculation, such as intravenous perfluorochemicals (Fluosol) or adenosine.—G.L. Schaer, M.D., and J.E. Parrillo, M.D.

Effect of Streptokinase on Left Ventricular Modeling and Function After Myocardial Infarction: The GISSI (Gruppo Italiano per lo Studio della Streptochinasi nell'Infarto Miocardico) Trial
Marino P, Zanolla L, Zardini P (Univ of Verona, Italy)
J Am Coll Cardiol 14:1149–1158, 1989   5–24

The GISSI trial has shown that thrombolysis with intravenous streptokinase lowers hospital mortality from acute myocardial infarction (MI). The relationship between treatment and left ventricular modeling was examined in 331 consecutive patients who underwent 2-dimensional echocardiography just before hospital discharge. Studies were repeated at 6 months in 232 patients. Infarct size was estimated semiquantitatively, and ventricular volumes were computed from an apical 4-chamber view.

Patients given streptokinase had smaller ventricular volumes and smaller regional wall motion indices (a semiquantitative measure of the number of dyskinetic or akinetic segments) at the time of discharge compared with those given routine care. No significant difference in ejection fraction was present. The differences in volume and regional dysfunction persisted at 6 months. As at the outset, end-systolic volume for comparably sized infarcts was smaller in patients given streptokinase than in control patients.

These echocardiographic findings support the hypothesis that streptokinase given to patients with acute MI lessens postinfarction left ventricular dilation and reduced regional wall motion abnormalities. Infarct expansion may be avoided as well. The beneficial effects of thrombolysis persist in the chronic phase and may help to explain the decrease in mortality observed.

▶ The benefit of thrombolytic therapy in acute MI has been well documented; what is interesting is that the rates of both in-hospital and late mortality are decreased. Presumably, this is attributable to opening of the infarct artery, but the precise mechanism of benefit is not entirely clear. Reestablishing a patent infarct artery may provide benefit by salvaging jeopardized myocardium, preventing infarct expansion, or both. Infarct extension refers to thinning and dilation of the infarct segment and goes under the general heading of ventricular remodeling. These results from the GISSI trial support the notion that acute reperfusion lessens subsequent left ventricular dilation, perhaps by preventing infarct expansion.—S. Hollenberg, M.D., and J.E. Parrillo, M.D.

The Spectrum of Death After Myocardial Infarction: A Necropsy Study
Stevenson WG, Linssen GCM, Havenith MG, Brugada P, Wellens HJJ (Univ of Limburg, Maastricht, The Netherlands)
Am Heart J 118:1182–1188, 1989   5–25

The frequency of various causes of death after myocardial infarction (MI) was studied by reviewing all autopsies performed at a university hospital during a 56-month period. Autopsies were done in 56% of the patients who died in the hospital and in 27% of those who were dead on arrival at the emergency room. An MI at any age was identified in 424 patients. Of these, 153 died of progressive noncardiac illness or complications of a major surgical procedure; the remaining 271 cases formed the study population.

Nineteen deaths occurred in the acute phase of a first infarction. Pump failure and cardiac rupture were the most frequent causes of death in this group. Among 80 patients who died 24 hours to 3 weeks after a first infarction, pump failure also was the predominant etiology, accounting for 44% of deaths. One third of the patients dying of arrhythmia or pump failure and 19% of those dying of cardiac rupture had recurrent acute MI. Three fourths of the deaths occurring more than 3 weeks after a first MI were caused by complications of a new acute or recent infarction.

Only 14% of out-of-hospital deaths occurring late after MI were caused by primary arrhythmia. Five percent or fewer of all deaths were ascribed to unexpected noncardiac causes.

It may be possible to lower mortality from MI by targeting treatment to specific causes of death according to the time elapsed after the event. Measures for lowering the risk of early infarct extension, myocardial rupture, and late recurrent infarction might be employed.

▶ The authors of this interesting study selected patients with autopsy-proven MI, either recent or remote, and attempted to determine the proximate cause of death. Their findings both confirm accepted wisdom and raise some provocative questions.

The inevitable constraint of such a study is patient selection. The Maastricht Academic Hospital is the only hospital in this Dutch city, and the proportion of autopsies performed was high, especially by current American standards. As one might expect, the proportion of postmortems done when patients died in the hospital was more than twice that done on out-of-hospital deaths; thus sudden, undiagnosed arrhythmias would be underrepresented. The brain was studied in only 9% of cases, which means that the incidence of a cerebrovascular accident was most likely underestimated. Within these limits, the study population probably comprised a reasonably representative sample of cardiac deaths in this area.

Certain findings were unsurprising. Patients with acute MIs who died before reaching the hospital were likely to have had arrhythmias. After admission to the coronary care unit, arrhythmic death was uncommon, and patients who died succumbed to pump failure. An appreciable proportion of the infarctions were clinically silent. Myocardial rupture occurred at a mean of 3.8 days after infarction, and most of these patients had only one area of infarction.

The more provocative findings concerned the cause of death in the early and chronic phase of MI; ischemia seemed to be a much more important problem that primary arrhythmias. Thirty-two percent of deaths between 24 hours and 21 days of an acute event were caused by recurrent acute infarction or infarct extension. In the chronic phase (after 21 days), primary arrhythmias accounted for only 14% of deaths, whereas 61% of deaths were attributed to recent or acute MI. It is also conceivable that myocardial ischemia may have been a contributing factor in some of the deaths caused by arrhythmias.

These findings suggest some strategies for improving mortality in acute MI. Out-of-hospital, arrhythmias are the main concern. In the early period one needs to worry most about infarct extension, pump failure, and myocardial rupture. In the chronic phase, reinfarction becomes a main concern.—S. Hollenberg, M.D., and J.E. Parrillo, M.D.

Meta-Analytic Evidence Against Prophylactic Use of Lidocaine in Acute Myocardial Infarction
Hine LK, Laird N, Hewitt P, Chalmers TC (Harvard School of Public Health, Boston)
Arch Intern Med 149:2694–2698, 1989   5–26

About half of the deaths from coronary heart disease in the United States result from ventricular arrhythmias that complicate acute myocardial infarction (MI). To prevent such arrhythmias, many coronary care units administer prophylactic lidocaine even though its value in preventing mortality has not been confirmed in randomized control trials. A meta-analysis was made of death rates in 14 such trials in which prophylactic lidocaine was given to patients with proved or suspected acute MI.

Six prehospital-phase and 8 hospital-phase randomized control trials were reviewed in blinded fashion. Patients in the prehospital-phase studies received a single bolus of lidocaine; those in the hospital-phase studies received a bolus of lidocaine plus continuous infusion. The 14 studies included more than 9,000 patients. Data on mortality were evaluated according to type of therapy, reporting interval, and patient category.

No meaningful effect on mortality was noted with the prehospital administration of lidocaine. Results in only those patients with subsequently confirmed acute MI were similar to those in the intention-to-treat group. During the treatment period patients who received lidocaine in the hospital-phase trials had a statistically significant increase in mortality (2.9%, with a confidence interval of .4% to 5.5% increase).

Lidocaine reduces episodes of primary ventricular fibrillation that can occur during and shortly after acute MI. This effect, however, apparently does not bring about improved survival.

▶ Meta-analyses have many shortcomings, but certain clinical issues cannot be resolved by more satisfactory means. This meta-analysis of Hine et al., addressing the use of prophylactic lidocaine in patients with known or suspected MI, confirms the conclusions of another meta-analysis published by MacMahon et al. in 1988 (1). In monitored environments, prophylactic lidocaine does not decrease, and probably increases, mortality in MI. This conclusion applies to both the prehospital and in-hospital administration of lidocaine, and to both suspected MI and proven MI.

In my judgment it is reasonable to reserve lidocaine for patients with ventricular tachycardia, couplets, or multifocal or frequent (more than 6 per minute) unifocal premature ventricular contractions. Such patients were excluded from the studies analyzed by Hine et al. and MacMahon et al.—R.E. Cunnion, M.D.

Reference

1. MacMahon S, et al: *JAMA* 260:1910, 1988.

Candidates for Thrombolysis Among Emergency Room Patients With Acute Chest Pain: Potential True- and False-Positive Rates
Lee TH, Weisberg MC, Brand DA, Rouan GW, Goldman L (Brigham and Women's Hosp, Boston; Harvard Med School; Yale-New Haven Hosp; Yale Univ; Univ of Cincinnati Hosp)
Ann Intern Med 110:957–962, 1989   5–27

In a prospective multicenter cohort study, 7,734 emergency room patients with acute chest pain were evaluated. True and false positive rates for eligibility for thrombolysis were calculated based on criteria used by previous randomized trials, such as age 75 years or younger, onset of pain within 4 hours of presentation, and an emergency room ECG showing probable acute myocardial infarction (MI).

Of the 1,118 patients (14%) who met criteria for acute MI, only 261 (23%) met eligibility criteria for thrombolysis. Sixty of the 6,616 patients without acute MI also met these criteria, for a positive predictive value of 81%. Thus for every 8 true positive patients eligible for thrombolytic therapy, 2 false positive patients also were eligible. However, if official hospital ECG readings were used instead of the readings by emergency room physicians, the postitive predictive value could increase to 88%.

If patients with contraindications to thrombolytic therapy are excluded, it is estimated that about 15% of emergency room patients with acute MI would meet eligibility criteria for thrombolysis as set by several previous clinical trials. False positive rates can be reduced if ECGS are reviewed by an experienced physician before treatment.

▶ This is one of a number of reports addressing the thorniest problem with thrombolytic therapy, namely, that most patients presenting with acute MI do not meet eligibility criteria. The proportion of patients eligible for thrombolysis will undoubtedly increase somewhat as more data are collected concerning its efficacy and safety in groups that now are customarily excluded (i.e., elderly patients, patients more than 4–6 hours beyond onset of chest pain, and patients with ECG features other than classic ST segment elevation). Nonetheless, even if indications for thrombolysis are gradually broadened, many or most patients with MI will probably remain ineligible, and we are already witnessing the evolution of alternative management strategies such as primary angioplasty for such patients.

The report of Lee et al. also underscores another significant problem with thrombolytic therapy—the inadvertent treatment of patients who appear to meet eligibility criteria but who in fact do not have an infarct. This problem can be minimized by careful analysis of ECGs by experienced interpreters and by recognizing other conditions that can mimic infarction (e.g., aortic dissection and pericarditis). Insofar as the mortality rate attributable to thrombolytic agents per se is probably less than 1%, the occurrence of thrombolytic complications among patients who do not have infarcts is unlikely to offset significantly the impressively improved survival rates among those who do have infarcts.—R.E. Cunnion, M.D.

The Natural History of Left Ventricular Thrombus in Myocardial Infarction: A Rationale in Support of Masterly Inactivity
Nihoyannopoulos P, Smith GC, Maseri A, Foale RA (Royal Postgrad Med School, Hammersmith Hosp; St Mary's Hosp, London)
J Am Coll Cardiol 14:903–911, 1989   5–28

The proper approach to left ventricular (LV) thrombus found after acute infarction remains uncertain. The incidence of thrombus formation was prospectively determined in 105 consecutive patients with a first myocardial infarction (MI), as well as the significance of thrombus for functional outcome and survival. Echocardiograms were suitable for serial evaluation in 87 patients, 53 of whom had anterior infarctions.

Left ventricular thrombi were found in 21 of the 53 patients with anterior infarction a median of 6 days after the acute event. None of the 34 patients with inferior infarctions had LV thrombi. Patients with mural thrombi had a lower hospital mortality rate than those without. Thrombi were present in 3 of 10 patients who had transient arm weakness or blurred vision. After 1 year, patients with LV thrombi were less symptomatic than the others. After 2 years only 5 of 21 patients still had evidence of thrombus. No patient had an embolic event after hospital discharge.

Mural thrombi are common after acute anterior MI, but clinical embolism is not and the presence of thrombus did not adversely influence the outcome in this series. Therefore, by itself, a thrombus should not be an indication for anticoagulation.

▶ Considerable uncertainty still surrounds the issue of anticoagulation after MI, with some authorities recommending full systemic anticoagulation for all patients presenting with large anterior infarctions. The report of Nihoyannopoulos et al. addresses itself specifically to the issue of whether LV thrombi, detected by echocardiography after infarction, represent an indication for anticoagulation. The report concludes that anticoagulation is not indicated and recommends "masterly inactivity."

Several shortcomings of these data need comment. First, all of the patients in the study were receiving heparin subcutaneously and aspirin and dipyridamole orally, and it is impossible to surmise what effect these agents may have had on the natural history of cardiogenic thromboembolism. Second, in a clinical sample of this size, only 2 or 3 embolic events would have been expected to occur, making it difficult to interpret the apparent innocuousness of LV thrombi. Third, in addition to the problem of LV thromboembolism, MI represents a complex situation in which antithrombotic therapy may have implications for the prevention of future coronary events.

The optimal approach to preventing both ventricular thromboembolism and complications of underlying coronary disease remains to be defined on the basis of a prospective clinical trial. At present, there are no sound data on which to base a noncontroversial recommendation, but it seems reasonable to administer full-dose heparin intravenously to patients early in the course of large anterior infarctions, independent of the present or absence of echocardiographic ventricular thrombi.— R.E. Cunnion, M.D.

Tolerance With Low Dose Intravenous Nitroglycerin Therapy in Acute Myocardial Infarction
Jugdutt BI, Warnica JW (Univ of Alberta, Edmonton)
Am J Cardiol 64:581–587, 1989   5–29

Tolerance is observed when nitroglycerin is given intravenously in high dosage to patients with coronary disease. Tolerance with the intravenous administration of low-dose nitroglycerin was examined in 154 patients with acute myocardial infarction (MI) who received prolonged low-dose treatment in a randomized, placebo-controlled study. The goal was to lower mean blood pressure by 10%, or by 30% in hypertensive patients, but not to less than 80 mm Hg.

The average initial nitroglycerin infusion rate required to achieve the target blood pressure was 45 µg/min. The infusion continued for an average of 39 hours. After 12 hours the mean blood pressure and rate-pressure product did not differ significantly between the groups. Nevertheless, these parameters increased within 1 hour of withdrawing nitroglycerin. Tolerance defined as the need to increase the nitroglycerin dose to maintain the target blood pressure effect, was identified in 24% of the patients. Ischemic injury, measured by ST segment scores, was decreased by nitroglycerin, compared with placebo, whether or not tolerance occurred. In contrast, the beneficial effect of nitroglycerin on infarct size was blunted in patients with tolerance.

Low-dose nitroglycerin, cautiously administered, is potentially helpful in salvaging cardiac muscle and function in patients with acute MI. Tolerance should not prevent the use of this treatment.

▶ This study has a number of clinical ramifications. First, progressive tolerance to prolonged low-dose nitroglycerin infusion does occur in some patients with acute MI, usually within the first 10 hours. Second, the incidence of significant tolerance is fairly low, fewer than 25% of patients. Third, even in patients in whom tolerance does not develop, the tolerance is only partial and can be combatted by increasing the dose. Fourth, patients with tolerance still benefit from nitroglycerin, with less ischemic injury and smaller infarct size than observed in placebo-treated patients, so that the occurrence of tolerance should not be a deterrent to using nitroglycerin. Whether nitrate-free intervals are beneficial in the setting of acute MI is not resolved by this study.—R.E. Cunnion, M.D.

Improved Prognosis Since 1969 of Myocardial Infarction Treated in a Coronary Care Unit: Lack of Relation With Changes in Severity
Hopper JL, Pathik B, Hunt D, Chan WWC (Univ of Melbourne, Australia)
Br Med J 299:892–896, 1989   5–30

Results of early studies indicated an improved outlook for patients with acute myocardial infarction (MI) after the introduction of coronary care units. Survival trends were examined over 1969–1983 for 4,253 patients with acute MI admitted to the coronary care unit of a tertiary referral hospital. Patients seen in the later years of the study were on average older and had less severe infarcts.

The hospital mortality rate in men declined from 16.7% in 1969–1973 to 8.5% in 1979–1983. The mortality rate in women remained constant at 19.2%. After adjusting for age and severity of infarction, the hospital mortality rate decreased by an average of 8% per year in men and remained constant in women. By 1983 men had only 60% of the mortality of women of similar age with comparably severe infarcts. Among hospital survivors, the 1-year mortality rate decreased by an average of 7% per year in both men and women. Although more recent patients have tended to have less severe infarcts, the trend toward an improved outlook is greater than can be ascribed to differences in the severity of infarction, especially for men.

▶ This interesting observational study demonstrates a clear-cut trend in acute MI toward lower in-hospital mortality among male patients and lower 1-year mortality among both male and female patients. Retrospective analysis implies that these improvements in survival cannot be explained entirely by a reduction in severity of the infarctions; hence, it seems likely that the better prognosis results from the myriad diagnostic and therapeutic advances made in acute coronary care in the past 2 decades. The persistent, disproportionately high in-hospital mortality rate among female patients is unexplained and disturbing. This study should serve as a cautionary note against the use of historical controls (rather than concurrent controls) in investigations of therapies for MI.—R.E. Cunnion, M.D.

Cardiac Morphologic Findings in Patients With Acute Myocardial Infarction Treated With Recombinant Tissue Plasminogen Activator
Gertz SD, Kalan JM, Kragel AH, Roberts WC, Braunwald E, and the TIMI Investigators (Natl Heart, Lung, and Blood Inst Bethesda, Md; Hebrew Univ, Jerusalem; Brigham and Women's Hosp, Boston)
Am J Cardiol 65:953–961, 1990   5–31

Treatment with thrombolytic agents can restore the patency of occluded coronary arteries. However, there has been concern that such treatment may increase the frequency of hemorrhagic infarcts. Myocardial hemorrhage after administration of recombinant tissue plasminogen activator (rt-PA) could increase the frequency of complications of infarction. The hearts of patients given rt-PA during the course of acute myocardial infarction were studied at necropsy to compare clinical and cardiac morphological findings in patients with hemorrhagic infarcts with those in patients with nonhemorrhagic infarcts.

The hearts of 52 patients who died a median of 2.7 days after the onset of chest pain were studied. All 52 patients had received rt-PA. Eight had percutaneous transluminal coronary angioplasty; another 6 had coronary artery bypass grafting. The infarcts were hemorrhagic in 23 cases, nonhemorrhagic in 20, and not grossly visible in 9. Comparisons between the patients with hemorrhagic and those with nonhemorrhagic infarcts showed similar frequencies of myocardial rupture, cardiogenic shock, and fatal hemorrhage; similar percentages of necrotic portions of the left ventricular wall among patients surviving longer than 18 hours from chest pain onset, with the hemorrhage confined to areas of necrotic myocardium in all cases; similar frequencies of thrombi in the infarct-related arteries, although all thrombi in those with hemorrhagic infarcts were nonocclusive whereas all thrombi in those with nonhemorrhagic infarcts wre occlusive; similar degrees of luminal cross-sectional area narrowing over all 5-mm segments of the 4 major epicardial coronary arteries in patients given only rt-PA; and similar numbers of patients in whom the infarct-related artery was narrowed by more than 75% in cross-sectional area at some point by plaque. There were also similar frequencies of plaque rupture and of hemorrhage into a plaque in patients without percutaneous transluminal coronary angioplasty. Fewer right ventricular infarcts were found in patients with hemorrhagic infarcts.

Hemorrhage occurs often in the infarcts of patients given rt-PA. Hemorrhage into an infarct does not seem to extend the infarct. Patients with hemorrhagic infarcts have no greater frequency of myocardial rupture or cardiogenic shock and no significant differences in coronary luminal narrowing, plaque rupture, or plaque composition.

▶ Before the widespread clinical use of thrombolytic agents and angioplasty, almost all myocardial infarctions (MIs) seen at autopsy were nonhemorrhagic. In recent years the number of hemorrhagic MIs observed at autopsy appears to have increased. This careful retrospective analysis of patients who died after rt-PA therapy confirms a high incidence of hemorrhagic infarction, 46%, but it also offers the reassuring finding that hemorrhagic infarction was not associated with an increased likelihood of infarct extension, myocardial rupture, or cardiogenic shock. Physicians who use rt-PA should be aware that it causes some infarctions to become hemorrhagic, but that this does not constrain its clinical usefulness.— R.E. Cunnion, M.D.

Doppler Color Flow Mapping in the Diagnosis of Ventricular Septal Rupture and Acute Mitral Regurgitation After Myocardial Infarction
Smyllie JH, Sutherland GR, Geuskens R, Dawkins K, Conway N, Roelandt JRTC
(Erasmus Univ, Rotterdam; Southampton Gen Hosp, England)
J Am Coll Cardiol 15:1449–1455, 1990   5–32

Doppler color-flow mapping is a sensitive diagnostic technique for defining congenital septal defects, chronic mitral regurgitation, and postinfarction ventricular septal rupture. However, there has been no large prospective study correlating Doppler color-flow findings with findings at catheterization or surgery in patients with complications of myocardial infarction (MI). The diagnostic accuracy of Doppler color-flow mapping to differentiate ventricular septal rupture from acute mitral regurgitation after recent MI was assessed in 50 patients who had post-MI pansystolic murmurs and cardiac decompensation.

Twenty-seven patients had anterior and 23 had inferior infarcts. All were evaluated by cardiac ultrasound that included 2-dimensional echocardiography, pulsed and continuous-wave spectral Doppler, and Doppler color-flow mapping. Diagnoses were confirmed subsequently by right heart catheterization/left ventriculography or surgical/pathologic inspection, or both. Forty-three patients had ventricular septal rupture, and 7 had severe isolated mitral regurgitation.

Two-dimensional echocardiography alone visualizes septal defects in 17 of 43 patients with ventricular septal rupture, and it correctly demonstrated the structural abnormalities of the mitral valve in 6 of 7 patients with mitral regurgitation. Doppler color-flow mapping greatly aided diagnosis in both groups. Doppler color-flow mapping demonstrated areas of turbulent transseptal flow and systolic flow disturbance within the right ventricular in all 43 patients with ventricular septal rupture. Doppler color-flow mapping demonstrated mitral regurgitation in the 7 affected patients, and it also identified the specific mitral leaflet abnormality by identifying the direction of the regurgitant jet. The procedure was less reliable in defining the severity of regurgitation, underestimating it by 1 or 2 grades in 4 patients as compared to angiography.

▶ Doppler color-flow imaging, when interpreted by an experienced echocardiographer, allows rapid, reliable, and precise bedside diagnosis of ventricular septal rupture and mitral regurgitation in patients in whom systolic murmurs develop after MI. This sensitive and specific information can be invaluable in guiding subsequent management. Before thoracotomy, coronary arteriography should still be performed in most cases, but the need for left ventriculography often can be eliminated.—R.E. Cunnion, M.D.

Acute Hemodynamic Changes During Intravenous Dipyridamole Thallium Imaging Early After Infarction

Miller DD, Scott RA, Riesmeyer JS, Chaudhuri TK, Blumhardt R, Boucher CA, O'Rourke RA (Univ of Texas, San Antonio; Audie L Murphy VA Hosp, San Antonio)

Am Heart J 118:686–694, 1989   5–33

Intravenous dipyridamole thallium-201 imaging, when performed early, can identify a subgroup of patients at high risk for adverse cardiac effects after myocardial infarction (MI). The safety and hemodynamic effects of intravenous dipyridamole infusion for thallium-201 scintigraphy were determined in 10 patients with recent uncomplicated MI. Dipyridamole thallium-201 imaging was performed within a mean of 7 days (range, 4–10 days) after MI. Central pressures and cardiac output values were measured serially in the coronary care unit during and after the administration of dipyridamole, .56 mg/kg over 4 minutes, and after aminophylline reversal of the dipyridamole effect. Cardiac medications were continued.

There were no serious ischemic responses during or after dipyridamole infusion, but 20% of the patients experienced noncardiac side effects and 30% had significant ST segment depression with associated angina in one third of them. The cardiac double-product did not change significantly. The systemic vascular resistance fell significantly and the cardiac index rose significantly, whereas pulmonary capillary wedge pressure (PCWP) increased significantly within 10 minutes of dipyridamole infusion. In 3 patients, new silent "V" waves in the PCWP tracing appeared (without angina) in association with anterior wall thallium-201 redistribution. All 3 patients with newly elevated wedge pressures (>15 mm Hg) had thallium-201 redistribution and multivessel coronary disease.

In all but 1 patient, hemodynamic changes, including new "V" waves, were promptly reversed by intravenously administered aminophylline (50–150 mg). Early postinfarction testing allowed time- and cost-effective risk stratification and saved an average of 4 hospital days and $1,843 per patient.

Dipyridamole induces significant hemodynamic changes similar to those that occur in spontaneous or exercise-induced angina that are not blunted by autonomically active drugs or reflexes in the early postinfarction setting. Early postinfarction intravenous dipyridamole thallium-201 imaging can be performed in most coronary patients. This test should be monitored cautiously, particularly in patients with recent acute ischemic syndromes. Angina and ST segment depression are rarely severe and can be reversed by the administration of aminophylline.

▶ After uncomplicated MI, stress testing before hospital discharge has become routine. If ischemia is induced, coronary arteriography generally is performed. Submaximal treadmill exercise is the most commonly used form of stress testing, although thallium imaging with oral dipyridamole is often used instead, particularly in patients who cannot exercise well. Intravenous dipyridamole, which is available for investigational use, may provide more accurate thallium imaging studies than oral dipyridamole.

In this study, Miller et al. demonstrated that use of intravenous dipyridamole for thallium imaging in 10 patients early after MI was associated with substantial changes in systemic vascular resistance, cardiac index, and wedge pressure. Even though none of their patients, studied in a very careful monitored setting, had serious ischemic events, it is apparent that this diagnostic procedure has significant potential for morbidity. Certainly, the relative safety of intravenous dipyridamole in this population of uncomplicated MI patients does not warrant any extrapolation of its use to patients with heart failure, angina, hypotension, or arrhythmias.—R.E. Cunnion, M.D.

Early and Late Results of Coronary Angioplasty Without Antecedent Thrombolytic Therapy for Acute Myocardial Infarction
O'Keefe JH Jr, Rutherford BD, McConahay DR, Ligon RW, Johnson WL Jr, Giorgi LV, Crockett JE, McCallister BD, Conn RD, Gura GM Jr, Good TH, Steinhaus DM, Bateman TM, Shimshak TM, Hartzler GO (St Luke's Hosp, Kansas City, Mo)
Am J Cardiol 64:1221–1230, 1989   5–34

Thrombolytic therapy in the treatment of acute myocardial infarction (MI) fails to recanalize the infarct vessel acutely in at least 25% of patients. Many institutions therefore have decided to perform coronary angioplasty routinely after thrombolysis. However, several recent studies suggest that morbidity and mortality are increased by this practice, suggesting that the routine use of angioplasty in conjunction with thrombolysis should be discontinued. There are few data available on the effectiveness of direct coronary angioplasty alone without antecedent thrombolytic therapy.

Direct coronary angioplasty without antecedent thrombolysis was performed in a large consecutive series of patients with acute MI—364 men and 136 women (mean age, 59 years). Of the 500 patients, 217 had anterior infarctions and 283 had inferior infarctions. Direct angioplasty was successful in 94% of these patients. The overall hospital mortality was 7.2%. Angiographic follow-up before hospital discharge, available for 307 patients, showed reocclusion of the infarct vessel in 15% of the patients. Significant bleeding complications occurred in only 3% of the patients. There were no strokes or myocardial ruptures. The mean global ejection fraction increased from 53% on preangioplasty ventriculography to 59% at 1 week. In 53% of the patients significant regional wall motion improvement was seen in the infact segments. The 1-year survival rate after hospital discharge was 95% and the 5-year survival rate, 84%.

Direct coronary angioplasty without antecedent thrombolysis in patients with acute MI was highly effective in reestablishing patency of the infarct vessel and salvaging ischemic myocardium. Both in-hospital and long-term mortality were low.

▶ Direct balloon coronary angioplasty is not available to most patients presenting with acute MI. Only 12% of hospitals in the United States have angioplasty facilities, and many of these do not keep interventional cardiologists and cardiac catheterization personnel on call for rapid emergency mobilization. Nonetheless, in hospitals with the capability, direct angioplasty is a promising technique in the management of acute MI, particularly in patients who have contraindications to thrombolytic therapy. The series of O'Keefe et al. is retrospective and uncontrolled, but the results are impressive in terms of restoration of coronary patency and long-term clinical outcomes. It is not likely that centers with less experienced operators and lower-volume catheterization laboratories would have similar success rates.

Thrombolytic therapy has been shown in controlled trials to reduce mortality from acute MI; direct angioplasty has not. There are no adequately controlled data comparing outcomes from direct angioplasty with those from thrombolytic therapy. Accordingly, for patients without contraindications to thrombolytic therapy, angioplasty should be substituted for thrombolytic therapy only in experienced high-volume centers that can accomplish the procedure without delay.—R.E. Cunnion, M.D.

Pulmonary Edema After Freebase Cocaine Smoking: Not Due to an Adulterant

Kline JN, Hirasuna JD (Univ of California, San Francisco; Valley Med Ctr, Fresno)
Chest 97:1009–1010, 1990   5–35

Freebase cocaine smoking has become a common abuse. Pulmonary edema after freebase use occurs rarely.

Man, 35, came to the emergency room with chest pain and shortness of breath. He had smoked freebase cocaine on the previous evening. He had inhaled only once or twice when a cough, chills, and chest pain developed. On the evening before this, he had smoked heavily. He had used "crack" 3–5 times a week for 6 years. He complained of exertional dyspnea, which had progressed to resting dyspnea at the time of examination. Chest radiographs showed bilateral pulmonary edema with a normal cardiac silhouette. The patient was hospitalized and given oxygen and erythromycin therapy. The dyspnea and cough rapidly disappeared. Forty-eight hours after admission, the radiographic pattern of pulmonary edema was virtually resolved.

In this patient, the mechanism of pulmonary edema after freebase cocaine smoking was not clearly established. However, the case is unique, because adulterants and contaminants were not found in the drug sample supplied by the patient.

▶ This case report is interesting for 2 reasons. First, it shows that pulmonary edema is another important cardiopulmonary complication of cocaine abuse. This possibility should be considered in the management of a patient with unexplained pulmonary edema. This report is also interesting in that no adulterant was found in the "crack" cocaine used by the patient, thereby excluding the possibility that a contaminant was responsible for the syndrome. Animal data have demonstrated that repeated dosing ("binging") with cocaine can produce progressive depression in global left ventricular function by a direct toxic effect on myocardial contractility (1). Thus a potential mechanism for cocaine-related pulmonary edema may be a direct negative inotropic effect.—G.L. Schaer, M.D., and J.E. Parrillo, M.D.

Reference

1. Johnson MN, et al: *Circulation* 80:II–15, 1989.

Acute Non-Q Wave Cocaine-Related Myocardial Infarction

Kossowsky WA, Lyon AF, Chou S-Y (Brookdale Hosp Med Ctr, Brooklyn, NY; State Univ of New York, Brooklyn)
Chest 96:617–621, 1989   5–36

Cocaine can produce myocardial ischemia and infarction in patients with or without preexisting coronary disease. An initial report in 1984 described 6 patients with acute myocardial infarction (MI) temporally related to cocaine use. Data were reviewed on 19 other patients in whom ischemic chest pain syndromes occurred after cocaine use.

The average patient age was 31 years. Non–Q-wave MI developed in 17 patients (89%) and Q-wave MI developed in 2 after the intranasal or intravenous use of cocaine or after smoking cocaine. Angina with marked ST segment elevation and associated ventricular tachycardia occurred in 1 patient. None of the patients had diabetes mellitus or hypertension, and all but 1 were cigarette smokers. The mean serum cholesterol level was 162 mg/dL. Of 5 patients who consented to coronary angiographic studies, 4 had normal coronary arteries and 1 had proximal stenosis of the right coronary artery. In none of 7 patients who underwent the cold pressor test was angina or an ECG change induced by cold stimulation. There were no deaths.

Cocaine-induced non–Q-wave infarction may be more prevalent than previously appreciated. Its pathogenesis may involve that of cocaine-induced coronary vasospasm.

▶ It is now firmly established that cocaine use, whether intranasally, intravenously, or by inhalation ("crack" smoking), occasionally results in MI. This paper emphasizes this association by reporting on a group of patients with cocaine-related MI, primarily of the non–Q-wave type. Because many patients with cocaine-related MI have subsequently been found to have angiographically normal coronary arteries, coronary vasospasm has been proposed as a possible mechanism. Animal (1) and human studies (2) have shown that cocaine produces mild coronary vasoconstriction (a sympathomimetic effect), but frank vasospasm has not been demonstrated experimentally. Indeed, clinical tests for coronary vasospasm such as the cold pressor test (in this series) and ergonovine testing (in previous investigations) have failed to provoke myocardial ischemia. Some reports have noted intracoronary thrombus associated with cocaine use and MI. Thus the precise mechanism responsible for cocaine-related MI remains to be fully clarified.—G.L. Schaer, M.D., and J.E. Parrillo, M.D.

References

1. Kuhn FE, et al: *J Am Coll Cardiol* 16:1481, 1990.
2. Lange RA, et al: *N Engl J Med* 321:1557, 1989.

Correlation Between Template Bleeding Times and Spontaneous Bleeding During Treatment of Acute Myocardial Infarction With Recombinant Tissue-Type Plasminogen Activator

Gimple LW, Gold HK, Leinbach RC, Coller BS, Werner W, Yasuda T, Johns JA, Ziskind AA, Finkelstein D, Collen D (Massachusetts Gen Hosp, Boston; Harvard Med School; State Univ of New York, Stony Brook; Univ of Vermont, Burlington)

Circulation 80:581–588, 1989   5–37

Early intravenous infusion of recombinant tissue-type plasminogen activator (rt-PA) in patients with acute transmural myocardial infarction (MI) can lyse coronary thrombi, improve left ventricular function, and reduce mortality. However, the use of intravenous rt-PA combined with heparin is associated with a variable, usually moderate, degree of systemic fibrinolytic activation and fibrinogen breakdown and a bleeding tendency. Bleeding complications during and after rt-PA treatment were correlated with serial template bleeding time measurements, adenosine diphosphate-induced platelet aggregation, clinical characteristics, and hemostatic parameters.

Of 55 consecutively admitted patients with acute MI and template bleeding time of less than 9.5 minutes, 52 were treated with rt-PA, 55 to 212 mg, over 90 to 360 minutes, combined with heparin. The mean bleeding time was significantly prolonged at 90 minutes. However, it returned toward baseline after 4 hours. Twenty-five percent of the patients had relatively minor but spontaneous bleeding that did not correlate with age, hypertension, smoking, partial thromboplastin time, platelet count, adenosine diphosphate-induced platelet aggregation, steady-state rt-PA level, or extent of fibrinogen degradation. On multivariate analysis, only the 90-minute bleeding time correlated with spontaneous bleeding. Prolongation of the 90-minute bleeding time to 9 or more minutes, occurring in 21 patients, correlated with spontaneous bleeding with a sensitivity and a specificity of 69%. In 14 patients taking aspirin, bleeding times at 90 minutes were significantly more prolonged and spontaneous bleeding significantly more frequent than in those not taking aspirin.

The template bleeding time may be a useful quantitative index of the hemorrhagic diathesis that occurs in some patients during thrombolytic therapy with rt-PA. It may represent a useful parameter for investigating the occurrence and mechanism of spontaneous bleeding. If confirmed in large prospective studies, bleeding time prolongation may be useful for the early detection of an increased bleeding risk, potentially allowing appropriate changes in the dose and duration of rt-PA treatment.

▶ When rt-PA was originally marketed, its supposed "clot-specific" mechanism was highly touted. The concept was that, by utilizing an exogenously administered plasminogen activator with a mechanism of action identical to that of endogenous plasminogen activators, bleeding complications associated with the use of thrombolytic therapy would be minimized.

As clinical experience with rt-PA and other lytic agents has become widespread, it is clear that no particular agent has any important biological advantage with respect to serious bleeding, because the bleeding incidence in numerous trials with all agents is on the order of .5% to 2%. Moreover, although bleeding occurs most frequently in association with vascular puncture and invasive procedures, suggesting that this is the primary causative factor, predicting its occurrence is otherwise an elusive hope. Although severe hypofibrinogenemia does predispose to bleeding, there is only a weak correlation between the degree of fibrinogen depletion and adverse events. This is entirely to be expected, as all currently used agents have complex effects on various hemostatic factors as well as on platelet function.

In this study of 52 consecutive patients with acute MI treated with rt-PA, 13 had identifiable, although non-major, bleeding events. There was a correlation with the template ((Ivy) bleeding time at 90 minutes after initiation of therapy. This is an important finding, if confirmed in a larger series of consecutive patients with more frequent serious bleeding, as there is a need for clinicians to be able to identify patients at risk. However, t-PA is often given concurrently with aspirin and a 24- to 72-hour infusion of heparin, and is itself administered as a prolonged infusion usually lasting for 3–6 hours, all of which may have adverse effects beyond 90 minutes. Thus it is not at all clear that this test will be widely applicable.— L.W. Klein, M.D., and J.E. Parrillo, M.D.

The Prognosis of Patients Suspected of Having Acute Myocardial Infarction Subsequent to Its Exclusion as the Diagnosis
Karlson BW, Herlitz J, Emanuelsson H, Karlsson T, Hjalmarson Å (Univ of Göteborg, Sweden)
Int J Cardiol 26:251–257, 1990   5–38

Most hospitals have well-defined routines for the care and follow-up of patients with acute myocardial infarction (MI). However, routines are lacking for those in whom this diagnosis is excluded. A literature review was done to investigate the prognosis of patients in whom the diagnosis of acute MI was considered but subsequently excluded.

Several studies showed a surprisingly poor prognosis for such patients, almost comparable with that of patients with a confirmed infarction. When the results of the various studies were pooled, however, a significant difference was noted between patients with true MI and those in whom this diagnosis was excluded. The overall mortality in the first group was 12%, compared with 7% in the second. Subsequent nonfatal infarction developed in 11% and 6%, respectively. The difference was significant even when both nonfatal and fatal MIs were considered during the 1-year follow-up. Electrocardiographic ST-T changes were a risk factor for coronary events. The results for other possible risk factors were conflicting.

Several studies have shown almost similar prognoses for patients hospitalized for chest pain, whether or not MI subsequently developed. When the results were pooled, those who sustained an infarction had a worse outcome in long-term mortality and further infarction. Research is urgently needed to identify subgroups of patients in whom MI has been ruled out but who are at high risk.

▶ The conventional clinical wisdom concerning the prognosis of patients suspected of having acute MI but in whom this diagnosis is subsequently excluded is that the in-hospital mortality rate is worse if the diagnosis is confirmed, but confirmed and nonconfirmed infarcts have similar long-term (i.e., 1 or 2 year) follow-up. This makes intuitive as well as pathophysiologic sense, as patients with unstable angina still often have critical coronary stenoses and multivessel coronary artery disease. Also, every major natural history study of the disease has documented that the ejection fraction is the most important clinical variable predicting prognosis.

This review pools a large number of such studies and concludes that there is actually a worse (1-year) long-term prognosis for those with a documented infarction, both with respect to mortality as well as to reinfarction.

Leaving aside the apparent statistical issues and the propriety of pooling studies with widely varying patient selection criteria and management, it is clear that to answer this question fully would require another large natural history study, which is unlikely in today's medical climate. Neither physicians, nor their patients, are likely to forego the perceived benefits of angioplasty and/or bypass surgery. Once these subgroups are excluded, no definitive study can be performed. Further, modern noninvasive as well as invasive testing has reached a level of sophistication such that the practicing physician can usually plan an intelligent strategy tailored for each patient. These factors probably render the whole question moot.—L.W. Klein, M.D., and J.E. Parrillo, M.D.

Relationship Between Myocardial Metabolites and Contractile Abnormalities During Graded Regional Ischemia: Phosphorus-31 Nuclear Magnetic Resonance Studies of Porcine Myocardium In Vivo

Schaefer S, Schwartz GG, Gober JR, Wong AK, Camacho SA, Massie B, Weiner MW (VA Med Ctr, San Francisco; Univ of California, San Francisco)
J Clin Invest 85:706–713, 1990   5–39

In previous studies it has been shown that changes in high-energy phosphates, especially in the ratio of phosphocreatine to inorganic phosphate (PCr/P_i), correlate strongly with changes in myocardial blood flow during steady-state regional ischemia. The hypothesis that changes in myocardial high-energy phosphates correlate with alterations in myocardial function during steady-state conditions of graded regional ischemia was examined. Phosphorus-31 nuclear magnetic resonance spectroscopy was used in an in vivo porcine model of graded coronary stenosis. Subendocardial blood flow was reduced by 16% to 94% and simultaneous measurements were made of regional subendocardial blood flow, high-energy phosphates, pH, and myocardial segment shortening.

As blood flow was reduced, myocardial segment shortening in the subendocardium decreased. The PCr/P_i ratio was directly related to myocardial segment shortening and was a sensitive marker of regional ischemia. Significant changes in P_i and hydrogen ion concentration $[H^+]$ were observed only during mild reductions in subendocardial blood flow. These changes in ion concentrations were relatively greater than the corresponding changes in contractility. Throughout the reductions of blood flow the concentration of adenosine triphosphate remained constant.

These findings demonstrate that changes in myocardial high-energy phosphates, especially PCr/P_i, are related to changes in myocardial contractility during steady-state regional ischemia in vivo. The data are consistent with the possibility that P_i or $[H^+]$ is an inhibitor of myocardial contractility during ischemia.

▶ This is a potentially important study, as it demonstrates that changes in myocardial high-energy phosphates, analyzed as the PCr/P_i ratio, are closely related to reductions in subendocardial blood flow, thus producing regional ischemia in this animal model. If the phosphorous-31 magnetic resonance spectroscopy technique were easily transferable to human disease, its applications could include any question of diagnosis with reference to myocardial flow distribution and the presence of ischemia. Issues such as stunned or hibernating myocardium, failure of thrombolytic therapy, the therapeutic effect of pharmacologic agents or even mechanical methods, and many others could be queried by this method.

The primary physiologic finding of interest is the close linear correlation observed between the PCr/P_i ratio and alterations in segmental shortening in ischemic myocardium. Another interesting characterization was the significant change in P_i and $[H^+]$ in the presence of only small reductions in flow and shortening. This latter observation not only indicates how sensitive myocardial metabolism is to ischemia, but also suggests a possible independent negatively inotropic effect.

The major limitations of this study relate directly to the difficulties of spatial localization and accurate measurements with the magnetic resonance technique. If such problems can be worked out, and the technology made available to clinical medicine, the exciting prospects raised in this paper have important implications.—W. Klein, M.D., and J.E. Parrillo, M.D.

Long-Term Effects of Intravenous Anistreplase in Acute Myocardial Infarction: Final Report of the AIMS Study
Chamberlain DA, for the AIMS Trial Study Group (Royal Sussex County Hosp, Brighton, England)
Lancet 335:427–431, 1990   5–40

Mortality data were reviewed after 12 months of follow-up in a randomized, double-blind, placebo-controlled study of 1,258 patients who received either intravenous anistreplase [anisoylated plasminogen streptokinase activator complex (APSAC)] or placebo within 6 hours of suspected acute myocardial infarction (MI). Only patients aged 70 years or younger were eligible for the ASPAC Intervention Mortality Study (AIMS trial). Anticoagulation with intravenous heparin followed administration of anistreplase or placebo after 6 hours.

Strongly significant improvements in survival after anistreplase treatment were apparent at 30 days, by which time only 40 patients (6.4%) who received anistreplase had died compared to 77 (12.1%) who received placebo (odds reduction in mortality, 50.5%). After 1 year significant improvements in survival after receiving anistreplase were still being observed: 69 patients (11.1%) who received anistreplase had died com-

AIMS Trial Study Group

	Placebo (n = 634)	Anistreplase (n = 624)	Absolute difference (%) (% anistreplase- % placebo)
Cardiovascular			
Cardiogenic shock	29	16	−2·0 (p = 0·07)
Cardiorespiratory arrest (died)	37	26	−1·7 (p = 0·2)
Sudden death: (0–14 days)	2	1	
(15–365 days)	19	12	
(0–365 days)	21	13	−1·2 (p = 0·2)
Cardiac rupture/VSD	13	5	−1·2 (p = 0·09)
Cardiac failure	154	131	−3·3 (p = 0·2)
Ventricular fibrillation	46	41	−0·7 (p = 0·7)
Ventricular tachycardia	67	98	5·1 (p = 0·006)
Other ventricular arrhythmia	92	124	5·3 (p = 0·01)
Sinus bradycardia (and unspecified)	63	107	7·2 (p < 0·001)
Supraventricular tachycardia	6	12	1·0 (p = 0·2)
Pericarditis	98	43	−8·6 (p < 0·001)
Reinfarction: in hospital (fatal and non-fatal)	30	38	1·4 (p = 0·3)
after discharge to 1 yr (non-fatal)	23	29	0·9 (p = 0·5)
Haemorrhage			
Gastrointestinal (all types)	9	19	1·6 (p = 0·06)
Haematoma/puncture site	6	46	6·4 (p < 0·001)
Haematuria/epistaxis/ haemoptysis	5	30	4·0 (p < 0·001)
Transfusion	5	5	0·0 (p = 1·0)
Total	26	86	9·7 (p < 0·001)
Allergy			
Anaphylaxis	0	4	0·6 (p = 0·06)
Other (pruritis/urticaria/rash/ asthma)	17	11	−0·9 (p = 0·3)
Cerebrovascular			
Stroke (excluding TIA)	4	8	0·7 (p = 0·4)
Stroke or TIA: within 24 h	0	5	
24 h–30 days	4	4	
31–365 days	1	4	
Total	5	13*	1·0 (p = 0·06)

Abbreviations: VSD, ventricular septal defect; *TIA*, transient ischemic attack.
*Excludes 1 patient who sustained residual impairment after resuscitation for cardiac arrest.

(Courtesy of AIMS Trial Study Group: *Lancet* 335:427–431, 1990.)

pared to 113 (17.8) who received placebo (odds reduction in mortality, 42.7%) (Fig 5–9).

The survival benefit of anistreplase was not related to time between onset of symptoms and thrombolytic treatment or to any patient characteristic assessed. Factors associated with reduced survival were more than 4 hours from onset of symptoms to treatment, older than 65 years, tachycardia, previous acute MI, previous angina, current nonsmoker, and an-

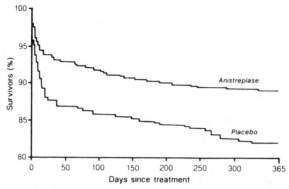

Fig 5–9.—Life-table survival curves up to 1 year after receiving anistreplase or placebo. (Courtesy of AIMS Trial Study Group: *Lancet* 335:427–431, 1990.)

terior MI. Major cardiovascular complications of acute MI were less frequent among patients who received anistreplase than among those who received placebo; bleeding was more common among patients who received anistreplase than among controls (table).

This study provides further evidence that thrombolytic treatment of acute MI is safe and effective in reducing long- and short-term mortality. If future studies should establish that thrombolytic treatment even before hospital admission is beneficial, anistreplase, which requires only a single intravenous injection, would have practical advantages over other available thrombolytic agents.

▶ Clearly, the most important study in the field of thrombolytic therapy for acute MI in the past year is the final report of the AIMS study. In this paper, the 1-year survival of patients treated with APSAC is shown to have an odds reduction of 43% as compared to a placebo-treated cohort. This observation represents a persistent beneficial effect derived from the 30-day follow-up data (50.5% odds reduction), which was reported previously.

These excellent mortality results, in combination with an adverse effect profile similar to other thrombolytic agents, has added a new drug to consider when choosing among therapeutic alternatives. As the GISSI-2 study found little therapeutic difference between streptokinase and recombinant tissue-plasminogen activator, a head-to-head trial with APSAC becomes necessary. The ISIS-3 study, already underway, compares all 3 agents in the same study design. Its results are anticipated to be crucial to the decision-making process.—L.W. Klein, M.D., and J.E. Parrillo, M.D.

A Randomized Pilot Trial of Brief Versus Prolonged Heparin After Successful Reperfusion in Acute Myocardial Infarction

Kander NH, Holland KJ, Pitt B, Topol EJ (Univ of Michigan)
Am J Cardiol 65:139–142, 1990   5–41

There is much controversy over whether and for how long intravenously administered heparin should be given after successful reperfusion in patients with acute myocardial infarction (MI). During a 14-month study period, 50 patients with acute MI who had angiographic evidence of successful reperfusion of an infarcted artery were randomly assigned to heparin, administered intravenously for 24 hours or less or prolonged infusion for at least 72 hours. Heparin was discontinued if significant bleeding occurred requiring 2 or more units of blood. The primary end points were 1-week patency confirmed by repeat cardiac catheterization or recurrent ischemia, or both.

Two patients in each group had documented reocclusions on follow-up catheterization, 3 of whom had recurrent symptoms. None of the patients in the brief infusion group, but 6 of the 25 patients in the prolonged infusion group, had significant bleeding requiring discontinuation of heparin therapy; 5 of the latter 6 had received thrombolytic agents before the initial cardiac catheterization. Prolonged heparin therapy for more than 24 hours does not appear to be justified in low-risk patients with acute MI in whom reperfusion is successful.

▶ The duration of the empiric use of intravenous heparin as adjunctive therapy with thrombolytic agents is controversial. Common clinical practice has been to continue the administration of heparin for up to 72 hours after successful reperfusion. However, there is a demonstrated bleeding risk with prolonged infusions, especially in patients who have had vascular punctures or have other medical problems. On the other hand, if anticoagulation is stopped too soon, reocclusion and reinfarction may occur.

This study shows that in a highly selected, low-risk group, prolonged therapy did not protect against rethrombosis and was associated with more bleeding in 6 of 25 vs. none of 25) as compared to a group receiving heparin for 24 hours or less. Although this conclusion may be justified in this small series of very carefully chosen subjects, and may in fact be the correct strategy in other, equally carefully chosen patients, one should be hesitant to generalize to a larger extent on the basis of this study. For one thing, reocclusion is a significant limitation of lytic therapy; in this series, 4 patients (8%) had reocclusion. It would take many more patients to conclude whether the undeniably increased bleeding risk was counterbalanced by preventing rethrombosis. These same authors have argued the crucial nature of concurrent heparin use with recombinant tissue-plasminogen activator, with its short half-life, and it seems somewhat inconsistent to suggest that after 24 hours the possibility of incompletely lysed thrombi suddenly becomes a non-issue. Another factor is that all 6 of the bleeding cases had an invasive procedure; although the precise number of access site complications is not given, the main study conclusion would fail to attain statistical significance if such cases were excluded.

Hence, a much larger, more appropriately designed trial with the statistical power to prove or disprove all hypotheses is needed to put this question to rest.—L.W. Klein, M.D., and J.E. Parrillo, M.D.

Intracoronary Thrombus and Complex Morphology in Unstable Angina: Relation to Timing of Angiography and In-Hospital Cardiac Events

Freeman MR, Williams AE, Chisholm RJ, Armstrong PW (Univ of Toronto)
Circulation 80:17–23, 1989   5–42

A randomized prospective study of coronary angiography in 78 patients with unstable angina was conducted to determine the significance of angiographic extent of disease, complex coronary morphology, and coronary thrombus on in-hospital outcome, and to assess the effect of timing of angiography on the frequency of coronary thrombus and complex coronary morphology. Forty-two patients were randomized to cardiac catheterization within the first 24 hours of admission and 36 to angiography to be performed later during the hospital admission.

Coronary thrombi were present in 18 of 42 early angiography patients and in 14 of 36 late angiography patients. Only 5 of 24 late elective angiography patients had coronary thrombi; 9 of 12 late urgent angiography patients had thrombi. No difference in the frequency of complex coronary morphology was observed among patients randomized to early angiography, late urgent angiography, or late elective angiography. Cardiac events, including death, myocardial infarction, and urgent revascularization, were more frequent in patients with coronary thrombus (73%), complex coronary morphology (55%), and multiple-vessel disease (58%) than in patients without these angiographic features. The corresponding percentages for those without angiographic features were 17%, 31%, and 7%. Thrombus was the most significant angiographic variable for predicting cardiac events.

That thrombus occurs more frequently in patients with early angiography within 24 hours of admission rather than later during hospital admission was not substantiated. However, the presence of coronary thrombus had an important temporal link to the presence of chest pain at rest. Intracoronary thrombi identified at coronary angiography were frequent in patients with unstable angina and may have also mediated the cardiac events associated with this syndrome.

▶ This study confirms the findings of Ambrose, Levin and Fallon, Meister, and their co-workers and many others who have recognized both the epidemiologic association and pathophysiologic correlation between thrombi, complex plaque morphology, and unstable angina. Although this hypothesis is by now an accepted and established one, all of the studies have the same limitation—the sensitivity and specificity of identifying thrombus or complex, ulcerated plaque by angiography is not known, and further, is surely not 100%. The elegant angioscopic work of Forrester et al. has demonstrated this fact, and ignoring its implications would be an error. A percutaneous study using the newer intravascular imaging techniques is necessary to sort out definitively the subtle differences in types of unstable angina and to recognize all of the components in its causation.—W. Klein, M.D., and J.E. Parrillo, M.D.

Clinical Correlates of Acute Right Ventricular Infarction in Acute Inferior Myocardial Infarction

Sinha N, Ahuja RC, Saran RK, Jain GC (Sanjay Gandhi Post-Graduate Inst of Med Sciences, Lucknow, India; KG's Med College, Lucknow)
Int J Cardiol 24:55–61, 1989   5–43

Acute myocardial infarction (MI) is generally viewed by clinicians as an infarction of part of the left ventricle. Isolated right ventricular (RV) infarction is extremely rare, and it has been of interest mainly to pathologists looking at autopsied specimens. Yet the clinical recognition of RV infarction is important as it occurs in 25% to 53% of patients with inferior MI. When present, RV infarction may dominate the clinical picture and hemodynamic consequences.

The ECG changes in 50 patients (mean age, 35–70 years) with RV infarction were correlated with the clinical features and course during hospitalization. The series included 42 men. None of the patients had a history of MI. A 16-lead ECG was recorded at the time of hospital admission and repeated at 24, 48, and 72 hours after onset of symptoms and daily thereafter until discharge. Right ventricular infarction was diagnosed by the presence of ST segment elevation of at least 1 mm in 1 or more right precordial leads. Clinical and ECG features of patients with RV infarction were compared with those having only inferior MI.

Twenty of the 50 patients with inferior MI had ECG evidence of RV infarction; 5 had ST elevation in a single right precordial lead and 15 had ST elevation in 2 or more right precordial leads. These ECG changes resolved within 72 hours in 90% of the patients. A comparison of the clinical features showed that giddiness and hiccups were significantly more common in patients with RV infarction. There was no difference between patients with and without RV infarction with regard to the occurrence of other symptoms (e.g., chest pain, referred pain, nausea, vomiting, restlessness, choking, suffocation, syncope, palpitation, or breathlessness). Signs of RV dysfunction-raised jugular venous pressure, Kussmaull's sign, hypotension excluding cardiogenic shock, and right-sided third heart sound in the absence of clinical left ventricular failure were seen either exclusively or more commonly in patients with RV infarction, as 11 of 20 patients had 2 or more of these signs. In most patients with hemodynamically significant RV infarction, the diagnosis can be made on the basis of a combination of clinical signs and ST elevation of at least 1 mm in 2 or more right precordial leads.

▶ The frequency with which RV infarction complicates the clinical course of inferior MI is being increasingly appreciated. This study reviews the clinical and ECG features in such patients and identifies several features that distinguish them from uncomplicated infarcts. Certainly, right precordial lead ECGs are not as commonly used diagnostically as their apparent clinical utility would dictate.—L.W. Klein, M.D., and J.E. Parrillo, M.D.

Cardiovascular Complications of Thrombolytic Therapy in Patients With a Mistaken Diagnosis of Acute Myocardial Infarction

Blankenship JC, Almquist AK (Geisinger Med Ctr, Danville, Pa; Minneapolis Heart Inst)
J Am Coll Cardiol 14:1579–1582, 1989   5–44

Thrombolytic drugs given to patients with syndromes that mimick acute myocardial infarction (MI) may result in unnecessary bleeding complications or exacerbation of underlying conditions. Two patients were treated with streptokinsae intravenously after a mistaken diagnosis of acute MI.

Acute MI was diagnosed by the primary physician from the ECG, but, in both cases, subsequent tests conclusively ruled out the diagnosis. Both patients received streptokinase intravenously; subsequently, pericardial tamponade developed, in 1 patient after aortic dissection and in the other after pericarditis. The administration of streptokinase delayed surgery in 1 patient and resulted in excessive bleeding during emergent aortic repair in the other. One patient died.

The potential for misdiagnosis of chest pain syndrome is clear, as well as the potential for adverse complications when thrombolytic therapy is administered to these patients. Physicians should adhere to more strict ECG criteria of acute MI before considering the patient for thrombolytic therapy. If the diagnosis remains uncertain, serial ECGs, emergent angiography, or echocardiography may be performed to exclude other syndromes causing chest pain.

▶ These reports highlight the dangers of misdiagnosis of acute MI in the thrombolytic era. In addition to these conditions, gastrointestinal bleeding from active peptic ulcer disease and other abdominal causes of pain have also been initially mistaken for acute MI, with potentially disastrous consequences. Strict ECG criteria of infarction must be insisted upon before thrombolytic therapy is administered.—L.W. Klein, M.D., and J.E. Parrillo, M.D.

Prognostic Significance of the Extent of Myocardial Injury in Acute Myocardial Infarction Treated by Streptokinase (the GISSI Trial)

Mauri F, Gasparini M, Barbonaglia L, Santoro E, Franzosi MG, Tognoni G, Rovelli F (DeGasperis Ctr, Milan, Italy; Mario Negri Inst, Milan)
Am J Cardiol 63:1291–1295, 1989   5–45

Clinical variables such as age, sex, and previous ischemic episodes influence the in-hospital prognosis of patients with acute myocardial infarction (MI). However, the role and interdependence of the site and extent of ischemic damage are less well defined. To evaluate the relative contributions of infarct site and extent in determining in-hospital outcome and efficacy of streptokinse therapy, 8,731 patients enrolled in the Gruppo Italiano per lo Studio della Streptochinasi nell'Infarto Miocardico (GISS) trial who had a first Q-wave acute MI were studied.

The first 4,372 patients underwent standard diagnostic and therapeutic interventions. The remaining 4,359 patients were treated with streptokinase. Electrocardiograms were analyzed by clinicians blinded to therapy and mortality. They recorded the presence of ST elevation or depression in each lead, the presence of Q waves of at least .03 second, major conduction disturbances, and infarct sites. Infarct location also was classified. In-hospital mortality was evaluated according to infarct size, location, and fibrinolytic treatment.

Anterior and inferior AMIs had nearly equal incidence rates, but the incidence of multiple-site and lateral AMIs was much lower. Overall mortality was 11.1%, slightly less than the 11.8% in the total GISSI group of 11,712 patients. Mortality varied according to site: 6.2%, inferior sites; 9.7%, lateral sites; 10.3%, multiple sites; and 16.3%, anterior sites. Streptokinase significantly reduced mortality in anterior and multiple-site infarcts, and there was a slight but not significant reduction in mortality from lateral acute MIs in streptokinase-treated patients.

More than 40% of the patients had small infarcts, 25.1% had modest-sized infarcts, 18.7% had large infarcts, and 8.9% had extensive infarcts. Overall mortality was directly correlated with infarct size. Streptokinase reduced mortality, but not significantly, in patients with small infarcts; however, mortality in patients with larger infarcts was significantly reduced with streptokinase.

The standard 12-lead ECG permits good evaluation of the extent of myocardial injury and therefore provides a good prognostic index in acute MI. The extent of myocardial injury appears to be more important than the site in determining in-hospital mortality and efficacy of streptokinase therapy. Streptokinase therapy has a more significant effect in larger myocardial injuries and appears not to be directly affected by the location of the acute MI.

▶ Attempts to establish precisely why anterior infarcts tend to have a worse prognosis than those in other locations inevitably are doomed because the peculiarities of coronary anatomy are such that the left anterior descending artery not only supplies 40% or more of the left ventricular (LV) myocardium, but also supplies important components of LV function, such as the interventricular septum, the anterolateral papillary muscle, and the apex. Trying to differentiate whether size or location is the most important determinant is, ultimately an academic exericse, because anterior infarcts also tend to be the largest.

This study puts a new twist on this old conundrum. The GISSI-1 study, as is widely appreciated, showed improved mortality only in anterior infarcts treated with streptokinase and not other locations. Is this because of the location or the size of anterior infarcts? This study not only uses a very insensitive indicator of infarct size (the number of ECG leads with ST elevation), but also ignores the fundamental difficulties in posing the question in the first place. In any case, it comes as no revelation that large infarcts should be treated aggressively.—L.W. Klein, M.D., and J.E. Parrillo, M.D.

An Analysis of Time Delays Preceding Thrombolysis for Acute Myocardial Infarction

Sharkey SW, Brunette DD, Ruiz E, Hession WT, Wysham DG, Goldenberg IF, Hodges M (Univ of Minnesota; Hennepin County Med Ctr, Minneapolis)
JAMA 262:3171–3174, 1989   5–46

Early administration of thrombolytic agents in acute myocardial infarction (MI) is essential to the success of treatment. Coronary artery thrombi are most susceptible to lysis if the thrombolytic drug is infused within 3 hours of onset of symptoms. As part of the Thrombolysis in Myocardial Infarction (TIMI) II trial, the time delays encountered when implementing intravenous tissue-plasminogen activator (t-PA) therapy were identified.

During a 2-year period, 236 patients with acute MI were treated with t-PA at 2 teaching hospitals and 2 private hospitals participating in the TIMI II trial. The average time from symptom onset to treatment with t-PA was 153 minutes, the average interval from symptom onset to arrival at the emergency department was 65 minutes, and the average interval from arrival at the emergency department to initiation of t-PA was 81 minutes. After arrival in the emergency department, patients waited an average of 19.9 minutes to have an initial ECG and an additional 70 minutes after the diagnosis of acute MI was confirmed by ECG before t-PA therapy was initiated.

A detailed analysis of time delays was performed for 50 patients with acute MI who were taken to 1 of the teaching hospitals. The interval between initial ECG and initiation of t-PA therapy was 46.8 minutes if t-PA was first administered in the emergency department and 82.1 minutes if the patient was first transferred to the coronary care unit. Thus most of the delay was encountered once the patient was already in the hospital. Factors identified as contributing to delay included securing additional peripheral intravenous access, determining arterial blood gas concentrations, obtaining blood samples for admission laboratory data, obtaining a chest radiograph, administering morphine and lidocaine, waiting for a cardiology staff member to approve administration of the thrombolytic agent, and waiting for the drug to arrive from the pharmacy. To overcome such delays, the decision to administer a thrombolytic drug should be made by the primary care physician in the emergency department without waiting for approval from a cardiologist.

▶ Despite the fact that more than 600,000 persons sustain acute MIs in the United States every year, only 25% receive thrombolytic agents. Undoubtedly, some of these patients have contraindications to lytic therapy, but most do not receive this therapy because they often come to the hospital close to, or after, the 6-hour window of benefit. Furthermore, to obtain optimum benefit, the earliest treatment possible within this window is mandatory.

In this analysis, performed at 2 private and 2 academic centers, the time delays from performance of the ECG to initiation of lytic therapy accounted for more than half of the total time from onset of symptoms to appropriate therapy. The factors identified in this study that caused the delays were primarily those of assessment, line placement, and blood drawing, which need to be done as quickly as possible in these patients. The finding that treatment in the emergency department (ED) would save 35 minutes vs. treatment in the coronary care unit leads to a highly controversial recommendation that "the decision to administer a thrombolytic drug should be made by the primary care physician in the ED and should not await the approval of a cardiologist unless the circumstances are uncertain." Each hospital and each physician will have to consider the impact of this study, and the ensuing recommendation, on their own practice.—L.W. Klein, M.D., and J.E. Parrillo, M.D.

Risk Stratification of Patients With Non–Q-Wave Myocardial Infarction: The Critical Role of ST Segment Depression
Schechtman KB, Capone RJ, Kleiger RE, Gibson RS, Schwartz DJ, Roberts R, Young PM, Boden WE, and the Diltiazem Reinfarction Study Research Group (Washington Univ; Brown Univ; Univ of Virginia; Baylor College of Medicine, Houston; Marion Labs, Kansas City, Mo; et al)
Circulation 80:1148–1158, 1989   5–47

The risk of recurrent infarction and sudden death is greatest during the first year after acute non–Q-wave myocardial infarction (MI). Although non–Q-wave MI is associated with less myocardial damage than Q-wave infarction, non–Q-wave patients are more likely to have residual ischemia and have a higher reinfarction rate. Thus stratification of post-MI patients into low- and high-risk subgroups is vitally important. In a fol-

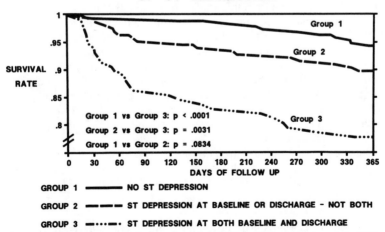

Fig 5–10.—Kaplan-Meier survival curves for patients with no ST depression (group 1), ST depression at baseline or discharge (group 2), and ST depression at baseline and discharge (group 3). Mortality was 5.5% in group 1 (n = 199), 10.1% in group 2 (n = 168), and 22.2% in group 3 (n = 117). (Courtesy of Schechtman KB, Capone RJ, Kleiger RE, et al: *Circulation* 80:1148–1158, 1989.)

low-up study of 515 patients who survived hospitalization with MB-creatine-kinase-confirmed acute non–Q-wave MI, analysis was made of factors related to mortality and late infarction.

The patients were enrolled in the Diltiazem Reinfarction Study, a randomized, double-blind, placebo-controlled clinical trial of the benefits of prophylactic diltiazem. Within 1 year, 57 deaths occurred; 19 were sudden and 10 were of noncardiac or unknown causes. Twenty-seven of the 64 patients who had reinfarctions died subsequent to that event.

Factors predictive of mortality were persistent ST depression, a history of congestive heart failure, older age, and ST elevation at hospital discharge. Both mortality and late reinfarction were strongly related to persistent ST depression, which may be a manifestation of "silent myocardial ischemia" and predispose non–Q-wave MI patients to a higher incidence of subsequent cardiac events (Fig 5–10).

Complete ECG data were available for 483 patients at both baseline and discharge. Of these, 203 (42%) were identified as high-risk patients, with a risk ratio for 1-year mortality more than 7 times that of patients with no risk factors. This high-risk group may benefit from aggressive therapy and may be considered for additional noninvasive testing or early coronary angiography.

▶ This retrospective study shows that patients with acute non–Q-wave infarcts who present with ST depression and have persistent changes at discharge have a worse 1-year outcome and a higher reinfarction rate than those with no ECG changes on admission or those in whom the ST changes at baseline do not persist. This particular finding was more significant than Killip class or left ventricular hypertrophy, which were also independently predictive.

This provocative conclusion is interesting, but the absence of uniformly performed noninvasive and invasive studies prevents any meaningful clinical strategy from being inferred from this study. To suggest that this subgroup be more aggressively managed or considered for earlier angiography in the absence of stress test data does not take into account the currently accepted clinical practice. Neither baseline ejection fraction nor regional function are considered as variables in the data analysis, and catheterization is almost considered to be an end point rather than part of the management strategy. Further, without some insight into changes in ejection fraction over the course of this study, one cannot begin to address the role of stunned or hibernating myocardium as either the cause of persistent ST depression or as an independent factor to consider in patient management.

Hence, except to suggest the need for a comprehensive, prospective trial, the clinician will have a difficult task finding a useful way to incorporate these data into daily practice.—L.W. Klein, M.D., and J.E. Parrillo, M.D.

Morphological Diagnosis of Congenital and Acquired Heart Disease by Magnetic Resonance Imaging
Sieverding L, Klose U, Apitz J (Univ Children's Hosp, Tübingen, Germany)
Pediatr Radiol 20:311–319, 1990   5–48

Magnetic resonance imaging (MRI) is an established method for the diagnostic imaging of a variety of organs. Its accuracy in defining cardiac anatomy and abnormalities was evaluated in 60 patients, mainly infants, with congenital or acquired heart disease. A multislice spin-echo tech-

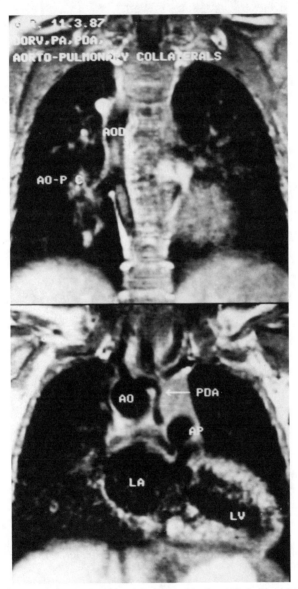

Fig 5–11.—Frontal sections of the heart of a 3-month-old infant with double-outlet right ventricle *(DORV)*, ventricular septal defect, and pulmonary atresia *(PA)*. No main pulmonary artery, normal left pulmonary artery *(AP)*, right aortic arch *(AO)*, and right descending aorta *(AOD)*. Aorticopulmonary collaterals *(AO-PC)* to the right pulmonic lobe, patent ductus arteriosus *(PDA)* to the left pulmonary artery *(AP)*; *LA*, left atrium; *LV*, left ventricle. (Courtesy of Sieverding L, Klose U, Apitz J: *Pediatr Radiol* 20:311–319, 1990.)

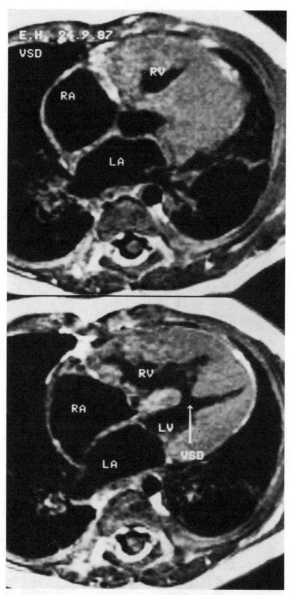

Fig 5–12.—Transverse sections of the heart of a 2-month-old infant suffering from a large muscular ventricular septal defect *(VSD)*. Myocardium of the left and right ventricle is hypertrophied as a result of coarctation of the aorta. *LA*, left atrium; *LV*, left ventricle; *RA*, right atrium; *RV*, right ventricle. (Courtesy of Sieverding L, Klose U, Apitz J: *Pediatr Radiol* 20:311–319, 1990.)

nique was used. The patients ranged in age from 10 days to 20 years; the mean age was 3.7 years. Findings with MRI were compared with the previous diagnoses made on the basis of echocardiography and angiocardiography.

The 66 anomalies of the vessels included 6 that were misdiagnosed. In

8 cases the previous diagnosis was amended. In 1 case an aorticopulmonary window was first detected by MRI. In another case MRI detected a recoarctation of the aorta. With MRI the extent of an aortic aneurysm could be defined and dissection of the aortic wall excluded. More information on the pulmonary vascular status was available with MRI in 5 patients. A diagnosis of atrial septal defect was established definitively in 2 cases, but MRI failed to detect atrial septal defect in 2 others. The diagnosis of partial anomalous pulmonary venous return was established by MRI, additional information was obtained about the pulmonary vein connections in a case of cor triatriatum. One alleged atrial tumor was recognized as a prominent eustachian valve. There were 35 ventricular anomalies in the series. Whereas MRI did not detect 2 membranous ventricular septal defects, it contributed to the diagnosis in 1 child with a double-inlet left ventricle and in 2 with ventricular aneurysms (Figs 5–11 and 5–12).

Magnetic resonance imaging proved superior to echocardiography and angiocardiography in the diagnosis of the vascular status in pulmonary vascular hypoplasia and anomalous pulmonary vein return. It was valuable in visualizing coarctations and aneurysms, and it also defined segmental anatomy and demarcated intra- and extracardiac tumors.

▶ Two-dimensional echocardiography remains the simplest, cheapest, and most accessible noninvasive tool for the diagnosis of heart disease in children. Despite the expense, inaccessibility of the patient, and the problems associated with the presence of a strong magnetic field, ECG-gated MRI may offer advantages in the diagnosis of specific lesions such as pulmonary hypoplasia, anomalous pulmonary venous return, and coarctation of the aorta.—D.G. Nichols, M.D.

Effects of Vasopressin and Catecholamines on the Maintenance of Circulatory Stability in Brain-Dead Patients

Iwai A, Sakano T, Uenishi M, Sugimoto H, Yoshioka T, Sugimoto T (Osaka Univ Hosp, Japan)
Transplantation 48:613–617, 1989   5–49

Long-term maintenance of the circulation after brain death may be helpful in basic and clinical research, particularly on organ transplantation. In a preliminary study, prolonged hemodynamic stability was achieved after brain death with combined administration of vasopressin and epinephrine. To investigate this process more extensively, 25 brain-dead patients were studied in 3 experiments.

In the first study the patients were randomly assigned to 1 of 3 groups on the basis of the dose of vasopressin. In group 1, 10 patients received epinephrine only to maintain systolic blood pressure above 100 mm Hg; in group 2, 2 patients received a diuretic dose of vasopressin, .1–.4 units per hour, in addition to epinephrine; and in group 3, 13 patients received a pressor dose of vasopressin, 1–2 units per hour, plus epinephrine. Despite an increasing dose of epinephrine, cardiac arrest and circulatory failure occurred within a short time in patients given no vasopressin or antidiuretic dose of the drug. In contrast, stable circulation was maintained in all patients who received a pressor dose of vasopressin plus epinephrine until infusion was discontinued.

In the second study the circulatory parameters in 5 group 3 patients with stable circulation were analyzed under 4 conditions: (1) neither vasopressin nor epinephrine (control), (2) vasopressin only, (3) epinephrine only, and (4) both vasopressin and epinephrine. Compared with the control condition, vasopressin alone increased the total peripheral resistance index (TPRI), whereas epinephrine alone increased the cardiac index. However, with infusion of both vasopressin and epinephrine, the mean arterial blood pressure (MAP) increased significantly with marked increases in the TPRI and cardiac index.

In the third study, 4 group 3 patients with stable condition were studied to determine the hemodynamic effects of the 3 catecholamines—epinephrine, norepinephrine, and dopamine—in combination with a pressor dose of vasopressin. The dose of norepinephrine required to maintain MAP above 90 mm Hg was 4 times that of epinephrine. In a dose sufficient to maintain MAP, epinephrine increased both the TPRI and cardiac index and norepinephrine increased the TPRI, whereas dopamine acted primarily on the heart by increasing the cardiac index.

Combined administration of vasopressin and epinephrine is an effective and reliable method of maintaining circulatory stability in brain-dead patients. A pressor dose of vasopressin is essential to maintain stable circulation. When given in combination with vasopressin, epinephrine maintains stable circulation through a mechanism of mutual interaction.

▶ In maintaining brain-dead patients for potential organ donation, certain physiologic needs must be met. This paper looks at the commonly required administration of vasopressin and catecholamine. The authors conclude that a pressor dose of vasopressin is important in maintaining circulatory stability in these patients, particularly if it is supplemented by a catecholamine. The authors also conclude that the vasopressin may be given in a standard fashion, but that the dose of catecholamine should be chosen after an understanding of the causes of the circulatory instability in the patients.—M.C. Rogers, M.D.

Rejection and Infection After Pediatric Cardiac Transplantation
Braunlin EA, Canter CE, Olivari MT, Ring WS, Spray TL, Bolman RM III (Univ of Minnesota Hosp and Clinic; Washington Univ)
Ann Thorac Surg 49:385–390, 1990   5–50

Orthotopic cardiac transplantation has only recently become an accepted treatment for end-stage cardiomyopathy in children and adolescents. The long-term survival, incidence of rejection, and incidence of infection were evaluated in 21 patients aged 6 months to 19 years (mean, 11.2 years) who underwent cardiac transplantation from 1985 to 1989. Eighteen patients survived the operative period, and all received triple-drug immunosuppression therapy consisting of cyclosporine, azathio-prine, and prednisone. The average follow-up period was 24 months (range, 5–49 months).

During follow-up acute myocardial rejection occurred in 7 patients on 12 occasions as documented by endomyocardial biopsy findings of dif-fuse lymphocytic infiltrate. Eight of the rejection episodes were associated with subtherapeutic blood levels of cyclosporine. Rejection episodes were more common in adolescents than in children, including 5 adolescents who stopped immunosuppressive therapy and/or started drinking alco-hol. Two of these adolescents died of arrhythmias related to myocardial dysfunction and ongoing rejection.

Actuarial freedom from rejection in the first 7 months after transplan-tation was 73%. There were no perioperative or late deaths from infec-tion. Bacterial sepsis was treated twice during follow-up, viral infection was treated 5 times, and fungal infection once. Actuarial freedom from serious blood borne infection was 83% at 1 year. The actuarial survival rates among the 18 operative survivors were 94% at 1 year and 78% at 3 years.

It appears that triple-drug immunosuppression has remarkably reduced the incidence of rejection and infection after cardiac transplantation in infants and children. Rejection episodes are common during the first year after transplantation but can also occur late. The majority of the rejec-tion episodes are associated with subtherapeutic cyclosporine levels. Bac-terial infections respond to standard antibiotic therapy, and viral infec-tions are well tolerated.

▶ The increasing use of heart transplants in infants has allowed analysis of the unique characteristics of posttransplant rejection in pediatric patients. These authors look at patients aged from 6 months to 19 years who underwent car-diac transplantation for cardiomyopathy. I am encouraged by the 1-year and 3-year survival of 94% and 78%, respectively. Furthermore, the incidence of bacterial infection appears to be relatively low, and the infections appear to re-spond to standard antibiotic therapy. What would be interesting in these pa-tients would be some analysis of how they do generally, beyond their cardiac and infectious disease status. This would be particularly useful in the infants because there has been some concern expressed that cyclosporine has the po-tential to be neurotoxic.— M.C. Rogers, M.D.

Value of Initial ECG Findings and Plasma Drug Levels in Cyclic Antidepres-sant Overdose

Lavoie FW, Gansert GG, Weiss RE (Univ of Louisville)
Ann Emerg Med 19:696–700, 1990   5–51

Cyclic antidepressants (TCAs) account for nearly 25% of all deaths from drug overdose. Because a number of ECG changes are seen with TCA overdose, the ability of initial ECG parameters to identify TCA in-gestion and predict later complications was assessed. The records of 401 overdose patients were reviewed. Of the 358 cases available for analysis, toxicologic screening showed 187 to be TCA positive and 171 TCA negative. The mean age was 33 years; 54.2% were women.

There were differences between the 2 groups in QRS duration, QTc, T40 axis, and heart rate. In 55 of the TCA-positive and 27 of the TCA-negative patients a far rightward deviation (130 to 270 degrees) was observed with respect to the T40 axis. The sensitivity of this parameter in predicting TCA ingestion was only 29%; its specificity was 83%. When all 4 parameters were combined, classification as TCA positive or TCA negative was correct in only 66% of the cases. Heart rate was the best single discriminator, followed by QRS duration. In all cases, correlation coefficients for plasma quantitative TCA levels by ECG parameter yielded an r of less than .33.

Although increased heart rate, prolonged QRS duration, increased QT interval, and rightward T40 axis were statistically different between TCA-positive and TCA-negative groups, reliance on 1 or all of these parameters would have misclassified approximately one third of the patients. Thus TCA levels do not correspond with ECG parameters, and ECG parameters cannot be used to include or exclude a diagnosis of TCA overdose.

▶ Although cardiac conduction abnormalities are common after TCA overdose, they are not sufficiently specific to aid in diagnosis except to confirm it.— R.W. McPherson, M.D.

Correlation Between Preoperative Ischemia and Major Cardiac Events After Peripheral Vascular Surgery
Raby KE, Goldman L, Creager MA, Cook EF, Weisberg MC, Whittemore AD, Selwyn AP (Brigham and Women's Hosp, Boston)
N Engl J Med 321:1296–1300, 1989   5–52

Ambulatory ECG monitoring can detect myocardial ischemia and may be able to predict the risk of cardiac events in patients with angina pectoris. To assess its value in predicting cardiac events after elective peripheral vascular surgery, monitoring was conducted for 24–48 hours within 9 days before surgery.

Preoperative ischemia was detected in 32 of the 176 patients (18%). There were 75 episodes, 73 of which were asymptomatic, that lasted for an average of 36 minutes. Major postoperative cardiac events occurred in 13 patients (7%). Among the 32 patients who had preoperative ischemia postoperative events occurred in 12, whereas only 1 of 144 patients without preoperative ischemia had an event after surgery. The sensitivity of preoperative ischemia was 92% and the specificity was 88%. A positive result had a 38% predictive value and a negative result had a 99% predictive value.

Preoperative ECG monitoring appears to be useful in assessing cardiac risk in patients undergoing elective peripheral vascular surgery. It is less expensive and more readily available than dipyridamole-thallium scintigraphy. Patients without preoperative ischemia should do well. Those with preoperative ischemia should be reevaluated and their medical regimen should be intensified. In the absence of improvement, more definitive action should be considered.

▶ Complications of coronary artery disease account for considerable morbidity and mortality following vascular surgical procedures. This report by Raby et al. demonstrates that preoperative ambulatory ECG monitoring can be used to identify patients at high risk for such complications. Ambulatory ECG monitoring is widely available and relatively inexpensive, and it is potentially of value for preoperative screening. Future studies must determine whether (1) alternative management strategies can be used to improve outcome in patients identified preoperatively as having increased risk for ischemic complications, and (2) whether clinical criteria can be used to identify certain low-risk patients and thus increase the cost effectiveness of ambulatory ECG monitoring.—M.J. Breslow, M.D.

Adverse Cardiac Effects of Combined Neuroleptic Ingestion and Tricyclic Antidepressant Overdose
Wilens TE, Stern TA, O'Gara PT (Massachusetts Gen Hosp, Boston)
J Clin Psychopharmacol 10:51–54, 1990   5–53

Both tricyclic antidepressants (TCAs) and neuroleptics each have adverse cardiac effects, but little is known about the combined effects of these agents. To identify the risk posed by neuroleptic-TCA overdose, the clinical course of 70 consecutive intensive care admissions for TCA overdose during a 5-year period was analyzed in a retrospective study.

Neuroleptics and TCAs were ingested by 12 patients. Amitriptyline was the TCA used by all patients. Compared with the 58 TCA-only patients, the TCA-neuroleptic patients had a markedly higher prevalence of first-degree atrioventricular block, a significantly higher prevalence of intraventricular conduction delay (QRS duration longer than .10 seconds), and a threefold increase in the prevalence of QTc prolongation. The mean levels of TCA were 14% greater in the TCA-neuroleptic group than in the TCA-only group; the difference was not significant.

These data show that the combination of a TCA and a neuroleptic in overdose may significantly increase the risk of adverse cardiac effects. A precise history should be obtained in all patients with suspected TCA overdose, and an ECG and/or TCA levels should be closely monitored in patients with combined TCA-neuroleptic overdose.

▶ Although TCAs are common causes of overdose and even suicide attempts, and the same can be said about neuroleptic agents, the frequent use of these drugs means that it is now possible to see significant numbers of patients who have ingested both. This co-ingestion appears to significantly increase the risk of important cardiac consequences, including first-degree block, prolongation of QRS duration, and prolongation of the QTc. Based on this study, it appears that

multiple drug injections represent a significant risk in this group of patients.—
M.C. Rogers, M.D.

Clonidine Poisoning in Young Children
Wiley JF II, Wiley CC, Torrey SB, Henretig FM (Children's Hosp of Philadelphia;
St Christopher's Hosp for Children, Philadelphia; Delaware Valley Regional Poison Control Ctr, Philadelphia)
J Pediatr 116:654–658, 1990   5–54

Clonidine is an α-adrenergic agonist that is used to treat hypertension, migraine headaches, Tourette's syndrome, and attention deficit disorder with hyperactivity. The course of clonidine poisoning, described in 47 consecutive inpatient records, was examined. The children, aged 9–84 months, were seen at 2 hospitals in a 5-year period. The mean age was 27 months.

The mean estimated dose of clonidine in 26 cases was 1.6 mg. All but 3 patients had CNS changes and nearly 80% had cardiovascular abnormalities. About one third of the patients had apnea or depressed breathing. Three fourths were symptomatic within an hour of ingesting clonidine. Routine toxicologic screening does not detect this drug, but specific serum studies detected it in 4 of 5 patients.

Eighteen patients received syrup of ipecac, and 33 underwent gastric lavage. All but 1 patient received activated charcoal. Six patients had to be intubated and ventilated; 7 were given atropine for bradycardia. Naloxone was given to 19 patients, but only 3 showed definite improvement. The mean duration of symptoms was about 10 hours, and the mean time in the hospital was 33 hours.

Delayed progression of symptoms from clonidine poisoning is not likely in a young child whose renal function is normal. Naloxone is not consistently effective as an antidote.

▶ Because of the frequent admission of critically ill children who present with a diagnosis of drug ingestion, it is always necessary to keep this potential cause of bizarre symptoms in mind. These authors review the presentation of clonidine poisoning in young children, which is a more frequently occurring event now that clonidine is so widely used in the treatment of hypertension. In particular, these authors review the potential use of naloxone and conclude that it is an inconsistent antidote to naloxone poisoning.—M.C. Rogers, M.D.

Positive Pleural Pressure Decreases Coronary Perfusion
Fessler HE, Brower RG, Wise R, Permutt S (Johns Hopkins Med Insts)
Am J Physiol 258:H814–H820, 1990   5–55

Maneuvers that increase pleural pressure raise pressure surrounding the heart (P_{SH}), and this may reduce left ventricular oxygen demand by increasing left ventricular afterload. However, coronary flow may also be directly impeded by positive P_{SH}. The effects of positive P_{SH} on coronary perfusion were assessed in an isolated canine heart-lung preparation with constant venous return, arterial pressure, and lung volume. Pressure surrounding the heart was raised in 10-mm Hg increments from 0 to 60 mm Hg.

Increased P_{SH} produced a rapid significant drop in left atrial transmural pressure (P_{LATM}) of up to a mean of 1.28 mm Hg. The decrease was interpreted as a reflection of reduced left ventricular afterload with constant venous return and lung volume. However, at P_{SH} levels of more than 30 mm Hg, initial drops in P_{LATM} were followed by sustained increases, which suggested deterioration in cardiac function despite the lower level of afterload. Increased P_{SH} was also associated with reductions in circumflex coronary artery flow. When the circumflex coronary artery was dilated maximally with adenosine, P_{SH} effects were amplified, suggesting that positive P_{SH} mechanically impeded coronary flow. The aortic-coronary sinus lactate concentration difference dropped from .71 to .1 mM when the P_{SH} was increased to 60 mm Hg for 90 seconds, suggesting myocardial ischemia.

When the P_{SH} was elevated at a constant cardiac output and arterial pressure, myocardial ischemia was produced. Thus, even in the absence of clinically apparent hemodynamic changes, increased pleural pressure may have unanticipated adverse effects on the balance of supply and demand for coronary perfusion.

▶ It is widely appreciated that diastolic blood pressure is the major upstream pressure in the coronary circulation, but there is considerable controversy regarding the determinants of downstream pressure. In the clinical arena the effects of various therapeutic interventions on coronary downstream pressure are not often considered. Fessler et al. have elegantly demonstrated that increases in intrathoracic pressure, i.e., positive end-expiratory pressure (PEEP), can result in decreased coronary blood flow, presumably by altering downstream pressure. As the authors point out, this effect on coronary blood flow was noted only when the intrathoracic pressure was very elevated. However, in patients with coronary artery lesions, PEEP-induced alterations in coronary perfusion pressure could precipitate myocardial ischemia. This study again highlights that PEEP is not without adverse effects, and optimal use of this therapeutic modality requires an in-depth appreciation of those potential problems.— M.J. Breslow, M.D.

Differential Regulation of Right and Left Ventricular β-Adrenergic Receptors in Newborn Lambs With Experimental Cyanotic Heart Disease
Bernstein D, Voss E, Huang S, Doshi R, Crane C, Peters R (Stanford Univ)
J Clin Invest 85:68–74, 1990   5–56

The sympathetic nervous system has a major role in cardiovascular adaptations to hypoxemia. Downregulation of the β-adrenergic receptor/adenylate cyclase system during chronic hypoxemia could contribute to declining myocardial performance and reserve. Myocardial β-adrenergic receptor regulation was studied in a newborn lamb model of cyanotic congenital heart disease. Hypoxemia was produced by gradually inflating a pulmonary arterial occluder balloon. An atrial septal defect was made, and oxygen saturation was lowered to between 65% and 74% for 2 weeks.

β-Receptor density decreased by 45% in the left ventricle during chronic hypoxemia but was unchanged in the right ventricle. Ligand affinity did not change in either ventricle. Isoproterenol-stimulated adenylate cyclase activity declined by 39% in the left ventricle and did not change in the right ventricle. Circulating epinephrine levels were increased fourfold; the myocardial norepinephrine concentration was unchanged.

Downregulation of the left ventricular β-adrenergic receptor/adenylate system was documented during chronic hypoxemia secondary to a right-to-left shunt in this newborn lamb model. Downregulation is associated with increased myocardial sympathetic stimulation mediated by circulating catecholamines. It may contribute to compromised left ventricular performance in patients with cyanotic congenital heart disease.

▶ Catecholamine-induced β-adrenergic receptor downregulation has been described in a variety of pathologic conditions associated with increased sympathetic nervous system activity. This study by Bernstein et al. documents a reduction in left ventricular β receptor number in lambs made chronically hypoxemic by creation of a right-to-left intracardiac shunt. Although no change in right ventricular β receptors was noted, chronic hypoxemia-induced downregulation may have offset the usual increase in receptor number seen with ventricular pressure overload. It is unclear, however, whether these changes in β receptor number are sufficient to affect ventricular function adversely, which was the original hypothesis of the investigators. This is an important question, because many clinical disease states are associated with high sympathetic activity and, probably, reduced β receptor number.—M.J. Breslow, M.D.

Cardiovascular Surgery

Circulatory Collapse Following Coronary Bypass Surgery: Multivessel and Graft Spasm Reversed in the Catheterization Laboratory by Intracoronary Papaverine
Gurley JC, Booth DC, Demaria AN (Univ of Kentucky)
Am Heart J 119:1194–1195, 1990   5–57

Sudden circulatory collapse shortly after successful coronary artery bypass grafting (CABG) is associated with high mortality because this complication is generally refractory to systemically administered drug therapy. Although coronary artery spasm has been suggested as an etiology, this diagnosis has rarely been demonstrated angiographically. One man with spasm was successfully treated with papaverine.

Man, 39, with disabling angina pectoris refractory to drug therapy underwent coronary arteriography, which revealed 3-vessel atherosclerotic disease, including subtotal occlusion of the right coronary artery. He underwent left internal mammary artery (LIMA) bypass grafting of the left anterior descending artery and saphenous vein grafting of the diagonal, circumflex marginal, and right coronary arteries. After his return to the surgical intensive care unit in stable condition, he suddenly went into cardiogenic shock with an ECG pattern of acute myocardial injury. The patient did not respond to intra-aortic balloon pumping and dopamine given intravenously. Intravenously administered nitroglycerin exacerbated the hypotension. Emergency coronary arteriography confirmed occlusive spasm of the LIMA, patency of all saphenous vein grafts, and severe diffuse spasm of all native coronary arteries. Papaverine in 10-mg bolus doses was administered directly into the LIMA and into each of the saphenous vein grafts via the angiographic catheters. Repeat arteriography showed a patent LIMA and the resolution of spasm in the native coronary arteries. There was marked hemodynamic improvement, and ECG abnormalities returned immediately toward baseline. Intravenous nitroglycerin and nasogastric nifedipine were administered subsequently. The patient's further postoperative recovery was uneventful.

Intracoronary papaverine may be useful in the treatment of coronary spasm in patients who experience hemodynamic collapse or acute myocardial infarction shortly after apparently successful CABG and are refractory to the intravenous administration of nitroglycerin.

▶ Papaverine is a vasodilator having potent effects on both epicardial conductance vessels as well as on resistance vessels. Although it has been used in the catheterization laboratory for patients with coronary artery disease, it is better known for its use in the treatment of acute mesenteric ischemia. This case represents its first use for diffuse spasm associated with cardiogenic shock after coronary artery bypass grafting. No doubt, the dramatic recovery this patient experienced will prompt others to examine this drug prospectively in patients with coronary artery spasm, as well as other vasospastic processes. The results of those studies will help us identify the most efficacious agent for acute coronary artery spasm.—A.C. Dixon, M.D., and J.E. Parrillo, M.D.

Acute Myocardial Dysfunction and Recovery: A Common Occurrence After Coronary Bypass Surgery
Breisblatt WM, Stein KL, Wolfe CJ, Follansbee WP, Capozzi J, Armitage JM, Hardesty RL (Univ of Pittsburgh)
J Am Coll Cardiol 15:1261–1269, 1990   5–58

Acute myocardial dysfunction is thought to be common in the early postoperative period after cardiopulmonary bypass operation, but its time course and frequency are not well defined. Twenty-four patients undergoing routine elective coronary bypass surgery underwent serial hemodynamic measurements and radionuclide evaluation of ventricular function before and after operation.

None of the patients sustained an intraoperative infarction, and there were no complications. In the immediate postoperative period 23 of the 24 patients had significant depression in the right and left ventricular ejection fractions, reaching a trough level at a mean of 262 minutes after operation. These findings were also associated with a depressed cardiac and left ventricular stroke work index, even though adequate ventricular filling pressures and mean arterial pressure were maintained.

The depression in ventricular function was partially reversible within 8–10 hours after operation, and complete recovery ensued within 48 hours. Depressed myocardial function was independent of bypass time, the number of grafts placed, preoperative medications, or postoperative core temperatures. The postoperative use of pressor or inotropic medications appeared to delay the timing of ventricular dysfunction but did not prevent its occurrence.

Left ventricular dysfunction in the early postoperative period continues to be common in patients undergoing coronary bypass procedures. The mechanism for this phenomenon is unclear, but reperfusion injury with oxygen free radicals has been suggested. The use of free radical scavengers to protect against this form of postoperative myocardial depression should be investigated.

▶ This study is helpful in that it defines the prevalence, time course, and extent of both the left and right ventricular dysfunction that is observed in postoperative coronary bypass surgery patients. Almost universal in this study, the ventricular depression appears to worsen progressively over the initial several hours after surgery and recovers slowly during the ensuing day.

Although the cardiac index remained within normal limits, a modest fall was observed that paralleled the fall in ejection fraction. Changes in ventricular volumes appeared to be the predominant cause of the reduction in ejection fraction. Whether the increase in ventricular compliance is related to myocardial edema, ischemic injury, a circulating myocardial depressant substance, or free oxygen radicals (as some have suggested) remains unknown. Additionally, the myocardial response of patients with a more complicated postoperative course remains to be further studied.—A.C. Dixon, M.D., and J.E. Parrillo, M.D.

First Human Use of the Hemopump, a Catheter-Mounted Ventricular Assist Device

Frazier OH, Wampler RK, Duncan JM, Dear WE, Macris MP, Parnis SM, Fuqua JM (Texas Heart Inst/St Luke's Episcopal Hosp, Houston; Nimbus Med Inc, Rancho Cordova, Calif)
Ann Thorac Surg 49:299–304, 1990   5–59

A previously developed left ventricular assist device had little success because its implantation required a major operative procedure. The Hemopump, a new device that can be implanted in minimal operative time, has had few complications associated with its use. Initial clinical data on use of the Hemopump in 7 patients were reviewed.

The study group included 5 men and 2 women (mean age, 59 years).

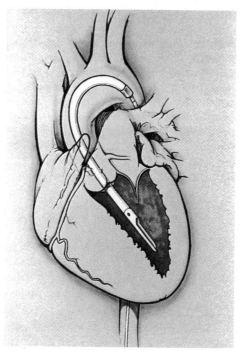

Fig 5–13.—The beveled, radiopaque tip of the inlet cannula facilitates placement across the aortic valve. (Courtesy of Frazier OH, Wampler RK, Duncan JM, et al: *Ann Thorac Surg* 49:299–304, 1990.)

All had multiple risk factors for early operative mortality; 5 patients could not be weaned from cardiopulmonary bypass and had no measurable cardiac output. The Hemopump was implanted in the left ventricle through the femoral artery in 4 patients and through the ascending aorta in 3. Operative time, including confirming the position of the pump by fluoroscopy, was approximately 15 minutes.

The catheter-mounted Hemopump has 3 basic elements: a disposable, intra-arterial axial-flow pump, a high-speed motor, and a control console. The inlet cannula is reinforced with a helical spring to prevent kinking and has a beveled radiopaque tip to ease its placement across the aortic valve (Fig 5–13). The Hemopump was used to support circulation for a mean of 66 hours.

Hemopump support immediately improved the hemodynamic status of all 7 patients. Inotropic drug therapy was reduced in 5 patients and afterload reduction therapy increased in 6. Five patients were alive for longer than 30 days after insertion of the Hemopump; 3 patients who were discharged from the hospital were alive and well at a follow-up of approximately 1 year.

▶ This report represents the first human experience obtained from the use of the Hemopump. If these clinical results are confirmed in larger trials, the Hemopump would be considered a significant technological advance in the care of the postoperative cardiovascular surgical patient who has pump failure. The ease and rapidity of insertion of the Hemopump comprise its most important advantage over previous ventricular assist devices, all of which need a thoracotomy for insertion. Perhaps this will lead clinicians to employ the Hemopump earlier in the course of cardiogenic shock, at a time when myocardial preservation can maximally benefit.

Despite these encouraging results, several problems with the device are evident from this report. Technical difficulties with the Hemopump itself occurred in a majority of patients. In 4 patients drive shaft fractures occurred, a problem that the authors state has prompted subsequent changes at the manufacturing level. In 2 patients the pump was unexpectedly ejected from the left ventricle, necessitating its remanipulation. Plasma free hemoglobins rose in most patients, leading one to be concerned about the development of renal failure. Lastly, although in this group of patients no clinical evidence of valvular or vascular injury was found, postmortem examinations in nonsurvivors are needed to better address this important issue.

These concerns will no doubt be addressed in the near future as clinical experience with the Hemopump broadens. Although its role in the failing postoperative cardiovascular surgical patient seems clear, the potential use of this device as a support while awaiting transplantation or in the management of cardiogenic shock from myocardial infarction remains to be defined.—A.C. Dixon, M.D., and J.E. Parrillo, M.D.

Arrhythmias

Suppression of Ventricular Arrhythmias in Man by *d*-Propranolol Independent of Beta-Adrenergic Receptor Blockade
Murray KT, Reilly C, Koshakji RP, Roden DM, Lineberry MD, Wood AJJ, Siddoway LA, Barbey JT, Woosley RL (Vanderbilt Univ)
J Clin Invest 85:836–842, 1990   5–60

Recent clinical studies have demonstrated that propranolol exerts electrophysiologic effects that are unrelated to its β-adrenergic receptor blocking action. Commercial propranolol is a racemic mixture of dextro- *(d)* and levo-rotatory *(l)* stereoisomers, with the *l*-isomer having far more potent β-adrenergic receptor blocking potential than the *d*-isomer.

The antiarrhythmic efficacy of *d*-propranolol was studied in 10 men aged 35–71 years with confirmed frequent ventricular ectopic depolarizations (VED) and nonsustained ventricular tachycardia (VT). After baseline data were obtained during an initial placebo phase, patients were given *d*-propranolol, 40 mg orally every 6 hours, with the dosage being increased every 2 days until suppression of arrhythmia, intolerable side effects, or a maximal dosage of 320 mg every 6 hours was reached.

Ventricular arrhythmias were completely suppressed in 6 patients and partially suppressed in 2 with *d*-propranolol dosages of 320–1,280 mg/ day. To determine whether the suppression of arrhythmia could be attributed to β-blockade, racemic propranolol was administered in dosages that produced the same or greater depression of the exercise heart rate.

Racemic propranolol did not suppress ventricular arrhythmias in 3 of the 8 patients in whom d-propranolol had been effective, indicating that d-propranolol exerted its antiarrhythmic effect by a non–β-adrenergic receptor-mediated action.

Propranolol suppresses ventricular arrhythmias by β-adrenergic and non–β-adrenergic receptor-mediated effects. The d-isomer of propranolol is also an effective antiarrhythmic agent that should be investigated further for use in patients who do not tolerate the β-adrenergic receptor blockade of racemic propranolol.

▶ The findings of Dr. Murray and colleagues that d-propranolol suppresses ventricular ectopy by β blockade and by another mechanism is interesting and provocative. Propranolol is normally given in racemic form (both d- and l-stereoisomers) with variable antiarrhythmic effects. The findings in the present study have implications for stereospecific antiarrhythmic effects of propranolol as well as other β blockers and antiarrhythmic drugs. This study suggests that there is a strong need to study the stereoisomers of these drugs further.—T.A. Buckingham, M.D., and J.E. Parrillo, M.D.

Signal-Averaged Electrocardiographic Late Potentials in Resuscitated Survivors of Out-of-Hospital Ventricular Fibrillation
Dolack GL, Callahan DB, Bardy GH, Greene HL (Univ of Washington)
Am J Cardiol 65:1102–1104, 1990   5–61

Recent reports suggest that the presence of late potentials on signal-averaged ECG in patients with ventricular fibrillation (VF) or ventricular tachycardia (VT) correlates with subsequent clinical arrhythmic events and inducibility during programmed electric stimulation. It has also been suggested that the electrophysiologic substrate in patients with VF differs from that in patients with clinical VT.

To compare the frequency of late potentials in patients with VF to that in patients with VT and correlate the findings with clinical and electrophysiological data, 25 patients with recurrent sustained VT and 46 survivors of out-of-hospital cardiac arrest secondary to documented VF were evaluated. After signal-averaged ECG all patients underwent electrophysiologic studies according to a standardized protocol. The end point of the study was completion of the protocol or induction of a sustained ventricular arrhythmia.

There were no significant differences between the 2 groups with regard to age, sex, presence of coronary artery disease, or ejection fraction. However, 80% of the patients with VT and 52% of those with VF had a myocardial infarction. This difference was statistically significant.

Twenty-one of the 25 patients with VT (83%) and 23 of the 46 patients with VF (50%) had late potentials on their signal-averaged ECG. Twenty-four patients with VT (96%) had inducible sustained VT on electrophysiologic study. However, sustained VT-VF was induced in only 27 patients with VF (59%). Ventricular fibrillation was induced in 24% of the patients with VF, but in none of the patients with VT. There was no significant association between the presence of late potentials and induced arrhythmias for either group of patients. Thus the inability of signal-averaged ECG to predict inducibility in patients with a history of out-of-hospital VF may constitute a significant limitation of this technique in identifying patients at risk for sudden cardiac death.

▶ This study showed a stronger correlation between late potential and inducible VT than inducible VF. Late potentials are caused by fragmentation and delay of the electrical impulse traveling through damaged myocardium, which may be closely related to areas of reentry. The results of this study, which are similar to those reported in a study published by our group in the *Journal of Electrophysiology* in 1988 (1), can be explained by the fact that VF is probably caused by mechanisms distinct from those causing VT.—T.A. Buckingham, M.D., and J.E. Parrillo, M.D.

Reference

1. Buckingham TA, et al: *J Electrophysiol* 2:424, 1988.

Effect of Empiric Antiarrhythmic Therapy in Resuscitated Out-of-Hospital Cardiac Arrest Victims With Coronary Artery Disease
Moosvi AR, Goldstein S, VanderBrug Medendorp S, Landis JR, Wolfe RA, Leighton R, Ritter G, Vasu CM, Acheson A (Henry Ford Hosp, Detroit; Univ of Michigan)
Am J Cardiol 65:1192–1197, 1990   5–62

In a previous outcome study of patients resuscitated after out-of-hospital cardiac arrest it was reported that a history of digoxin or quinidine therapy was the most significant clinical predictor of mortality. The increased mortality was thought to be either the result of adverse drug effects or the presence of heart failure. The effect of empiric therapy with antiarrhythmic drugs on survival in patients with coronary artery disease (CAD) who were resuscitated after out-of-hospital cardiac arrest was reviewed retrospectively.

From July 1975 through June 1982, 274 patients were successfully resuscitated after out-of-hospital cardiac arrest; 227 had significant CAD. Of 209 patients for whom complete data on drug therapy were available, 116 did not receive antiarrhythmic therapy; 45 were given procainamide, and 48 were treated with quinidine after hospital discharge. Digoxin therapy was initiated in 101 patients. Sudden death was defined as death within 1 hour of new or accelerating symptoms. Follow-up ranged from 6 to 93 months (average, 35 months).

The 2-year cumulative total survival rates were 61% for quinidine-treated patients, 57% for procainamide-treated patients, and 71% for those not treated with antiarrhythmic drugs. The 2-year sudden death survival rates were 69% for quinidine, 69% for procainamide, and 89% for no antiarrhythmic therapy. The effect of concomitant digoxin and antiarrhythmic drug therapy on total survival was not asociated with a statistically significant difference among the 3 treatment groups.

Empiric antiarrhythmic therapy with quinidine or procainamide failed to provide protection against sudden death in this group of high-risk survivors of out-of-hospital cardiac arrest. Patients who did not receive antiarrhythmic drug therapy fared better than treated patients with respect to sudden death.

▶ The value of this retrospective study is limited because the sudden death survivors were not randomized to antiarrhythmic drugs (procainamide or quinidine) or no therapy. However, the study is interesting in that it gives us a rough idea of the mortality rates and sudden death rates in sudden death survivors. These data failed to show a benefit of antiarrhythmic drugs used in an empiric fashion.—T.A. Buckingham, M.D., and J.E. Parrillo, M.D.

Surgical Coronary Revascularization in Survivors of Prehospital Cardiac Arrest: Its Effect on Inducible Ventricular Arrhythmias and Long-Term Survival
Kelly P, Ruskin JN, Vlahakes GJ, Buckley MJ Jr, Freeman CS, Garan H (Massachusetts Gen Hosp, Boston; Harvard Med School)
J Am Coll Cardiol 15:267–273, 1990   5–63

The effects of coronary revascularization on arrhythmia were ascertained in 50 survivors of cardiac arrest who were followed for a mean of 39 months after coronary artery bypass surgery. All underwent electrophysiologic testing with programmed ventricular stimulation. None had acute myocardial infarction at the time of cardiac arrest, but 24 had a history of infarction.

Preoperative assessment demonstrated inducible ventricular arrhythmia in 33 of the 41 patients tested (80%). Nineteen of 42 who were studied after operation when not receiving antiarrhythmic drugs had inducible arrhythmias. Thirty patients with inducible arrhythmias before operation had postoperative testing when not taking antiarrhythmic drugs and induction of arrhythmia was suppressed in 14. None of 11 patients with inducible ventricular fibrillation before operation exhibited it after revascularization, but inducible ventricular tachycardia persisted in 80% of cases.

Four patients had recurrent arrhythmia during follow-up and 1 of them died. Three nonsudden cardiac deaths occurred. Both depressed left ventricular function and advanced age predicted cardiac deaths.

Coronary revascularization abolishes inducible ventricular arrhythmia in some survivors of cardiac arrest, even when infarction does not occur at the time of arrest. Patients with inducible ventricular fibrillation whose ventricular function is well preserved are especially likely to do well after revascularization.

▶ Dr. Kelly and co-authors present interesting data on the effect of coronary revascularization on the results of electrophysiology studies. In particular, inducible ventricular fibrillation was eliminated by revascularization but not inducible ventricular tachycardia. This suggests that ischemia is important in the genesis of inducible ventricular fibrillation. The long-term follow-up suggests that specific treatment of ischemia in patients with inducible ventricular fibrillation may be beneficial and sufficient.— T.A. Buckingham, M.D., and J.E. Parrillo, M.D.

Adenosine for Paroxysmal Supraventricular Tachycardia: Dose Ranging and Comparison With Verapamil. Assessment in Placebo-Controlled, Multicenter Trials
DiMarco JP, Miles W, Akhtar M, Milstein S, Sharma AD, Platia E, McGovern B, Scheinman MM, Govier WC, and the Adenosine for PSVT Study Group
Ann Intern Med 113:104–110, 1990   5–64

Adenosine is an endogenous nucleoside that inhibits sinus node automaticity and depresses atrioventricular nodal conduction and refractoriness. Two prospective double-blind, placebo-controlled trials were conducted in a total of 359 patients with ECG findings of paroxysmal supraventricular tachycardia (PSVT) to compare the effects of adenosine with those of verapamil.

In the first study the effects of sequential intravenous boluses of 3, 6, 9, and 12 mg of adenosine were compared with the effects of equal amounts of saline. In the second study patients received 6 mg of adenosine (or 12 mg if needed) or 5 mg of verapamil (or 7.5 mg if needed).

Intravenous boluses of adenosine ended episodes of PSVT in 91% of the patients given the 12-mg dose. A maximum of 16% of patients responded to administration of placebo. In the second trial more than 90% responded to the maximum doses of both adenosine and verapamil. Thirty-six percent of patients had adverse effects from adenosine, but these were brief and usually mild. Various transient arrhythmias followed the termination of tachycardia in all groups.

Adenosine can terminate episodes of PSVT reliably when the atrioventricular node is an integral part of the reentrant circuit. Its overall effectiveness is similar to that of verapamil, but it acts more rapidly.

▶ The above study shows that the use of a rapid bolus injection of adenosine (6–12 mg) is effective in terminating more than 90% of episodes of PSVT. Side effects were brief and self-limited because of the extremely short half-life of this drug.— T.A. Buckingham, M.D., and J.E. Parrillo, M.D.

Prognosis of Late vs. Early Ventricular Fibrillation in Acute Myocardial Infarction

Jensen GVH, Torp-Pedersen C, Køber L, Steensgaard-Hansen F, Rasmussen YH, Berning J, Skagen K, Pedersen A (Glostrup County Hosp, Copenhagen)
Am J Cardiol 66:10–15, 1990   5–65

Ventricular fibrillation (VF) occurs in 10% to 15% of patients hospitalized for acute myocardial infarction (MI). The prognostic significance of VF is thought to depend on the time of occurrence (earlier or later than 48 hours after MI) and the absence (primary) or presence (secondary) of signs of heart failure. Early primary VF was assumed not to influence short- and long-term mortality, but study results have been contradictory. The length of the monitoring period after acute MI was extended to determine the importance of late VF.

During a 9-year period, 422 of 4,269 patients admitted with acute MI had an episode of in-hospital VF; 281 patients (68%) had early VF and 132 had late VF. The monitoring period was for 18 days. In-hospital mortality was similar in the 2 groups: 50% of those with early VF and 54% of those with late VF. Patients with early VF had a better survival after discharge, but this difference was explained by the presence of heart failure. When VF was not associated with heart failure, early and late VF had the same prognosis after 1, 3, and 5 years. Both heart failure and cardiogenic shock were significant risk factors for in-hospital death.

With long-term monitoring, there is no special risk for patients with late VF compared to patients with early VF after acute MI. Patients with late VF, especially when it is not associated with heart failure, will benefit from such long-term monitoring.

▶ This study is interesting because it contradicts the conventional teaching that VF occurring during the acute phase of an MI does not indicate a poor prognosis. This study suggests that VF in the postinfarction patient should always be taken as a serious prognostic sign.—T.A. Buckingham, M.D., and J.E. Parrillo, M.D.

Efficacy and Tolerance of High-Dose Intravenous Amiodarone for Recurrent, Refractory Ventricular Tachycardia
Mooss AN, Mohiuddin SM, Hee TT, Esterbrooks DJ, Hilleman DE, Rovang KS, Sketch MH Sr (Creighton Univ, Omaha)
Am J Cardiol 65:609–614, 1990   5–66

The necessity for a rapid antiarrhythmic effect in patients with life-threatening ventricular arrhythmias prompted a study of high-dose amiodarone intravenously administered to 35 such patients whose recurrent sustained ventricular tachycardia (VT) was resistant to conventional drugs. Twenty-three patients had coronary artery disease, and all but 4 patients had signs of overt heart failure. After withdrawing oral treatment, amiodarone was given in a loading dose of 5 mg/kg, followed by 20–30 mg/kg daily for 5 days. Added bolus doses of 150 mg were given if sustained VT recurred.

Overall, 63% of the patients responded to intravenously administered amiodarone. Ten of the 13 nonresponders died of arrhythmia. Thirteen patients continue to receive amiodarone orally after an average follow-up of 19 months. Six of them required hospitalization for recurrent sustained VT. Four short-term responders died suddenly out of hospital. Electrocardiographic changes during treatment were not predictive of the clinical response. Thirteen patients required a dose reduction or withdrawal of treatment because of side effects, most frequently hypotension.

Intravenously administered amiodarone effectively terminates recurrent, refractory VT in most patients. The present recommendation is for a bolus of 5 mg/kg given over 30 minutes, followed by infusion of 10–20 mg/kg daily for 3 days.

Intravenous Amiodarone for the Rapid Treatment of Life-Threatening Ventricular Arrhythmias in Critically Ill Patients With Coronary Artery Disease
Ochi RP, Goldenberg IF, Almquist A, Pritzker M, Milstein S, Pedersen W, Gobel FL, Benditt DG (Minneapolis Heart Inst; Univ of Minnesota)
Am J Cardiol 64:599–603, 1989   5–67

The effectiveness of intravenously administered amiodarone for rapid control and prevention of recurrent life-threatening ventricular arrhythmias associated with cardiovascular collapse was investigated in 22 critically ill patients with coronary artery disease. The mean ejection fraction was 27%. In these patients, recurrent ventricular tachyarrhythmias proved refractory to about 4 (range, 2–6) conventional antiarrhythmic drugs.

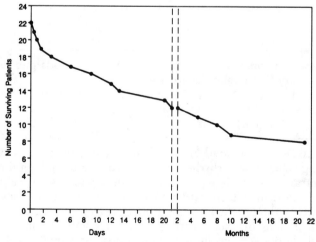

Fig 5–14.—Line graph shows patient mortality after intravenous amiodarone therapy over time measured initially in days and later in months. Twelve patients survived to hospital discharge. (Courtesy of Ochi RP, Goldenberg IF, Almquist A, et al: *Am J Cardiol* 64:599–603, 1989.)

In the 24 hours before intravenous amiodarone therapy, the patients had a mean of 2 (range, 1–9) episodes of life-threatening ventricular tachycardia, ventricular fibrillation, or both, that required 4 direct current (DC) cardioversions. All patients received a continuous infusion of amiodarone, 900–1,600 mg/day for about 4 days. Within 24 hours after initiation of amiodarone therapy, the 20 patients who remained alive had a mean of 1 episode of life-threatening ventricular arrhythmia that required a mean of 2 DC cardioversions. By the second day of amiodarone infusion, 19 patients remained alive and had .4–.7 episodes of life-threatening arrhythmias that required DC shocks. Overall, arrhythmias were controlled in 50% of the patients within 24 hours and in 64% within 48 hours of initiation of amiodarone infusion. At a mean follow-up of 22 months, 12 patients had been discharged from the hospital and 8 were alive (Fig 5–14). Adverse hemodynamic effects, including hypotension, did not occur during amiodarone infusion, although preexisting congestive heart failure worsened in 2 patients.

Intravenously administered amiodarone may be effective for the rapid control of spontaneous, refractory, life-threatening ventricular tachyarrhythmias in critically ill patients with coronary artery disease. The drug is well tolerated despite the severely depressed left ventricular function in these patients.

► Sustained ventricular tachycardia refractory to conventional antiarrhythmics can be life-threatening and is of concern to the critical care physician. There is a need for new, more effective, agents that can be administered intravenously. This study shows promise for the intravenous use of amiodarone in such patients. At the time of this writing, clinical studies are underway that may lead to the FDA approval of the intravenous form of amiodarone for such patients.— T.A. Buckingham, M.D., and J.E. Parrillo, M.D.

Heart Block as a Predictor of In-Hospital Death in Both Acute Inferior and Acute Anterior Myocardial Infarction
McDonald K, O'Sullivan JJ, Conroy RM, Robinson K, Mulcahy R (St Vincent's Hosp; Univ College Dublin)
Q J Med 74:277–282, 1990   5–68

Myocardial infarction (MI) can be complicated by atrioventricular block. The occurrence of block worsens the prognosis in both anterior and inferior wall infarction. The prognostic effect of atrioventricular block in acute anterior and inferior MI was assessed in 705 successive patients hospitalized with a first Q-wave MI of the anterior or inferior wall.

Second- or third-degree atrioventricular block developed in 8.6% of the patients, being more common in inferior than anterior infarctions. According to multiple logistic regression analysis, 3 factors were independently correlated with block: inferior infarction, older age, and larger infarct size as determined by cardiac enzymes. The death rate was 27.9%

in patients with block and 9.3% in those without block. It was significantly higher in both anterior and inferior infarction groups. Block was a significant independent prognostic factor when age, infarct size, infarct site, and block were analyzed simultaneously as predictors of death. The relative risk of death in patients with block was similar for anterior and inferior infarction. There was a higher incidence of unheralded death in inferior infarcts associated with high-degree block.

Atrioventricular block is an ominous predictor of death in inferior and anterior wall infarctions. Its effect is independent of infarct size. It appears to exert an adverse effect on survival even in smaller inferior infarctions. Patients with inferior infarction complicated by atrioventricular block are at a higher risk of dying suddenly.

▶ This study shows that the occurrence of second- or third-degree atrioventricular block after an acute MI was associated with a higher in-hospital mortality and sudden death rate. In this study, block was a predictor independent of other factors. Unfortunately, the mechanism of sudden death was not determined. In addition, it is not clear whether thrombolytic agents were used in this patient population and what role they may have played.—T.A. Buckingham, M.D., and J.E. Parrillo, M.D.

Association of Intravenous Erythromycin and Potentially Fatal Ventricular Tachycardia With Q-T Prolongation (Torsades de Pointes)
Schoenenberger RA, Haefeli WE, Weiss P, Ritz RF (Univ Hosp, Basle, Switzerland)
Br Med J 300:1375–1376, 1990   5–69

Treatment with erythromycin can be complicated by ventricular arrhythmias. Potentially life-threatening ventricular arrhythmias were associated with prolongation of the Q-T interval induced by erythromycin in 1 patient.

Woman, 61, was hospitalized with fever, pneumonia, and severe respiratory distress. She had long-standing pulmonary hypertension secondary to pulmonary embolism. The ECG demonstrated sinus tachycardia, right atrial hypertrophy, and a normal rate-corrected Q-T interval. Ceftriaxone and erythromycin lactobionate treatment was begun. During the fifth erythromycin infusion, pronounced prolongation of the Q-T interval, multiform ventricular extrasystoles, and an episode of nonsustained torsades de points were noted. In the eighth and tenth infusions there was an increase in Q-T_c intervals, with a gradual return to normal over the next 5–6 hours. Torsades de pointes occurred again with maximal prolongation of the Q-T_c interval. Therapy was changed to ciprofloxacin, and no further arrhythmia occurred. The patient was discharged 3 weeks later.

Rapid injections of erythromycin should be avoided to minimize the danger of toxic plasma concentrations. Close Q-T_c and rhythm monitoring should be considered for patients at risk. Patients with impaired hepatic drug metabolism or preexisting cardiac disease may need a smaller dose or an alternative antibiotic.

▶ The authors present a reasonably well-documented case of erythromycin-induced torsades de pointes. Erythromycin, particularly in intravenous form, must be added to the long list of drugs already known to cause torsades. Caution should be used when giving this drug to patients with underlying heart disease.—T.A. Buckingham, M.D., and J.E. Parrillo, M.D.

Implications of Sustained Monomorphic Ventricular Tachycardia Associated With Myocardial Injury

Woelfel A, Wohns DHW, Foster JR (Univ of North Carolina)
Ann Intern Med 112:141–143, 1990   5–70

Patients with sustained monomorphic ventricular tachycardia occasionally have elevated serum levels of creatine kinase that are indicative of myocardial injury. However, the implications of this finding with regard to subsequent susceptibility to ventricular tachycardia and the need for chronic antiarrhythmic therapy are uncertain.

Twelve men with sustained monomorphic ventricular tachycardia and elevated total serum levels of creatine kinase and MB isoenzyme fraction were studied retrospectively. All had a history of myocardial infarction and left ventricular dysfunction, and 4 patients had previous arrhythmias. Presenting ventricular tachycardia lasted from 30 minutes to 12 hours, and the rate ranged from 145 to 210 beats per minute.

Sinus rhythm was restored by electric countershock in 10 patients and by intravenously administered lidocaine or procainamide in 2. Serial ECGs after conversion showed no new Q waves in any patient. Two patients had transient ST segment depression after cardioversion. The highest total serum level of creatine kinase was 8.83 μkat/L and the overall mean peak level of creatine kinase was 4.85 μkat/L, with a mean MB fraction of .12. Peak elevation of the enzyme occurred 4–10 hours after admission. All 12 patients eventually had electrophysiologic studies to guide the selection of antiarrhythmic therapy; however, testing was delayed in 5 of the 8 patients who had no previous episodes of ventricular tachycardia. These patients were tested only after experiencing subsequent episodes 5–15 months later. After testing, 11 patients received drug therapy and 1 had surgery. During a mean follow-up of 37 months 1 patient had another episode of sustained ventricular tachycardia and 2 died suddenly.

Management of patients with previous myocardial infarction who present with sustained monomorphic ventricular tachycardia should not be based on the detection of myocardial injury by enzyme elevation alone. These patients are at high risk for recurrent episodes of ventricular tachycardia and should receive definitive, prolonged antiarrhythmic therapy.

▶ The authors note that sustained ventricular tachycardia associated with a cardiac enzyme rise has some clinical significance as ventricular tachycardia without an enzyme rise. This suggests that acute ischemia and injury are not important precipitating factors for sustained ventricular tachycardia not occurring the setting of a clear acute myocardial infarction. Management should be the same for sustained ventricular tachycardia regardless of an accompanying (usually mild) enzyme rise.—T.A. Buckingham, M.D., and J.E. Parrillo, M.D.

Miscellaneous

Renal and Hemodynamic Effects of Intravenous Fenoldopam Versus Nitroprusside in Severe Hypertension
Elliott WJ, Weber RR, Nelson KS, Oliner CM, Fumo MT, Gretler DD, McCray GR, Murphy MB (Univ of Chicago)
Circulation 81:970–977, 1990   5–71

Nitroprusside is preferred for the acute reduction of blood pressure in hypertensive emergencies because of its rapid onset of action and long history of efficacy. However, nitroprusside can cause deterioration in renal function. Fenoldopam mesylate is a novel dopamine-1 receptor agonist that lowers blood pressure while enhancing renal blood flow. To compare the renal and hemodynamic effects of fenoldopam and nitroprusside administered intravenously in the treatment of hypertensive emergencies, studies were made in 18 men and 10 women (average age, 49 years) whose average blood pressure was 219/137 mm Hg. Twenty-six patients were black. All patients were thought to have acute target organ damage caused by severe hypertension and were admitted to the intensive care unit.

During the open-label part of the trial, 5 patients received fenoldopam

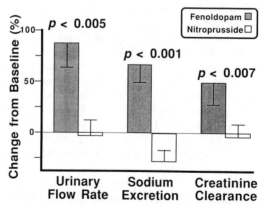

Fig 5–15.—Bar graphs of relative effects of infusion of fenoldopam or nitroprusside on renal parameters, measured for each patient as percent change from baseline (before infusion) and then averaged. Error bars represent standard errors; statistics were generated by nonpaired t test. (Courtesy of Elliott WJ, Weber RR, Nelson KS, et al: *Circulation* 81:970–977, 1990.)

and 6 were given nitroprusside. The remaining 17 patients were randomized between the 2 treatment drugs according to a predetermined schedule. Thirteen patients received fenoldopam and 15 were treated with nitroprusside.

Both fenoldopam and nitroprusside lowered blood pressure safely to an average of 176/105 mm Hg for at least 1 hour during drug infusion at a constant dose. A small increase in heart rate was seen with both drugs. There was a clear dose-response relationship between blood pressure and drug dose. Renal function parameters, including urinary flow, sodium excretion, and creatinine clearance, increased significantly in fenoldopam-treated patients but decreased nonsignificantly in nitroprusside-treated patients (Fig 5–15). A direct comparison of the 2 treatment groups revealed that the percentage change in each of these parameters was significantly greater in fenoldopam-treated patients.

Fenoldopam and nitroprusside are both effective in the treatment of severe hypertension. The beneficial effect on renal function when fenoldopam is used appears to be an advantage over the use of nitroprusside.

▶ This study is of particular interest because black patients constitute a small minority of subjects previously studied under treatment with fenoldopam. Dopamine-1 agonists may be playing an increasing role in the armamentarium of antihypertensive agents, especially in light of their effects in maintaining or increasing sodium and water excretion. Blacks appear to have reduced salt and water excretion rates, independent of the degree of renal dysfunction (1). Although hypertension is coming under more pharmacologic control than previously, hypertensive crisis is still not uncommon in the emergency rooms. The key to effective therapy is minute to minute blood pressure control by the intravenous infusion of agents such as nitroprusside, labetalol, or fenoldopam to insure that precipitous hypotension does not develop. Of equal importance is the smooth transition to oral therapy to maintain adequate blood pressure regulation. This dopamine-1 agonist may become a preferred agent for treating severely hypertensive patients with significant renal dysfunction.—P.R. Liebson, M.D., and J.E. Parrillo, M.D.

Reference

1. Gillum RF: *Hypertension* 1:468, 1979.

Clinical Predictors of Myocardial Damage After High Voltage Electrical Injury
Chandra NC, Siu CO, Munster AM (Johns Hopkins Med Insts)
Crit Care Med 18:293–297, 1990   5–72

Patients with electrical burns from high-voltage sources may also have sustained myocardial damage. Because the clinical presentation of myocardial damage is variable and patients rarely have typical ischemic chest discomfort or other cardiac symptoms, the diagnosis of myocardial injury is often missed initially. To identify early clinical predictors of myocardial damage in high-voltage electrical injury, 24 patients so injured were studied over a 32-month period.

None of the patients had evidence of arc burns. The voltage they had been exposed to was verified from industrial sources. Wounds of exit and entrance were entered on a standard burn diagram to identify the pathway of injury. To assess myocardial damage, 3 serial ECGs were obtained daily on each patient. Blood samples for the measurement of total creatine kinase (CK) and its MB isoenzyme (CK-MB) were drawn on admission and every 8 hours for 24 hours thereafter. If these were elevated, measurement continued daily until CK normalized. None of the patients had a history of myocardial ischemia.

The total CK concentration in 13 patients ranged from 1,373 to 52,544 mU/mL and all were MB positive, indicating myocardial damage. Ten of these 13 had changes on ECG. The other 11 patients also had evidence of CK elevation with ranges from 227 to 640 mU/mL, but all were MB negative, indicating the absence of myocardial damage. Four of these 11 patients had changes on ECG.

The pathways of electricity through the body were vertical in all 13 patients with myocardial damage but were vertical in only 5 of the 11 without myocardial damage. The mean percent of body surface burns was 16% in patients with confirmed myocardial damage and 4% in those without, a statistically significant difference. Thus the presence of a vertical pathway of injury and the magnitude of body surface burns are significant clinical predictors of myocardial damage in patients who sustain high-voltage electrical injuries.

▶ Electrical injury is an occasional cause of sudden cardiac death. Frequently, cardiac resuscitation at the time of electrical injury can be successful, providing that defibrillation capabilities are available. There are 3 broad categories of electrical injury: lightning and distribution lines of power companies, both more than 7,000 volts, and household circuitry, where individuals electrocuted usually become part of a ground circuit, a potential of 120 volts. Low-voltage electrocution can be as low as 30 volts, provided that skin resistance is decreased by moisture, for example. A low-voltage shock may not produce ventricular fibrillation but can cause loss of skeletal muscle control, which, for example, could paralyze a person swimming and lead to drowning.

Burn marks from electrocution are fairly punctate, well circumscribed, and frequently subtle. Physiologic conditions that may lower the threshold to ventricular fibrillation include adrenergic stimulation and acidosis.—P.R. Liebson, M.D., and J.E. Parrillo, M.D.

Acute Myocardiotoxicity During 5-Fluorouracil Therapy
Misset B, Escudier B, Leclercq B, Rivara D, Rougier Ph, Nitenberg G (Inst G Roussy, Villejuif, France)
Intensive Care Med 16:210–211, 1990   5–73

The incidence of myocardial ischemia as a complication of 5-fluorouracil (5-FU) chemotherapy is 1.2%. One man had acute reversible cardiac failure without coronary ischemia that was associated with 5-FU monotherapy.

Man, 38, with no evidence of coronary artery disease, underwent rectosigmoid resection for adenocarcinoma. Because of peritoneal metastases, chemotherapy with 5-FU was given intravenously and intraperitoneally by continuous infusion. On the fourth day of chemotherapy the patient became dyspneic and hypotensive. A chest radiograph showed cardiac enlargement with pleural effusion and infiltrates in the right lower lobe. The next day 5-FU was discontinued and the patient was transferred to the intensive care unit. Right-sided catheterization of the heart revealed a pulmonary wedge pressure of 37 mm Hg with a cardiac index of 2.3 L/min/m². Two-dimensional echocardiography showed a slightly dilated and diffusely hypokinetic left ventricle. There was no increase in cardiac enzymes, and infarction did not occur. Dobutamine and furosemide given intravenously rapidly improve the patient's clinical and hemodynamic status. All symptoms resolved after 8 days of drug therapy. Because of the severity of cardiogenic shock, rechallenge was not attempted.

Previous experimental studies have suggested that this adverse effect could be caused by accumulation of 5-FU in the myocardium, leading to depletion of high-energy phosphate compounds. The metabolic and clinical changes seen in these studies were all reversible. Thus the myocardiotoxicity that occurs in some patients who undergo 5-FU chemotherapy may represent a direct effect of 5-FU on myocardial cells.

► This report underscores the rapidity with which myocardial dysfunction can occur even in a younger individual treated with cytotoxic drugs. Of note is the role of echocardiography in demonstrating noninvasively the selective structural and functional abnormalities of the cardiac chambers. Although inotropes and diuretics are effective in sustaining left ventricular function, angiotensin-converting enzyme inhibitors are also useful by decreasing peripheral vascular resistance in situations in which the left ventricle is globally hypokinetic and dilated. Although left ventricular dysfunction was associated with overt symptomatology in this individual, clinical manifestations after chronic administration of chemotherapy may be more subtle, requiring periodic monitoring of left ventricular function, especially with chronic administration of anthracycline derivatives. This report also underscores the ability of 5-FU to produce myocardial toxic effects in addition to the better known cardiotoxic anthracycline derivatives. Echocardiography or gated blood pool scans are useful for periodic ventricular function monitoring.—P.R. Liebson, M.D., and J.E. Parrillo, M.D.

Hemodynamics During PEEP Ventilation in Patients With Severe Left Ventricular Failure Studied by Transesophageal Echocardiography
Schuster S, Erbel R, Weilemann LS, Lu W, Henkel B, Wellek S, Schinzel H, Meyer J (Univ School of Medicine, Mainz, Germany)
Chest 97:1181–1189, 1990   5–74

Although positive end-expiratory pressure (PEEP) ventilation benefits the lungs, the cardiac index and systemic oxygen transport are lowered. The effects of PEEP ventilation on hemodynamics and ventricular function were examined in 5 patients with normal cardiopulmonary function and 11 with severe left ventricular failure. The latter patients required ventilation after myocardial infarction. Transesophageal echocardiography was performed during administration of PEEP at levels up to 16 cm water.

In both groups of patients the end-diastolic area of the right atrium decreased significantly with PEEP ventilation and right atrial pressure increased. The cardiac index declined in both groups in relation to decreased right ventricular filling volume. Positive end-expiratory pressure ventilation with 8–10 cm of water did not impair left ventricular function further in patients with congestive heart failure. The decrease in cardiac index was caused by a decrease in stroke index.

Ventilation with PEEP can enhance left ventricular performance in patients with a dilated left ventricle and pulmonary congestion. Careful hemodynamic monitoring is necessary when levels of more than 8 cm of water are used. Lower levels of PEEP have minimal hemodynamic effects.

▶ This intriguing study demonstrated that PEEP produces effects on the right and left heart different from what we might expect, i.e., the right heart volume is decreased but the left heart volume is sustained, the later primarily by blood pooling from the lungs. The rapidity of such shifts, and the opposite effect after discontinuance of PEEP, are reasons for special vigilance to underlying pressure/volume relationships of the heart in candidates for PEEP. Although 2-dimensional echocardiography can be useful in such evaluations, transthoracic echocardiography is frequently suboptimal in such patients. Transesophageal echocardiography (TEE), especially when biplane probes become generally available, will allow evaluation of chamber volumes and provide valuable focal information in selected patients. Under these circumstances, however, TEE requires special skills by the operator. Passage of the endoscopic probe is made easier by temporary deflation of the endotracheal tube balloon. Reproducibility of the TEE echocardiographic volumes requires meticulous technique.—P.R. Liebson, M.D., and J.E. Parrillo, M.D.

Differing Responses in Right and Left Ventricular Filling, Loading, and Volumes During Positive End-Expiratory Pressure
Schulman DS, Biondi JW, Matthay RA, Zaret BL, Soufer R (Yale Univ; West Haven VA Med Ctr, New Haven, Conn)
Am J Cardiol 64:772–777, 1989   5–75

Twenty patients on mechanical ventilation who required positive end-expiratory pressure (PEEP) underwent studies of ventricular function. Multisystem disease was frequent. Thirteen patients met the criteria for adult respiratory distress syndrome.

Seven patients had a rise in left ventricular (LV) end-diastolic volume when PEEP was administered (group 1), and 13 (group 2) had a fall in LV end-diastolic volume. The group 1 patients more often had coronary artery disease, and they had a lower cardiac output, LV and right ventricular (RV) ejection fractions, and peak filling rate compared with the group 2 patients. Ventricular volumes increased as the peak filling rate declined in group 1 patients given PEEP. In group 2 patients, LV volume decreased, whereas RV volume and peak filling rate were unchanged. Changes in the peak filling rate on PEEP correlated inversely with changes in RV end-diastolic volume.

Volume infusion is not appropriate for all patients who have a fall in cardiac output on PEEP. Ventricular performance should be monitored during PEEP in patients who have biventricular dysfunction at baseline or a history of coronary artery disease and congestive heart failure. Such patients may appropriately receive arterial vasodilators, nitrates, or inotropic agents as adjunctive measures.

▶ The effect of PEEP on LV performance is complex. Although in most instances PEEP results in preload reduction, in other instances it results in depressed myocardial systolic and diastolic performance. The purpose of this study was to identify which subset of mechanically ventilated patients requiring PEEP would manifest deterioration in LV function. This is of interest because, when the clinical application of PEEP results in diminished cardiac output, it would be helpful to discern whether the deterioration was attributable to preload reduction or to worsening myocardial performance. The latter scenario would not be expected to improve with volume expansion, whereas the former would.

The authors found that patients with depressed baseline biventricular function (reduced RV and LV ejection fractions) responded to PEEP with increased LV volume, decreased LV ejection, and worsening LV filling. This set of patients had a higher frequency of coronary artery disease and previous heart failure than did the set of patients who responded to PEEP with decreased LV volume and no change in LV ejection or filling rate. The authors postulate that LV function deteriorated in the former set of patients because of PEEP-induced myocardial ischemia. If cardiac output falls in response to PEEP, the authors suggest that these patients would be better managed by administration of vasodilators or inotropes rather than by conventional treatment with volume expansion. The results of their study would seem to support the recommendation. To identify which patients would fall into which of the 2 groups, it is necessary to consider the patients' cardiac history; baseline indices of LV and RV function would also be needed.—J.T. Barron, M.D., Ph.D., and J.E. Parrillo, M.D.

Comparative Effects of Verapamil and Nitroprusside on Left Ventricular Function in Patients With Hypertension
Brush JE Jr, Udelson JE, Bacharach SL, Cannon RO III, Leon MB, Rumble TF, Bonow RO (Natl Heart, Lung, and Blood Inst, Bethesda, Md)
J Am Coll Cardiol 14:515–522, 1989   5–76

Congestive heart failure is a common complication of chronic systemic hypertension. Left ventricular (LV) systolic dysfunction is usually the underlying cause, but LV diastolic dysfunction also occurs in systemic hypertension, and frank congestive heart failure may develop in the presence of preserved systolic function. Calcium-channel antagonists can improve LV function in several cardiac disorders. Their effect on LV function in systemic hypertension was examined using verapamil and nitroprusside in 10 patients aged 43–62 years with symptomatic systemic hypertension. All had symptoms of angina pectoris but no coronary artery disease.

The patients underwent cardiac catheterization with simultaneous radionuclide angiography and micromanometer pressure measurements to assess LV pressure-volume relationships. Nitroprusside and verapamil were administered sequentially and titrated to achieve a 20% reduction in mean arterial pressure to allow direct comparison of drug effects on cardiac function at matched mean arterial pressures and heart rates.

At equihypotensive doses, verapamil and nitroprusside had markedly different effects on LV function. Nitroprusside caused a significant decrease in cardiac index and stroke volume index related to a significant decrease in the LV end-diastolic volume index but did not alter systemic arterial resistance. Thus nitroprusside mainly reduced the LV preload. Verapamil caused a negative inotropic effect as confirmed by a downward and rightward shift in the pressure-volume relationship in 8 of the 10 patients. However, peripheral vasodilation and apparent improvement in LV filling balanced the negative inotropic effects, and cardiac index and stroke volume index were maintained during verapamil infusion.

The primary hypotensive effect of verapamil is a decrease in systemic vascular resistance. The primary hypotensive effect of nitroprusside is a decrease in cardiac index resulting from a reduction in LV preload.

▶ When blood pressure must be decreased rapidly, such as in hypertensive emergencies, the diastolic volume of the LV must be maintained to assure that hypotension does not develop. This study indicates that, although nitroprusside is useful intravenously for lowering blood pressure, it may lead to marked decreases in LV end-diastolic volume (LVEDV) when the initial LV diameter is small, especially in elderly patients with hypertrophic small LVs (1). Documentation of the LV dimension at baseline before antihypertensive therapy can be achieved simply with 2-dimensional echocardiography. The study also demonstrates that calcium-channel blockers can be useful in maintaining LVEDV. β-Blockers also tend to maintain LVEDV by slowing the heart rate and by minimally changing or increasing the peripheral vascular resistance. Diuretics and vasodilators, including α blockers, tend to decrease LVEDV. These considerations are important in both acute and more chronic therapy of hypertension.—P.R. Liebson, M.D., and J.E. Parrillo, M.D.

Reference

1. Topol EJ, et al: *N Engl J Med* 312:277, 1985.

Acute Epstein-Barr Virus Myocarditis Simulating Myocardial Infarction With Cardiogenic Shock

Tyson AA Jr, Hackshaw BT, Kutcher MA (Bowman Gray School of Medicine, Winston-Salem, NC)

South Med J 82:1184–1187, 1989   5–77

Acute Epstein-Barr virus myocarditis may mimic acute myocardial infarction (MI). A patient was seen with Epstein-Barr virus myocarditis that closely resembled acute MI complicated by cardiogenic shock.

Woman, 38, was admitted for emergency cardiac catheterization after complaining of substernal chest pain, shortness of breath, and near syncope. Additional history revealed that the patient and her family had had a viral syndrome of sore throat, fever, and cough during the week preceding her cardiac decompensation. Electrocardiographic findings were consistent with a diagnosis of acute MI (Fig 5–16). The chest radiograph was normal. Baseline laboratory data were within the normal range except for an elevated leukocyte count. Cardiac catheterization revealed no pathologic changes of the coronary artery, but severe global hypokinesia was seen on the left ventriculogram. Endomyocardial biopsy revealed myocytic degeneration and mononuclear cell infiltration consistent with acute viral myocarditis. Viral serology studies confirmed a recent Epstein-Barr virus infection.

▶ Myocarditis may be a subtle diagnosis in a patient presenting with findings suggesting an infarction. A clue to possible diagnosis is global left ventricular hypokinesis and dilatation seen on echocardiographic study or nuclear ventriculography in a patient who has a possible MI with no history of previous infarction. If cardiogenic shock is present, as was the case with this presentation, cardiac catheterization will usually be performed and the diagnosis of coronary artery disease ruled out. Although there is a possibility of infarction caused by

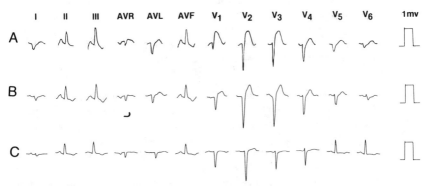

Fig 5–16.—**A**, at presentation on January 7, ECG 1986 revealed prominent anterior ST segment elevation and pathologic Q waves; **B**, on January 11, 1986, ECG revealed slightly lowered anterior ST segments with persistent Q waves; **C**, later on January 11, 1986, ECG revealed total resolution of anterior ST segment elevation with substantial improvement in anterolateral R wave voltage. (Courtesy of Tyson AA Jr, Hackshaw BT, Kutcher MA: *South Med J* 82:1184–1187, 1989.)

small-vessel coronary artery disease not apparent on coronary angiograhy, an endomyocardial biopsy and titers for common viral pathogens (e.g., Epstein-Barr virus, coxsackie virus) that can produce acute myocarditis must be considered.—P.R. Liebson, M.D., and J.E. Parrillo, M.D.

Effect of Flosequinan in Patients With Acute-Onset Heart Failure Complicating Acute Myocardial Infarction
Schneeweiss A, Wynne RD, Marmor A (Geriatric Cardiology Research Found, Geneva, Tel Aviv, Israel; Boots Co PLC, Nottingham, England; Zive Med Ctr, Safed, Israel)
Crit Care Med 17:879–881, 1989   5–78

Flosequinan is a synthetic direct-acting vasodilator having a balanced effect on the venous and arterial vascular beds. Flosequinan is indicated for patients with severe heart failure complicating acute myocardial infarction (MI) resistant to conventional drug therapy.

The drug trial was done in 8 men and 2 women (mean age, 64 years) hospitalized with severe acute-onset heart failure complicating MI that had not responded to high intravenous doses of furosemide, nitroglycerin, or isosorbide mononitrate or dinitrate. Eight patients had also received dobutamine, which had not improved their condition. Hemodynamic parameters were monitored by a pulmonary artery thermodilution catheter from the onset of heart failure. After a mean of 3.8 days of unsuccessful conventional therapy, a single 100-mg dose of flosequinan was administered orally. Hemodynamic measurements were obtained every hour for 4 hours after administration of flosequinan. No other changes in any other drug doses were made during the 4-hour evaluation.

Nine patients survived and 1 died of cardiac shock 4 days after the single flosequinan dose. However, the death was not considered treatment related. Flosequinan was well tolerated, and symptomatic hypotension, cardiac arrhythmias, or other adverse drug effects did not occur. Hemodynamic improvement peaked within 1–2 hours after administration of flosequinan and remained at this level at 4 hours.

▶ This study indicates that dramatic hemodynamic improvement in patients with heart failure complicating acute MI can be achieved by the administration of a single oral dose of flosequinan. What is surprising is that this benefit was achieved in patients with heart failure refractory to appropriate therapy with intravenous nitroglycerin and intravenous dobutamine. Larger, better-controlled trials studying the benefits of this new agent are needed to evaluate its role more precisely in the management of acute heart failure. It will also be of interest to determine whether it is effective in the long-term management of chronic congestive heart failure.—J.T. Barron, M.D., Ph.D., and J.E. Parrillo, M.D.

Acute Preload Effects of Furosemide

Krasus PA, Lipman J, Becker PJ (Baragwanath Hosp; Univ of Witwatersrand, Johannesburg, South Africa)
Chest 98:124–128, 1990   5–79

Furosemide has been thought to induce rapid diuresis in patients with pulmonary vascular congestion, thereby reducing plasma volume and pulmonary capillary pressure. A number of studies, however, have suggested other mechanisms for the drug's effect. It was proposed that bolus doses of intravenously administered furosemide initially increase pulmonary capillary wedge pressure (PCWP). To determine the acute PCWP effects of an intravenously administered bolus dose of furosemide, 33 patients in an intensive care unit were studied.

Most of the patients were in acute left ventricular failure (LVF) after myocardial infarction or chronic LVF caused by cardiomyopathy, or had adult respiratory distress syndrome. The patients were divided into 3 groups according to their use of vasodilator drugs at the time of study. The dose of furosemide was 20 mg with a PCWP of 20 mm Hg or less, and 40 mg with a PCWP of 21–25 mm Hg. After administration of the drug, PCWP was measured every 5 minutes for the next hour.

There were 12 patients in group 1 (furosemide only), 10 in group 2 (furosemide plus preload reduction), and 11 in group 3 (furosemide plus preload and afterload reduction). In group 3 patients an immediate and sustained drop in PCWP occurred after administration of furosemide. In the other 2 groups there was an initial increase in PCWP up until 15 minutes, followed by a diuresis-induced decrease in PCWP below baseline levels at 1 hour.

These trends were independent of underlying pathology or the dose of furosemide used. To prevent an increase in PCWP before onset of furosemide-induced diuresis, the concomitant use of a "mixed" vasodilator is recommended. Pre- and afterload reducing agents may eliminate the initial and possibly adverse effects of furosemide.

▶ It is to be noted, even though furosemide administered alone (without preload or afterload reduction) initially caused a rise in mean PCWP, the magnitude of this increase (.7 mm Hg from baseline) was trivial and, in our opinion, not of clinical import. What is of interest in this study is the purported mechanism for this small and transient rise in PCWP with the bolus administration of furosemide. The authors postulate that furosemide administration causes a deleterious release of endogenous vasoconstrictors that results in acute elevation of ventricular preload and afterload. Francis et al. (1) were the first to expound the hypothesis that furosemide results in activation of the neurohumoral axis, including the renin-angiotensin system. If correct, this may explain why congestive heart failure patients taking furosemide are particularly prone to hypotension when an angiotensin-converting enzyme inhibitor is administered.—J.T. Barron, M.D., Ph.D., and J.E. Parrillo, M.D.

Reference

1. Francis GS, et al: *Ann Intern Med* 103:1, 1985.

Effects of Endothelin on the Coronary Vascular Bed in Open-Chest Dogs
Clozel J-P, Clozel M (F Hoffmann-La Roche & Co, Basel, Switzerland)
Circ Res 65:1193–1200, 1989   5–80

Endothelin is a peptide that is the most potent vasoconstrictor known. Its effects on the coronary vascular bed by intracoronary injection were examined in open-chest anesthetized dogs. The circumflex coronary artery was perfused at a constant pressure of 100 mm Hg. Coronary flow distribution was measured using radioactive microspheres.

Endothelin decreased coronary blood flow by 30% at a dose of 1 μg, and by 61% at a dose of 3 μg; a 10-μg dose was lethal. Flow decreased more in the subepicardium that in the subendocardial region. The circumflex arterial surface area decreased by 20% with the 3-μg dose of endothelin. α-Adrenergic blockade, serotonergic blockade, angiotensin-converting enzyme inhibition, and cyclooxygenase inhibition all failed to modify the effects of endothelin.

Endothelin produces dose-related coronary vasoconstriction in dogs, occurring preferentially in the subepicardial region. It is possible that, when arterial thrombus or plaque rupture injures the coronary artery wall, endothelin secretion is induced, leading to coronary vasospasm.

▶ Since its discovery in 1988, our understanding of the physiologic and potential pathophysiologic role of endogenously produced endothelin has advanced significantly. Elevated circulating levels of endothelin have been found in many disease states, including essential hypertension, unstable angina, acute myocardial infarction, congestive heart failure, acute or dialysis-dependent chronic renal failure, and endotoxic shock. Most exciting from a therapeutic standpoint, monoclonal antibodies to endothelin-1 have been found to limit infarction size in a left coronary artery ligation model of acute myocardial infarction in rats (1).

This study by Clozel et al., although using doses of endothelin much higher than the levels found in human disease, demonstrates the very potent effect of endothelin on coronary artery resistance and flow in dogs. It is interesting to hypothesize, as the authors have done, that disruption of the coronary endothelium by activated platelets or atherosclerotic plaque rupture leads to the production and local release of endothelin. This would then constrict the underlying vascular smooth muscle, causing a diminution of flow, with resultant thrombosis and the development of an acute ischemic syndrome. One can anticipate that, with the current level of interest in this peptide, we will soon know whether this hypothesis holds true.—A.C. Dixon, M.D., and J.E. Parrillo, M.D.

Reference

1. Watanabe T, et al: *Nature* 344:114, 1990.

Cardiac Tamponade Associated With Drug-Induced Systemic Lupus Erythematosus

Mohindra SK, Udeani GO, Abrahamson D (South Chicago Community Hosp, Chicago)
Crit Care Med 17:961–962, 1989   5–81

Cardiac tamponade developed as the initial symptom of procainamide-induced systemic lupus.

Woman, 45, had worsening shortness of breath for 6 weeks and low-grade fever for 2 weeks, as well as joint and muscle pains. She had a history of ventricular arrhythmias and had received procainamide for 3 years, along with phenytoin for a seizure disorder, and indomethacin and aspirin for osteoarthritis. Her blood pressure was 70/58 mm Hg with 12 mm Hg of pulses paradoxus. Significant venous distention was present, along with pitting edema. The patient was in severe metabolic and respiratory acidosis, and she was placed on a ventilator. An echocardiogram showed a large pericardial effusion and classic signs of tamponade. The patient was given hydrocortisone intravenously and underwent pericardiocentesis. Peripheral perfusion improved rapidly, with correction of the acidosis. The pericardial effusion was markedly reduced in size and a study performed 6 months later showed no effusion.

Cardiac tamponade is a rare presentation of drug-induced lupus. Management includes rapid decompression and administration of high-dose steroids. It is important to maintain adequate intravascular volume. When drug-induced lupus is suspected, it is best to withdraw the offending drug.

▶ Pericarditis and pericardial effusions are frequent findings in patients with primary systemic lupus erythematosus (SLE), occurring in about 20% to 30% of patients. Cardiac tamponade develops only rarely as a result of SLE-induced pericardial effusion. In one series of 150 primary SLE cases, 29 patients had pericarditis and in 2 of these tamponade developed. Procainamide causes a lupus-like syndrome in about 30% of patients receiving this drug on a long-term basis. This is the first report of procainamide-induced SLE leading to cardiac tamponade. When this occurs, the authors recommend pericardiocentesis, corticosteroid administration, and immediate discontinuation of the drug.—J.T. Barron, M.D., Ph.D., and J.E. Parrillo, M.D.

Recognition of Cardiac Tamponade in the Presence of Severe Pulmonary Hypertension

Frey MJ, Berko B, Palevsky H, Hirshfeld JW Jr, Herrmann HC (Hosp of the Univ of Pennsylvania)
Ann Intern Med 111:615–617, 1989   5–82

Patients with pulmonary hypertension typically have increased systemic venous pressure with dyspnea. Consequently, it may be difficult to recognize cardiac tamponade.

Woman, 44, had primary pulmonary hypertension for 1 year; increased peripheral edema and progressive dyspnea recently developed. Her blood pressure was 120/60 mm Hg without paradox. The jugular venous pressure was 12 cm water. The patient had a tender, enlarged liver, distal cyanosis, and marked pitting ankle edema. Echocardiography showed a markedly hypertrophied, dilated, hypokinetic right ventricle and abnormal septal motion suggesting right ventricular (RV) pressure overload. A large pericardial effusion also was noted. The posterior left ventricular (LV) wall collapsed in diastole. The RV pressure was 110/28 mm Hg and the intrapericardial pressure was 12 mm Hg, exceeding the LV end-diastolic pressure. Removal of 350 mL of pericardial fluid decreased the LV end-diastolic pressure from 10 mm Hg to 5 mm Hg. Cardiac output increased from 2.3 L/min to 2.8 L/min. Left ventricular wall motion became normal.

Intrapericardial pressure exceeded the LV diastolic pressure in this patient, explaining the echocardiographic finding of isolated LV diastolic collapse. The presence of severely increased right-sided cardiac pressure precluded typical clinical and echocardiographic signs of cardiac tamponade.

▶ This case report is curious because it describes an echocardiographic sign of cardiac tamponade that ordinarily applies to motion of the right ventricle. Collapse of the right ventricle is seen as inward motion of the RV free wall toward the interventricular septum during diastole. Under normal circumstances, the free wall should move away from the septum as blood fills the right ventricle, distending it. The right ventricle collapses during diastole in tamponade when intrapericardial pressure exceeds the RV end-diastolic pressure. The left ventricle does not undergo collapse because the elevated intrapericardial pressure is not as easily transmitted across the much thicker-walled ventricle. In the present case, the right ventricle was markedly hypertrophied and dilated secondary to pulmonary hypertension. The end-diastolic pressure was 28 mm Hg. It is likely that, in this patient, the left ventricle was more compressible than the right.—J.T. Barron, M.D., Ph.D., and J.E. Parrillo, M.D.

Two-Dimensional Echocardiography and Doppler Color Flow Mapping in the Diagnosis and Prognosis of Ventricular Septal Rupture
Helmcke F, Mahan EF III, Nanda NC, Jain SP, Soto B, Kirklin JK, Pacifico AD
(Univ of Alabama, Birmingham)
Circulation 81:1775–1783, 1990   5–83

Rupture of the interventricular septum after acute myocardial infarction (MI) is life-threatening. Early and accurate diagnosis is essential for successful treatment. Doppler color flow mapping was used in conjunction with 2-dimensional echocardiography to assess ventricular septal rupture (VSR) after acute MI and to correlate these findings with cardiac catheterization and surgical or autopsy data.

Fifteen patients, 7 with anterior and 8 with inferior acute MI, were studied. Turbulent flow traversing the ventricular septum was used to diagnose VSR. Color M-mode and conventional Doppler techniques determined the direction and velocity of shunt flow.

Doppler color flow mapping correctly defined the site of septal rupture in all cases. Rupture occurred at areas of discordant septal wall motion or "hinge points." Death occurred in all 3 patients with moderate tricuspid regurgitation and 3 of 4 patients with right-to-left shunting during diastole. All had an elevated right ventricular end-diastolic pressure. The right ventricular wall motion index was significantly increased in the patients who died compared with survivors. However, there was no difference in left ventricular wall motion index. Rupture size measured by Doppler color flow imaging correlated with the size determined during surgery or autopsy and the pulmonic-to-systemic shunt flow ratio by cardiac catheterization. Color-guided continuous-wave Doppler estimates of right ventricular systolic pressure and cardiac catheterization measurements were correlated.

Two-dimensional echocardiography combined with Doppler color flow mapping is useful for assessing ventricular septal rupture. The latter method permits rapid, accurate detection and characterization of VSR and its differentiation from mitral regurgitation. These methods also permit assessment of right ventricular dysfunction, tricuspid regurgitation, and shunt direction, which seems to be important prognostic indicators.

▶ Rapid decompensation of cardiac function can occur in the acute MI period with VSR, papillary muscle rupture with acute mitral regurgitation, or rupture of the free wall of the left ventricle, the latter causing rapid hemodynamic compromise and (if untreated) early mortality but sometimes producing an acute pseudoaneurysm. All of these conditions require early surgery. As shown in this study, diagnosis and prognosis can be obtained rapidly by 2-dimensional echocardiography in correlation with Doppler color flow mapping. Especially in complex acute ventricular septal defect, or pseudoaneurysm, transesophageal echocardiography is a useful diagnostic adjunct.—P.R. Liebson, M.D., and J.E. Parrillo, M.D.

Treatment of 150 Cases of Life-Threatening Digitalis Intoxication With Digoxin-Specific Fab Antibody Fragments: Final Report of a Multicenter Study
Antman EM, Wenger TL, Butler VR Jr, Haber E, Smith TW (Brigham and Women's Hosp, Boston; Burroughs Wellcome Co, Research Triangle Park, NC; Columbia Univ; Massachusetts Gen Hosp, Boston)
Circulation 81:1744–1752, 1990   5–84

Advanced digitalis intoxication can be fatal, especially in patients who have underlying cardiac dysfunction or have ingested massive doses. A multicenter clinical trial was undertaken using purified digoxin-specific Fab fragments in 150 patients with potentially life-threatening digitalis toxicity. The Fab fragments were purified from immunoglobulin G produced in sheep. The dose given was equal to the amount of digoxin or digitoxin in the patient's body. Patients ranged in age from only a few hours to 94 years.

Fifty percent of the patients were receiving long-term digitalis treatment, 10% had taken a large overdose accidentally, and 39% had suicidal intent. Of the 148 assessable patients, 80% had resolution of all signs and symptoms, 10% improved, and 10% had no response. The median time to initial response was 19 minutes after termination of the Fab infusion. Most of the patients (75%) had some evidence of a response within 60 minutes.

Fourteen patients had adverse events that may have been related to Fab treatment. The most common events were rapid development of hypokalemia and exacerbation of congestive heart failure. There were no allergic reactions. Fifty-four percent of the patients who had cardiac arrest as a manifestation of digitalis toxicity survived hospitalization. The reasons for partial and no responses were underlying heart disease that was the true cause of some of the presumed manifestations of suspected digitalis toxicity, too low a Fab dose, and treatment of patients who were already moribund.

A treatment response can be expected in 90% or more of patients with solid evidence of advanced and potentially life-threatening digitalis toxicity. This trial supports the theoretical advantages of using Fab fragments instead of whole antibodies in human beings.

▶ Of note in this study is evidence that digoxin-specific Fab fragments may be useful in digitoxin toxicity as well, that hypokalemia following such intervention should be guarded against, and that reinstitution of digitalis preparations within at least 7 days is usually unnecessary. Purified digoxin-specific Fab fragments (Digibind) have been available commercially in the United States since 1986. A postmarketing surveillance study of more than 700 additional patients should provide further insight into the use of Fab fragments for digitalis toxicity.—P.R. Liebson, M.D., and J.E. Parrillo, M.D.

Relation Between Extent of Left Ventricular Hypertrophy and Occurrence of Sudden Cardiac Death in Hypertrophic Cardiomyopathy
Spirito P, Maron BJ (Natl Heart, Lung, and Blood Inst, Bethesda, Md)
J Am Coll Cardiol 15:1521–1526, 1990   5–85

Sudden unexpected death can be the first clinical manifestation of hypertrophic cardiomyopathy. Left ventricular hypertrophy may be an important determinant of many clinical features of hypertrophic cardiomyopathy, but the relationship between its magnitude and the occurrence of sudden cardiac death is not well understood. The magnitude of hypertrophy was assessed in 29 asymptomatic or mildly symptomatic patients with hypertrophic cardiomyopathy who subsequently died suddenly or had cardiac arrest with documented ventricular fibrillation. The findings on 2-dimensional echocardiography in this group were compared with those in a group of 95 surviving patients of similar age and symptomatic state.

Maximal left ventricular wall thickness was significantly greater in the patients who died suddenly than in controls. The left ventricular wall thickness index, a quantitative expression of the overall extent of hypertrophy, was also greater in those who died suddenly. Marked and diffuse hypertrophy was 8 times more common in patients who died suddenly than in the controls. The prevalence of mild and localized hypertrophy was similar in the 2 groups. However, of the 4 patients with mild hypertrophy who died suddenly, only 1 was an adult; 3 were preadolescents whose hypertrophy would have been considered more substantial had it been corrected for body surface area.

Most asymptomatic or mildly symptomatic patients with hypertrophic cardiomyopathy who died suddenly have marked and diffuse left ventricular hypertrophy. There is a relationship between the extent of hypertrophy and the occurrence of sudden and unexpected death in this disease. Sudden cardiac death is not common in asymptomatic or mildly symptomatic adults with hypertrophic cardiomyopathy and relatively mild left ventricular hypertrophy.

▶ The importance of this study is the implication that asymptomatic or mildly symptomatic young individuals may be at risk for sudden death based on a subclinical finding, i.e., evidence of left ventricular wall thickening, diagnosed by meticulous 2-dimensional echocardiographic measurement techniques. Clearly, echocardiography is not a screening procedure in a supposedly healthy individual. How would such a diagnosis with its ominous prognostic implications be considered? Electrocardiographic evidence for left ventricular hypertrophy would be suggestive, as would an ejection systolic murmur, S_4 gallop at the apex, an early systolic ejection click best heard at the base, and a double systolic apical impulse. Should significant left ventricular hypertrophy be found in a nonhypertensive individual without valvular heart disease and a small cardiac chamber, fitting the picture of hypertrophic cardiomyopathy, it is possible that β blockers may be protective against life-threatening arrhythmias and at least alleviate some of the nonspecific symptoms. Unfortunately, presently there is no evidence that any pharmacologic intervention can decrease sudden death from hypertrophic cardiomyopathy.—P.R. Liebson, M.D., and J.E. Parrillo, M.D.

Mechanism of Cocaine-Induced Myocardial Depression in Dogs
Fraker TD Jr, Temesy-Armos PN, Brewster PS, Wilkerson RD (Med College of Ohio, Toledo)
Circulation 81:1012–1016, 1990   5–86

Numerous clinical reports of cardiovascular toxicity in humans suggest that cocaine depresses myocardial function. To determine whether the observed myocardial depression occurs secondary to myocardial ischemia, or is attributable to a direct myocardial depressant action of cocaine, studies were made in 14 dogs. The animals were anesthetized with intravenously administered sodium pentobarbital and instrumented with arterial and venous catheters and a Doppler blood flow transducer on the left circumflex coronary artery. Two weeks later, heart rate, blood pressure, coronary blood flow, and the regional left ventricular ejection fraction (LVEF) were measured at baseline and 1, 2, 5, and 10 minutes after intravenous cocaine infusion at doses of 4 mg/kg.

The dogs were left fully conscious during cocaine infusion. However, to minimize the effects of cocaine on myocardial oxygen demand, a subset of 6 dogs from the original 14 was studied a second time 1 week later after receiving the same dose of cocaine while sedated with pentobarbital. Two-dimensional echocardiographic images were recorded continuously on videotape throughout each experiment. All dogs tolerated the experiments without incident.

Mean blood pressure, heart rate, coronary blood flow, and rate-pressure product increased significantly after cocaine treatment in conscious dogs. However, with the exception of coronary blood flow, these parameters did not change significantly in the sedated dogs. After cocaine treatment, the mean regional LVEF in conscious dogs was depressed by 50% at 1 minute, 35% at 2 minutes, and 21% at 5 minutes. By 10 minutes after cocaine treatment, the regional LVEF had recovered to a level not significantly different from baseline values. In sedated dogs, the mean regional LVEF was depressed by 44% at 1 minute and 36% at 2 minutes after cocaine treatment. Thus the effect of cocaine on regional LVEF was remarkably similar in both conscious and sedated dogs. Cocaine causes myocardial depression, and myocardial depression after cocaine administration is not related to an increase in myocardial oxygen consumption. Rather, it is consistent with a direct myocardial depressant action.

▶ Although the results of this study suggest that cocaine depresses myocardial function by a direct toxic effect on the myocardium, it is important to keep in mind that cocaine can also provoke coronary artery vasospasm. Myocardial infarction associated with cocaine use has been reported, and vasospasm induced by cocaine has been demonstrated.—J.T. Barron, M.D., Ph.D., and J.E. Parrillo, M.D.

Outcome of 290 Patients With Aortic Dissection: A 12-Year Multicentre Experience
Chirillo F, Marchiori MC, Andriolo L, Razzolini R, Mazzucco A, Gallucci V, Chioin R (Universita' di Padova, Padova, Italy)
Eur Heart J 11:311–319, 1990   5–87

There are at least 2,000 new cases of spontaneous aortic dissection per year in the United States. The availability of more accurate diagnostic methods and the refinement of surgical procedures have dramatically changed the prognosis in these patients. The clinical, hemodynamic, and

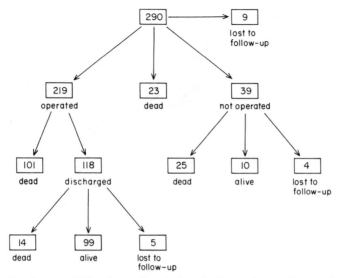

Fig 5–17.—Outcome of 290 patients with aortic dissection diagnosed over a 12-year period. (Courtesy of Chirillo F, Marchiori MC, Andriolo L, et al: *Eur Heart J* 11:311–319, 1990.)

angiographic data collected by questionnaire from 11 catheterization laboratories in northern Italy were studied retrospectively.

During a 12-year study period, 290 patients had an angiographic diagnosis of aortic dissection, including 217 (mean age, 55 years) who had dissection involving the ascending aorta and 73 (mean age, 61 years) who had distal dissection. Emergency catheterization was performed in 199 patients and elective aortography in 91. Shock, tamponade, acute myocardial infarction, renal failure, or heart failure was present in 68 of the 199 patients who underwent emergency aortography and 11 of the 91 patients who had elective catheterization.

Of 290 patients, 9 were lost to follow-up, 23 died before any therapy could be given, 39 were not operated on, and 219 underwent emergency operation (Fig 5–17). Of 219 patients operated on, 101 died within 30 days and 118 were discharged alive. Fourteen of the latter group died subsequently, 5 were lost to follow-up, and 99 were still alive. Ten of the nonsurgical patients were still alive, 25 died, and 4 were lost to follow-up. Only 2 of the 39 patients not operated on were referred for medical treatment; the other 37 did not have surgery because of their overall poor condition. Most survivors were symptom free, but all were monitored at regular intervals and took drugs to control hypertension and reduce inotropism.

During the 12-year period there was a significant increase in the number of diagnosed cases, a significant increase in the number of operations, and a significant decline in operative mortality. Acute myocardial infarction, persistent shock, and persistent CNS deficit were significant independent predictors of operative mortality in patients with dissection involving the ascending aorta. Persistent shock was the only independent predictor of operative mortality in those with distal aortic dissection. The overall late mortality related to aortic dissection in patients who underwent surgical treatment was 8.8%.

▶ This is a comprehensive description of the outcome of recognized aortic dissection. The authors subclassified patients into Stanford types A and B. Type A dissections involve the ascending aorta regardless of the site of the primary intimal tear and extent of distal propagation, whereas type B dissections involve the descending aorta only. Unfortunately, they identified the preoperative risks factors affecting mortality for types A and B but did not give data on the perioperative mortality of the 2 types. They also did not distinguish between acute and chronic dissections because they believe that such a classification is arbitrary and frequently difficult to assess. It is unfortunate that some attempt at this distinction was not made because more information is needed on the natural course of dissections not operated on, especially type B.—J.T. Barron, M.D., Ph.D., and J.E. Parrillo, M.D.

6 Neurologic Disease

A Randomized, Controlled Trial of Methylprednisolone or Naloxone in the Treatment of Acute Spinal Cord Injury: Results of the Second National Acute Spinal Cord Injury Study
Bracken MB, Shepard MJ, Collins WF, Holford TR, Young W, Baskin DS, Eisenberg HM, Flamm E, Leo-Summers L, Maroon J, Marshall LF, Perot PL Jr, Piepmeier J, Sonntag VKH, Wagner FC, Wilberger JE, Winn HR (Natl Acute Spinal Cord Injury Study, Yale Univ)
N Engl J Med 322:1405–1411, 1990   6–1

There is evidence from animal studies that methylprednisolone and naloxone both may be beneficial in the management of acute spinal cord injury, but their clinical efficacy remains uncertain. In a multicenter double-blind, placebo-controlled study, 487 patients with acute cord injury were studied; 95% of them were treated within 14 hours of injury. Methylprednisolone was given in a bolus dose of 30 mg/kg, followed by an infusion of 5.4 mg/kg/hr for 23 hours. Naloxone was given in a bolus dose of 5.4 mg/kg, followed by 4 mg/kg/hr for 23 hours. Half of the study patients had spinal fracture-dislocation.

By 6 months, patients given methylprednisolone within 8 hours of injury had improved significantly, compared with those given placebo. Motor function, pinprick sensation, and touch sensation were all improved. Both patients with neurologically complete lesions and others with incomplete lesions improved with steroid administration. Patients treated later and those given naloxone had an outcome similar to that of placebo patients. Major morbidity and mortality were similar in all groups.

Methylprednisolone, but not naloxone, may improve the neurologic outcome when given in the first hours after acute spinal cord injury. The steroid may act by suppressing breakdown of membrane through inhibiting lipid peroxidation and hydrolysis at the injury site. When lipid peroxidation is inhibited, the vasoreactive products of arachidonic acid metabolism are reduced, improving blood flow at the site of injury.

▶ The efficacy of steroids in neural injury has been debated and studied for 2 decades. This clinical study was well organized from a scientific perspective, and those patients who received steroids but not naloxone had a better outcome. The complexity of control of oxygen and substrate delivery to neural tissue makes determination of the mechanism difficult to delineate. Durg-produced hemodynamic improvement at critical times during the injury process might be statistically small or insignificant but physiologically important. Because the entire sequence of injury is as yet unclear, clinical investigators are unable to focus investigative efforts sufficiently to detect those small but important drug effects.— R.W. McPherson, M.D.

Anemia in Acute Phase of Spinal Cord Injury

Huang C-T, DeVivo MJ, Stover SL (Univ of Alabama, Birmingham)
Arch Phys Med Rehabil 71:3–7, 1990   6–2

Anemia is a frequent medical complication of multiple trauma, even without detectable blood loss. The incidence and clinical characteristics of anemia were investigated in 28 patients the first weeks after spinal cord injury. The patients, whose mean age was 32 years, had injuries from the C3 to C7 level. All but 4 had neurologically complete cord lesions. No patient had a personal or family history of hematologic disorders.

More than 80% of the patients had a subnormal red blood cell mass and one fourth had subnormal serum erythropoietin levels. The blood volume was below normal in 9%, and about the same proportion had low reticulocyte counts. The hemoglobin and hematocrit were below normal in more than two thirds of the patients. Low total iron-binding capacity was the rule. The serum transferrin level was depressed in nearly 80%. Most patients had a normochromic, normocytic anemia, but 14% had microcytic changes. Many nutritional abnormalities were noted, most frequently a low serum albumin concentration.

The red blood cell mass is substantially lowered in most patients with cord injury, but erythropoiesis usually is normal. Packed cells may be preferable to whole blood, and overhydration should be avoided. Possible factors in this anemia include nutritional deficiencies, endocrine changes, immune system changes that alter marrow cell maturation, and the effects of stress.

▶ The authors describe the hematologic profiles and nutritional status up to 45 days after cervical cord injury. The authors found that normochromic, normocytic anemia was frequent in patients following spinal cord injury, even though the process of erythropoiesis usually did not appear altered. The etiology of the anemia appears to be multifactorial and includes nutritional deficiencies and possible changes in the endocrine and immune systems. No patient required blood transfusion. Because of their findings, the authors suggest that transfusion with red blood cells rather than with whole blood is most appropriate when the anemia becomes too severe. They also suggest that overhydration should be avoided. However, it should be remembered that most patients with cervical cord injury are young and can tolerate relatively severe anemia. A major issue in this group of patients is how to decide when the risks of severe anemia outweigh the risks associated with blood transfusion. In addition, overhydration is frequently used as an important means of blood pressure support after acute injury.—J.R. Kirsch, M.D.

Polyneuropathy: Potential Cause of Difficult Weaning

Coronel B, Mercatello A, Couturier J-C, Durand P-G, Holzapfell L, Blanc P-L, Robert D (Hôp de la Croix-Rousse, Lyon, France; Hôp Edouard Herriot, Lyon)
Crit Care Med 18::486–489, 1990   6–3

Critical illness polyneuropathy (CIP) is a new neurologic syndrome that may occur as a complication of sepsis and multiple organ failure in patients on respiratory support systems. These peripheral motor neuropathies have dramatically increased nursing time, the duration of artificial ventilation, weaning, and the need for physiotherapy.

Between 1981 and 1987, 12 men and 3 women aged 20–76 years had CIP while they were in the intensive care unit and receiving respiratory support. The mean duration of ventilation was 77 days, and the mean duration of weaning was 22 days. Clinical signs included weakness, predominantly of the lower legs. Patients could not move easily or stand up. Thirteen patients had decreased muscle mass. Deep tendon reflexes were absent in 7 patients, normal in 7, and hyperactive in 1. Two patients had dysesthesia. Electromyograms (EMGs), obtained at various times during hospitalization, showed fibrillations in the distal muscles of both legs in 12 patients and only on the right side in 3 patients. Motor nerve conduction velocities were near normal or normal.

Long-term clinical and EMG follow-up data were available for 4 patients. At 4–8 years after hospitalization, amyotrophy had disappeared in 3 of the 4 patients. Two patients still had dysesthesia. One patient needed assistance to sit and walk. Recovery was delayed and incomplete in all 4 patients.

Critically ill polyneuropathy is a new disease that occurs in patients with sepsis and multiorgan failure and requires respiratory support. It can be diagnosed early in the course by EMG. A specific mechanism to explain CIP has not yet been identified.

▶ When CIP was described almost a decade ago, many intensivists doubted that they had ever seen a case. This report adds 15 more patients to an increasngly large and now unquestionable collection of victims. The pathogenesis of this syndrome is not known; the patients seem to share only the need for prolonged mechanical ventilation. No other risk factor appears to be shared among the reported cases or those that we have seen. The electrophysiologic disturbances are indicative of damage to the lower motor neurons or their axons. There is no evidence of demyelination.

The disorder itself appears to be reversible, in that all patients who have survived the underlying disorder appear to have been weaned successfully. A predilection for motor nerves is unexplained. Perhaps a comparable disorder of autonomic nerves may explain some cases of intractable hypotension.—T.P. Bleck, M.D., and J.E. Parrillo, M.D.

Intracranial Hemorrhage After Use of Tissue Plasminogen Activator for Coronary Thrombolysis

Kase CS, O'Neal AM, Fisher M, Girgis GN, Ordia JI (Boston Univ; Univ of Massachusetts, Worcester; Waltham-Weston Hosp, Mass)
Ann Intern Med 112:17–21, 1990   6–4

Six patients—none of them hypertensive when admitted—had intracranial hemorrhage after receiving tissue plasminogen activator (t-PA) for thrombolysis. Three patients were from a center where 60 patients received t-PA in a 1-year period.

Woman, 67, previously treated for hypertension, had an inferior myocardial infarct diagnosed. After normal coagulation values were documented, the patient was given 6 mg of t-PA 4 hours after onset of chest pain and a total of 100 mg over 6 hours. An intravenous bolus of 5,000 units of heparin was given, followed by an infusion of 1,000 units per hour. The heparin dose was reduced when a partial thromboplastin time (PTT) of 81 seconds was found. Dysarthric speech and right hemiparesis were seen 8 hours after the start of t-PA treatment. The highest blood pressure had been 164/100 mm Hg. Computed tomography showed several areas of intracerebral hemorrhage. Blood was evacuated at craniotomy; no vascular malformation was seen. The patient was left with moderate spastic hemiparesis.

Up to one third of the patients given t-PA have hemorrhagic complications, usually bleeding at vascular accession sites. All of the present patients bled after receiving a full dose of 100 mg of t-PA. All had an excessively prolonged PTT. Hemorrhages predominated in the subcortical white matter of the hemispheres, as in anticoagulant-related intracerebral hemorrhage. No patient had received aspirin before or after t-PA. The combined use of t-PA and heparin may raise the risk of intracerebral bleeding.

▶ The authors summarize the clinical details of 6 patients who sustained intracranial hemorrhage as a consequence of t-PA and heparin therapy, which was administered for thrombolysis after acute myocardial infarction. We are left to assume that none of these patients had a history of strike, which would have contraindicated the administration of t-PA. In each case, the PTT after heparin administration was well beyond the therapeutic range, raising the question that the heparin, rather than the t-PA, was responsible for the hemorrhages. Most of the hemorrhages in these 6 patients were in locations that would be uncommon for hemorrhages related to chronic hypertension. Bleeding in these locations usually is a consequence of an underlying vascular or neoplastic lesion, or a bleeding diathesis. As the authors suggest, the loading dose of heparin used may have contributed to the hemorrhagic tendency.

Currently, t-PA is in phase II trials as an agent for the treatment of thrombotic stroke. In this trial, it is not followed by heparin. In a pilot study, 10% of patients had an intracerebral hemorrhage. Most of these patients were treated more than 2 hours after onset of symptoms. Thus it is unlikely that intracerebral hemorrhage occurred in the patients reported by Kase et al. so a result of undetected cerebral emboli. Although the complications documented in this report suggest that following t-PA with heparin may not be wise, we do not believe it argues against the use of t-PA in either acute myocardial infarction or acute cerebral infarction. Studies with t-PA in the latter condition remain quite preliminary, thus the drug should not be used outside of a study protocol.—
T.P. Bleck, M.D., and J.E. Parrillo, M.D.

Measured Energy Expenditure in Severe Head Trauma
Moore R, Najarian MP, Konvolinka CW (Conemaugh Valley Mem Hosp, Johnstown, Pa; Temple Univ)
J Trauma 29:1633–1636, 1989   6–5

The Harris-Benedict equation for estimating basal energy expenditure is commonly used to calculate energy requirements in severely injured patients who require parenteral nutrition. Caloric requirements can also be calculated by indirect calorimetry that involves measuring oxygen consumption and carbon dioxide production. A retrospective review was done to determine the energy requirements of patients with severe closed head injury, using both the Harris-Benedict equation and indirect calorimetry.

The study population consisted of 20 patients aged 3–67 years (mean, 29 years) who had been admitted with Glasgow Coma Scale scores of 7 or less and required initial mechanical ventilation. All 20 patients had major closed head injury with only minor associated injuries. A metabolic profile to assess resting energy expenditure was recorded within 48 hours of admission, after which enteral feeding was initiated.

The measured oxygen consumption was on average 166% of predicted values, and it was at least 112% of the predicted value in all patients. The measured resting energy expenditure was 160% of values predicted by the Harris-Benedict equation, with no value less than 112% (Fig 6–1). Only 2 patients had received a short course of steroids, but their hypermetabolic response did not differ significantly from that in the other 18 patients.

Patients with severe head trauma are physiologically in an early hypermetabolic state. Critically ill patients receiving inappropriate calories

Measured Versus Predicted Energy Expenditure

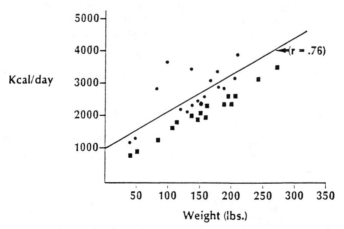

Fig 6–1.— Measured vs. predicted resting energy expenditure: *circles* represent measured via indirect calorimetry, *squares* represent predicted via Harris-Benedict equation. (Courtesy of Moore R, Najarian MP, Konvolinka CW: *J Trauma* 29:1633–1636, 1989.)

have serious sequelae. Resting energy expenditure values derived from the Harris-Benedict equation are grossly inaccurate, thus their use may lead to inadequate nutritional support. The use of indirect calorimetry in severely head-injured patients provides an accurate alternative approach to the management of the caloric needs of these patients.

▶ The metabolic requirements of critically ill patients have been a source of investigation for more than 20 years. Many critically ill patients have displayed a hypermetabolic state, and these authors demonstrate exactly the same thing in patients with severe head injury.—M.C. Rogers, M.D.

Dexamethasone Treatment for Bacterial Meningitis in Children and Adults
Girgis NI, Farid Z, Mikhail IA, Farrag I, Sultan Y, Kilpatrick ME (Abbassia Fever Hosp, United States Naval Med Research Unit; Egyptian Ministry of Health, Cairo)
Pediatr Infect Dis J 8:848–851, 1989   6–6

Dexamethasone may have value in addition to standard antibacterial therapy in patients with bacterial meningitis. In this open prospective study, 429 patients having organisms isolated from the CSF or present on a gram-stained smear of CSF were assigned to receive either ampicillin and chloramphenicol alone, or antibacterial therapy with dexamethasone added (table). Steroid was given twice daily for 3 days in a dose of 8 mg to children younger than age 12 years and 12 mg to adults.

The case fatality rate was significantly less in patients with pneumococcal meningitis who received dexamethasone. Overall neurologic sequelae, including hearing impairment and paresis, were less frequent in patients given dexamethasone, but the effect was significant only for those with *Streptococcus pneumoniae* meningitis. None of 45 survivors given steroid had hearing loss, but 4 of 32 who did not receive dexamethasone had severe hearing loss. Steroid therapy did not alter the time to defervescence or to return of consciousness, the CSF leukocyte count, or the CSF

Cerebrospinal Fluid Findings on Hospital Admission and After 24–36 Hours of Therapy

CSF Finding	Dexamethasone and Antibiotics		Antibiotics Only	
	Admission	24–36 hours	Admission	24–36 hours
Leukocytes (cells/mm³)	24 000 ± 15 200*	3180 ± 2800	20 500 ± 17 300	4100 ± 3200
Glucose (mg/dl)	12.5 ± 10.1	22.2 ± 17.1	18.2 ± 14.3	35.3 ± 26.5
Protein (mg/dl)	310 ± 214	295 ± 228	270 ± 180	250 ± 170

*Mean ± SD.
(Courtesy of Girgis NI, Farid Z, Mikhail IA, et al: *Pediatr Infect Dis J* 8:;848–851, 1989.)

glucose or protein content. Dexamethasone, when added to antibacterial therapy for bacterial meningitis, improves survival, especially in pneumococcal meningitis, and lowers the incidence of neurologic sequelae, including hearing loss.

▶ This paper adds to the growing and convincing body of literature that supports the early use of dexamethasone in the treatment of bacterial meningitis to increase survival and prevent neurologic sequelae. Dexamethasone appears to work by decreasing the production of interleukin-1, tumor necrosis factor, CSF lactate, and prostaglandin E_2, as well as decreasing neutrophil adhesion to cerebral capillary endothelium, all of which contribute to blood-brain barrier disruption and meningeal inflammation. Future studies will have to determine the precise timing of dexamethasone administration (before or concurrent with antibiotic administration) and the optimal dose, which may differ depending on the organism.— D.G. Nichols, M.D.

Somatosensory and Auditory Brain Stem Conduction After Head Injury: A Comparison With Clinical Features in Prediction of Outcome
Lindsay K, Pasaoglu A, Hirst D, Allardyce G, Kennedy I, Teasdale G (Southern Gen Hosp, Glasgow; Univ of Glasgow)
Neurosurgery 26:278–285, 1990   6–7

Assessment with evoked potentials correlates well with clinical features and outcome in patients with recent head injuries. Measurement of evoked potentials may be valuable in patients in whom neurologic examination is impaired or impossible. Central somatosensory pathways (CCT) and brain stem auditory conduction (BCT) were examined in 101 patients, and these results were compared with clinical features as predictors of outcome.

The patients all had severe head injury and remained in a coma for at least 6 hours. Central somatosensory pathways were recorded in all patients and BCT was recorded in 92. The Glasgow Coma Score was used to record the level of consciousness.

Forty patients had no spontaneous eye movements, and in 28 patients both pupils were fixed. Seventy-five patients had a coma score of 8 or less. These clinical indices correlated with outcome at 6 months and with results of both the BCT and CCT studies. The strongest correlation with outcome was produced by the CCT in the "best" hemisphere. With CCT the correlation with outcome was stronger when patients were examined within 2–3 days, rather than 24 hours, after the injury. This was not true for BCT.

Of the 24 patients with an absent CCT, 22 died and 1 remained in a vegetative state. Five patients had an absent BCT but a normal CCT. One of these patients died, 1 remained in a vegetative state, and 3 are severely disabled. The addition of evoked potentials did not, however, significantly improve the predictive accuracy of clinical data. Thus when neurologic examination is feasible, the extra time and effort involved in record-ing evoked potentials does not appear to be justified.

▶ This study is reassuring in validating the usefulness of clinical examination (Glasgow Coma Score) in predicting the outcome of the head-injured patient. If sedation and paralysis of the patient cannot be interrupted to perform a clinical examination, somatosensory or brain stem auditory-evoked potentials are good predictors of outcome.—D.G. Nichols, M.D.

Myocardial Infarction With Normal Coronary Arteries After Acute Expo-sure to Carbon Monoxide
Marius-Nunez AL (Edgewater Med Ctr, Chicago)
Chest 97:491–494, 1990   6–8

Studies have shown that myocardial ischemia after carbon monoxide poisoning occurs with levels of carbon monoxide in hemoglobin of more than 25%. In such cases the ECG is a useful screening test. One patient with angiographic evidence of myocardial infarction had normal coro-nary arteries.

Man, 46, sustained an acute myocardial infarction after carbon monoxide ex-posure that was demonstrated by ECG and serum enzymes. The coronary angio-gram obtained 1 week after hospitalization showed no evidence of coronary ob-structive lesions. The patient had been found unconscious, and his medical profile was negative for risk factors for coronary heart disease.

During carbon monoxide exposure myocardial damage may be ex-plained by 2 factors. First, decreased oxygen transport capacity of the blood leads to a reduced amount of oxygen available to tissues. Second, impaired mitochondrial function results from reversible inhibition of the intracellular respiration by the formation of cytochrome a, a_3-CO ligand.

▶ This case report demonstrates myocardial infarction in a patient without cor-onary artery obstruction. Cyanide is a common product of combustion, and cy-anide intoxication frequently accompanies carbon monoxide intoxication. It is unclear whether cyanide intoxication played a role in this patient's cardiac problem.—R.W. McPherson, M.D.

Cardiac Abnormalities Demonstrated in Four Cases of Accidental Electro-cution and Their Potential Significance Relative to Nonfatal Electrical Inju-ries of the Heart
James TN, Riddick L, Embry JH (Univ of Texas, Galveston; Univ of South Ala-bama, Mobile; Alabama Dept of Forensic Sciences, Mobile and Birmingham)
Am Heart J 120:143–156, 1990   6–9

Death from accidental electrocution is usually attributed to fatal cardiac arrhythmias, especially ventricular fibrillation. However, relatively little is known about the anatomical changes in the heart, particularly about the cardiac conduction system. The hearts of 4 men who died in electrical accidents were studied with particular attention to the cardiac conduction system, coronary arteries, and neural structures of the heart.

All 4 hearts exhibited widespread focal necrosis that involved the myocardium and included the specialized tissue of the sinus and atrioventricular nodes. Contraction band necrosis of smooth muscle cells in the tunica media of the coronary arteries was prominent in all 4 hearts. Cells in the His bundle and bundle branches were less affected. The neural structures of the heart were minimally involved. In 3 hearts there were significant cardiac abnormalities of a chronic or preexisting nature that could have predisposed to fatal arrhythmias. Two hearts showed slight cardiomegaly, a factor well known to facilitate the development of ventricular fibrillation and to make treatment more difficult. One heart showed chronic focal fibromuscular dysplastic narrowing of small coronary arteries, including the artery that supplied the coronary chemoreceptor. Another heart exhibited extensive fatty deposition within and around the sinus and atrioventricular nodes.

The consistently abnormal morphological findings in the conduction system in all 4 hearts may explain the pathogenesis of electrical instability after electrical injuries. In addition, there were preexisting chronic cardiac abnormalities that, when combined with the effects of electrocution, may be fatal.

▶ Demonstration of injury to the cardiac conduction system in patients who have received electrical injury suggests that, in nonfatal shocks, cardiac abnormalities may contribute to long-term patient management problems.—R.W. McPherson, M.D.

Echocardiographic Observations in Survivors of Acute Electrical Injury
Homma S, Gillam LD, Weyman AE (Massachusetts Gen Hosp, Boston)
Chest 97:103–105, 1990   6–10

Cardiovascular sequelae in survivors of acute electrical injury have rarely been studied. Two-dimensional echocardiographic findings were reviewed in 2 young men who experienced cardiac arrest when they touched high-tension wires.

Man, 25, healthy, lost consciousness when a ladder he was holding contacted a 7,200-volt electric line. Cardiopulmonary resuscitation was begun immediately. The patient was in ventricular fibrillation when he arrived at the hospital, but stable sinus rhythm was achieved after 7 direct current countershocks were given over 30 minutes. On the next day, results of neurologic and cardiac examinations were normal. The ECG showed sinus rhythm with diffuse nonspecific ST and T

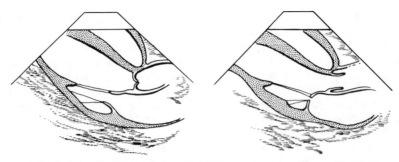

Fig 6–2.—End-diastolic (**left**) and end-systolic (**right**) appearances in a 15-year-old patient resuscitated from an acute electrical injury. Note the severe left ventricular hypokinesis. (Courtesy of Homma S, Gillam LD, Weyman AE: *Chest* 97:103–105, 1990.)

changes. Initial creatine kinase values were 4,295 units per liter; the 12-hour post-admission values were 4,275 units per liter. Echocardiography at admission revealed globally severe biventricular hypokinesis with dyskinesis of the left ventricular apex. Repeat echocardiography showed slightly improved left ventricular function after 2 days and marked improvement after 3 weeks, but apical dyskinesis persisted. On a stress test 2 months later, the patient reached the predicted maximum heart rate without symptoms; however, the resting ECG showed T wave abnormalities that had been noted previously. There was no change with exercise. Thallium imaging showed a fixed apical defect consistent with scar.

In this patient and another who received electrical injury, left ventricular dysfunction was irreversible (Fig 6–2). Other findings suggest an ischemic basis for the abnormalities.

▶ This report describes the long-term follow-up of 2 patients with persistent left ventricular dysfunction who survived electrical injury. The fact that these patients sustained long-term, irreversible injury is in contrast to the totally reversible left ventricular dysfunction that had been suspected. As a result of these considerations, long-term follow-up of cardiac function in electrical injury appears warranted.—M.C. Rogers, M.D.

7 Infectious Disease

Conservative Management of Adult Epiglottitis
Wolf M, Strauss B, Kronenberg J, Leventon G (Tel-Aviv Univ, Israel)
Laryngoscope 100:183–185, 1990   7–1

Acute epiglottitis is considered to be a mainly pediatric emergency, but recent reports have suggested an increasing incidence among adults. Some authors have reported a rapid and aggressive course in adults with epiglottitis, whereas others have reported a more benign outcome. Furthermore, there is controversy over the need for intubation or tracheotomy, or both. Identification of specific risk factors that might contribute to the development of a compromised airway in adult epiglottitis was sought in a review of 30 adults with a diagnosis of acute epiglottitis during a 10-year period.

At presentation, all patients had pain, 28 had dysphagia, 8 complained of hoarseness, and 6 were dyspneic, 3 of whom had experienced dyspnea of sudden onset. Two patients had hemoptysis. The onset of epiglottitis was gradual in 15 patients, abrupt in 8, and unclear in 7. Acute disease developed in 2 distinct forms—either gradually, usually beginning as an upper respiratory tract infection, or accelerated, within hours.

Eight patients had epiglottic abscesses, 3 on the free edge of the epiglottis, 1 on the laryngeal surface, and 4 on the lingual surface of the epiglottis. All patients were given antibiotics intravenously, and 15 were given steroids. None of the patients required intubation or tracheotomy. No age-related or sex-related differences in symptoms and signs were noted. Patients with dyspnea showed no characteristic features.

The course of epiglottitis in adults differs from that usually seen in children. In contrast to the interventionist approach in children, a noninterventionist and conservative approach is recommended for adults with acute epiglottitis.

▶ Adult epiglottitis is being increasingly recognized, and this retrospective analysis of 30 adults with epiglottitis highlights several important features of the adult form of this disease. Whereas *Hemophilus influenzae* is the most frequent causative pathogen in the pediatric age group, streptococci and staphylococci are more prevalent in the adult form. However, *H. influenzae* has been found in up to 26% of adults with epiglottitis in other series (1). More important, unlike pediatric patients, adults are much less likely to have acute upper airway obstruction requiring intubation and tracheostomy. The reasons for this are not entirely known but may be related to the difference in pathogens that affect each age group. Further, the adult compared to the pediatric upper airway has a larger cross-sectional diameter relative to the size of the epiglottis. Although adults generally respond to the prompt institution of antibiotics and expectant management, complications such as bacteremia, abscess formation, and acute airway obstruction can occur.—A.L. VanDervort, M.D., and R.L. Danner, M.D.

Reference

1. Mustoe T, Strome M: *Am J Otolaryngol* 4:393, 1983.

Improved Survival in Patients With AIDS, *Pneumocystis carinii* Pneumonia, and Severe Respiratory Failure
Friedman Y, Franklin C, Rackow EC, Weil MH (Cook County Hosp, Chicago; Univ of Health Sciences/Chicago Med School, North Chicago)
Chest 96:862–866, 1989   7–2

The mortality among patients with AIDS who have *Pneumocystis carinii* pneumonia (PCP) causing acute respiratory failure reportedly ranges between 84% and 100%. The mortality associated with a single PCP episode has been reported to be 28% to 43%. A prospective study was undertaken because of an impression of increased survival of these patients in the present institution's intensive care unit (ICU).

During a 2-year period from 1987 through 1988, 58 patients with AIDS were admitted to the ICU to receive positive pressure ventilation with continuous positive airway pressure by mask, or endotracheal intubation and mechanical ventilation. All patients underwent diagnostic fiberoptic bronchoscopy with bronchoalveolar lavage and/or transbronchial biopsy.

Thirty-three of the 58 patients were identified as having PCP and acute respiratory failure. Twelve of these 33 were discharged home from the hospital and 21 died during hospitalization. The mean duration of survival after discharge was 7.9 months. This survival rate is higher than that reported in the literature.

On the basis of the previously published mortality rate for AIDS patients with PCP and acute respiratory failure admitted to the ICU, it has been recommended that that patients not be given intensive care or mechanical ventilation. In view of the availability of newer treatment modalities and considering the improved survival seen in this group of patients, it is suggested that competent patients with AIDS who have PCP and acute respiratory failure should be allowed to have a choice regarding intensive care and mechanical ventilation.

▶ Specific antiviral therapy (anti-HIV) and earlier diagnosis of and prophylaxis for opportunistic infections have led to an increase in the longevity of patients with AIDS. Mortality from *Pneumocystis carinii* pneumonia (PCP), a major cause of death in these patients, has decreased because of these measures, although the prognosis for patients with AIDS and PCP requiring mechanical ventilation has remained exceptionally high. The value of corticosteroids, recently found to be beneficial in PCP (1), has not been defined in this subgroup.

In fact, many centers, because of early recognition, better care, and newer therapies, are experiencing an increased survival in AIDS patients with PCP admitted to the ICU for acute respiratory failure (ARF). In this prospective analysis of 33 consecutive patients with AIDS, PCP, and ARF there was a 36% survival rate (12 survivors vs. 21 nonsurvivors); this is considerably better than the 16% survival reported by others. In this study no predictive factors were identified that could differentiate survivors from nonsurvivors, and both survivors and nonsurvivors had a similar severity of illness. Further, in patients for whom follow-up was available (10 of 12 patients), the mean survival was about 8 months. The prognosis of AIDS continues to evolve with the introduction of new therapies. Patients with AIDS, PCP, and ARF should not be categorically excluded from or advised against intensive care.—A.L. VanDervort, M.D., and R.L. Danner, M.D.

Reference

1. Bozzette SA, et al: *N Engl J Med* 323:1451, 1990.

Prognosis of Patients With AIDS Requiring Intensive Care
Smith RL, Levine SM, Lewis ML (New York VA Med Ctr, New York City; New York Univ)
Chest 96:857–861, 1989   7–3

The Acute Physiology and Chronic Health Evaluation (APACHE) II classification accurately predicts mortality in patients who require intensive care. However, the APACHE II classification was designed before the rapid expansion of the AIDS epidemic. The applicability of the APACHE II system to certain subgroups of patients with AIDS known to have a poor prognosis was determined.

During a 57-month study, 106 patients with AIDS and 166 controls without AIDS were admitted to the intensive care unit. Complete data were available for 83 patients with AIDS; 37 of them had *Pneumocystis carinii* pneumonia (PCP) requiring mechanical ventilation for respiratory failure. Of the 166 patients without AIDS, 39 had respiratory failure, 25 of them requiring mechanical ventilation.

Based on the APACHE II scores, the predicted mortality for the patients without AIDS was 34% and the observed death rate was 31%. Thus the APACHE II system accurately predicted the in-hospital death rate for this group of patients. The predicted mortality for the patients with AIDS was about 46%, whereas the observed death rate was 64%. The difference was statistically significant. The observed mortality among the 37 AIDS patients with PCP requiring mechanical ventilation was 86.5%, whereas the predicted mortality was 44%. The observed mortality among the 46 AIDS patients without PCP was 47%, compared with a predicted mortality of 46%. The APACHE II system is not useful for assessing disease severity in AIDS patients with PCP requiring mechanical ventilation, and a new diagnostic category for this subgroup of AIDS patients should be added to the APACHE II system.

▶ Both real and artifactual increases in the longevity of AIDS patients have occurred since the clinical syndrome was first described a decade ago. This has been achieved through improvement in diagnosis and in early recognition and management of opportunistic infections, and through the introduction of new antiviral therapies. *Pneumocystis carinii* pneumonia remains a serious problem, although identification of subpopulations at high risk for this complication, prophylaxis, and early diagnosis have affected the incidence and mortality of this infection. Recent trials have shown that corticosteroids can further reduce the risk of respiratory failure and death in moderate to severe PCP, although steroid therapy may not benefit patients who require mechanical ventilation (1).

Overall, the prognosis of intubated patients with AIDS and PCP is poor, but may be improving (2). The study cited here suggests that the APACHE II system may not accurately predict mortality in this subgroup of patients. In this investigation, however, APACHE II scores were assigned retrospectively to 65% of the patients; 20% of eligible patients were excluded because charts were incomplete. Clearly, other centers must confirm the need for a new APACHE II diagnostic category for this subgroup of AIDS patients. The epidemiologic usefulness of the APACHE II classification would be diminished if it fails to perform adequately in patients with a specific diagnosis (that may not be known at the time of scoring), or who have a disease that has an evolving prognosis. The authors correctly point out that the APACHE II system can make statistical predictions about groups but cannot be applied to individual patients. In this study the APACHE II score could not distinguish between survivors and nonsurvivors of PCP pneumonia.— R.L. Danner, M.D.

Reference

1. Bozzette SA, et al: *N Engl J Med* 323:1451, 1990.
2. Friedman Y, et al: *Chest* 96:862, 1989.

Risk Factors for Hospital-Acquired Candidemia: A Matched Case-Control Study
Wey SB, Mori M, Pfaller MA, Woolson RF, Wenzel RP (Univ of Iowa Hosps and Clinics)
Arch Intern Med 149:2349–2353, 1989   7–4

Nosocomial candidemia is an increasingly common infection associated with high fatality rate. To determine independent predictors for these infections, 28 potential risk factors were analyzed through a matched case-control study involving 88 pairs of patients hospitalized between July 1983 and December 1986.

Univariate analysis showed that the strongest single risk factor for nosocmial candidemia was the number of antibiotics administered previously, with an estimated exposure odds ratio of 12.5 for those who took

3–5 antibiotics, compared to those who received none to 2 antibiotics. Multiple logistic regression analysis by a conditional likelihood method showed that the best predictor of the disease was a model composed of 4 variables: number of antibiotics received before infection, isolation of *Candida* species from sites other than blood, previous hemodialysis, and previous use of a Hickman catheter. Controlled clinical trials are warranted to determine whether limiting the number of antibiotics or instituting prophylaxis or early treatment, or both, for high-risk patients will reduce the incidence of nosocomial candidemia.

▶ Nosocomial candidemia is a dreaded complication of medical devices, immunosuppression, and antibiotic therapy. These interventions should be used judiciously and for only as long as they are necessary. Antibiotics should always be limited to those that are clinically indicated. The administration of multiple antibiotics could be a cause of nosocomial candidemia or simply an associated factor that identifies a high-risk patient group. Notably, controlled studies comparing single antibiotics with multiple-drug regimens in neutropenic patients have not shown a decreased risk of fungal injections (1). Surprisingly, the duration of neutropenia, a previously identified risk factor for invasive fungal infections, was not strongly associated with candidemia in this study. This may be because of the practice of instituting empiric antifungal therapy in neutropenic patients who have persistent fever despite antibacterial therapy. The recent development of new antifungal agents with improved toxicity profiles offers the hope of effective prophylaxis or early empiric treatment in other high-risk patient populations.— R.L. Danner, M.D.

Reference

1. Pizzo PA, et al: *N Engl J Med* 315:552, 1986.

Sensitivity and Specificity of Blood Cultures Obtained Through Intravascular Catheters
Wormser GP, Onorato IM, Preminger TJ, Culver D, Martone WJ (New York Med College, Valhalla; Ctrs for Disease Control, Atlanta)
Crit Care Med 18:152–156, 1990   7–5

Authors disagree on the reliability of blood cultures obtained through indwelling intravascular catheters. The results of a large series of catheter blood cultures were compared with those of an equal number of peripheral blood cultures drawn at the same time in patients being assessed for suspected sepsis.

Two hundred catheter blood cultures and 200 peripheral blood cultures were studied. The blood cultures were obtained from an upper extremity, cervical, or thoracic catheter, or from a femoral catheter. Peripheral arterial blood cultures were obtained from 55 different catheters in 24 patients on 101 occasions.

Catheter blood cultures had a sensitivity of 96% and a specificity of

Comparison of Blood Cultures Obtained Through Intravascular Catheters and by Venipuncture

Catheter Type	Comparison of Catheter Culture/ Peripheral Culture*				Total	Sensitivity†	Specificity†
	+/+	-/-	+/-	-/+			
Peripheral arterial	8	92	1	0	101	100 (75-100)	99 (97-100)
Central venous	9	24	2	1	36	90 (71-99)	92 (82-100)
Pulmonary artery	6	26	1	0	33	100 (54-100)	96 (89-100)
Hickman/Broviac	4	26	0	0	30	100 (50-100)	100 (92-100)
All catheters	27	168	4	1	200	96 (89-100)	98 (96-100)

*Isolation of the same organism from both cultures is indicated by +/+. Sterile cultures are indicated by -. Isolation of organisms from 1 of the cultures only is indicated by +/- or -/+.
†95% confidence intervals in parentheses. Values shown are %.
(Courtesy of Wormser GP, Onorato IM, Preminger TJ, et al: Crit Care Med 18:152-156, 1990.)

98% in the detection of septicemia. Sensitivity and specificity varied among catheter groups but not significantly (table). Factors believed to have influenced these favorable results included the relatively short duration of catheter placement and the particular emphasis on aseptic technique.

Blood obtained for culture through indwelling intravascular catheters can be a convenient, sensitive, and specific means of detecting septicemia if ample attention is given to methodological detail. The use of a well-trained phlebotomist and vigorous stopcock disinfection is important.

▶ Indwelling intravascular catheters are frequently used in critically ill patients to provide information on hemodynamic status, to administer medications, and to draw blood specimens from patients with limited vascular access. This well-designed study found that catheter-obtained blood culture specimens were sensitive (96%) and specific (98%) when compared to specimens obtained simultaneously by venipuncture. Most culture specimens were obtained from indwelling catheters in place for 4 days or less; catheters used to administer hyperalimentation were excluded from analysis. This study suggests that indwelling catheters of short duration (4 or fewer days) may be used to obtain blood cultures in patients with limited vascular access if rigorous aseptic technique is observed. Because the meticulous methods used in this study are unlikely to be duplicated in clinical practice, catheter-drawn blood specimens cannot be generally recommended.—A.L. VanDervort, M.D., and R.L. Danner, M.D.

Increasing Frequency of Staphylococcal Infective Endocarditis: Experience at a University Hospital, 1981 Through 1988
Sanabria TJ, Alpert JS, Goldberg R, Pape LA, Cheeseman SH (Univ of Massachusetts Med Ctr, Worcester)
Arch Intern Med 150:1305–1309, 1990   7–6

Both the presentation and causes of infective endocarditis (IE) have changed in the past 50 years. To determine the characteristics of IE, all 113 patients discharged with that diagnosis from the University of Massachusetts Medical Center in Worcester between 1981 and 1988 were reviewed.

Fifty-six patients had staphylococcal endocarditis. The in-hospital mortality rate was 25% despite aggressive medical and surgical treatment. Eighty percent of these 56 cases involved *Staphylococcus aureus;* the mortality rate was 28%, compared with 9% in the non–*S. aureus*-infected group. Death rates were higher in patients with congestive heart failure, atrioventricular block, atrial fibrillation, and prosthetic valve endocarditis. Of those with congestive heart failure, 76% needed surgery. The mortality rate among patients with congestive heart failure and *S. aureus* infection was 45%. Overall, 64% of the patients were alive at late follow-up a mean 28.6 months after treatment. Death rates were highest in the first 3 months after the diagnosis of staphylococcal endocarditis.

The frequency of staphylococcal endocarditis is increasing. This form of endocarditis is associated with a high hospital case fatality rate and often requires urgent surgery. Mortality is higher in patients with heart failure, *S. aureus* infection, and atrial fibrillation. Most patients with this entity die within 3 months of admission.

▶ Anatomical cardiac valvular abnormalities, prosthetic valvular surgery, and intravenous drug use are factors that are known to predispose individuals to the development of IE. Interesting features in this report include a higher proportion of IE caused by *Staphylococcus* at this institution than has been previously reported (50% of cases). Other series have reported that staphylococci cause 20% to 30% of IE, with 80% to 90% secondary to *S. aureus*. This organism frequently produces a fulminant course characterized by metastatic infection and an approximate mortality of 40%. This report found the overall acute mortality rate from *S. aureus* IE to be 28% with appropriate antibiotics and surgery, compared to 9% in the non–*S. aureus* group. Patients with IE as a consequence of intravenous drug abuse had lower mortality as a group, as has been reported previously. However, because of inadequate follow-up and noncompliance, this group had recurrence rates of IE as high as 46%. This study is in agreement with many of the prognostic factors for IE that have been identified in other reports. A broader-based, multicenter sample of data is necessary to confirm the findings of this study from a single tertiary care hospital that the frequency of staphylococcal IE is increasing.—A.L. VanDervort, M.D., and R.L. Danner, M.D.

Aggressive Intensive Care Treatment of Very Elderly Patients With Tetanus Is Justified
Jolliet P, Magnenat J-L, Kobel T, Chevrolet J-C (Geneva Univ Hosp, Switzerland)
Chest 97:702–705, 1990   7–7

Tetanus has declined in developed countries, but many elderly persons lack adequate immunity against the disease. Most patients are older than 60 years. Three patients older than age 80 years who recently had tetanus were studied. A comparison of reported patients older than age 70 years with younger ones showed no difference in duration of intubation, hospital stay, or frequency of cardiovascular complications. Infectious complications were fairly frequent in both groups. Of the 10 reported patients, 2 died; both were younger than 70 years.

Aggressive intensive care is warranted for elderly patients with generalized, severe tetanus. Complete recovery is possible even after prolonged total neuromuscular blockade. The quality of life can be comparable to what it was before tetanus occurred.

▶ This retrospective study examines the impact on outcome of aggressive intensive care in elderly patients with tetanus. The decreased mortality of all patients with tetanus now admitted to the intensive care unit (ICU) is most likely attributable to improvements in mechanical ventilation and neuromuscular paralysis. These supportive measures have all but eliminated respiratory failure caused by muscle spasms, a frequent cause of death before the institution of specialized critical care units. Also contributing to this decrease in mortality is better nursing care and medical surveillance with early recognition and treatment of potentially life-threatening complications. Notably, elderly patients with tetanus had just as favorable an outcome as younger patients. These results argue strongly against the rationing of ICU care in elderly patients with tetanus simply on the basis of age.—A.L. VanDervort, M.D., and R.L. Danner, M.D.

Long-Term Respiratory Support and Risk of Pneumonia in Critically Ill Patients
Langer M, Mosconi P, Cigada M, Mandelli M, and the Intensive Care Unit Group of Infection Control (Istituto Ricerche Farmacologiche Mario Negri, Milan, Italy; Ospedale Maggiore, Milan)
Am Rev Respir Dis 140:302–305, 1989   7–8

Patients in intensive care are at high risk for infection because they have serious underlying disease and because they are exposed to respiratory care devices. However it is difficult to distinguish the patient's own risk from device-related risk.

To determine how much the duration of respiratory assistance increases the risk of pneumonia, 1,475 patients admitted to 23 intensive care units (ICs) were studied. Only patients with no pulmonary infection at admission who were not in the terminal stage of an illness and had an ICU stay of longer than 48 hours were included. The incidence of pneumonia vs. the duration of ventilatory support was plotted, and the same

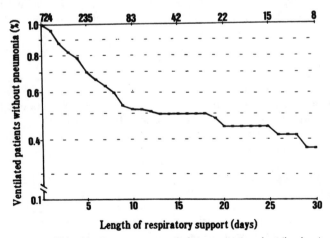

Length of respiratory support (days)

Fig 7–1.—Actuarial life-table. Curve represents cumulative proportion of ventilated patients "free of pneumonia" at each day of respiratory support. On top line number of patients on ventilation and free of pneumonia at correspondent day of respiratory support as indicated on bottom. Patients lost between points are those who acquired pneumonia (terminal event) or stopped ventilation (censored observations), or both. (Courtesy of Langer M, Mosconi P, Cigada M, et al: *Am Rev Respir Dis* 140:302–305, 1989.)

data were computed as an actuarial life-table in which the day of onset of pneumonia was considered the terminal event.

Overall, 724 patients received ventilatory assistance on admission to the ICU, and 603 patients had ventilatory assistance for more than 24 hours. The mean ICU stay was 11.5 days. Of the ventilated patients, 168 contracted pneumonia (23%). The incidence of pneumonia in nonventilated patients was 7%, and in patients with respiratory assistance for 24 hours or less the incidence was 5.5%. In patients with respiratory assistance for more than 24 hours the incidence of pneumonia was 27%. A plotted "survival curve" showed that the rate of pneumonia acquired during ventilation was constant throughout the first 8–10 days of ventilation, after which it decreased (Fig 7–1). Only 10% of ventilated patients who contracted pneumonia did so after day 10.

The incidence of pneumonia during ventilatory support rises from approximately 5% in patients receiving up to 24 hours of respiratory assistance to 68.8% in those assisted for more than 30 days. Pneumonia occurs early in patients receiving ventilatory support; there is a high and constant risk for the first 8–10 days. Late development of pneumonia is rare, and the risk after 10 days of ventilatory support is low.

▶ Critically ill patients who require mechanical ventilation for prolonged periods of time are at risk for acquiring nosocomial pulmonary infections. This study confirms previous observations that the risk of nosocomial pneumonia increases with the duration of mechanical ventilation. Further, using an actuarial life-table analysis, the authors show that the risk of acquiring pneumonia is highest in the first 10 days of respiratory support and decreases to a low level thereafter. A likely explanation is that patients who do not contract pneumonia before 10 days of ventilatory support are a self-selected subpopulation that may have always been at low risk for this complication. We agree with the authors that "the length of respiratory assistance and (with it) the 'device-related risk' are more a contributory, rather than primary, cause of pulmonary infection."—A.L. VanDervort, M.D., and R.L. Danner, M.D.

Handwashing Practices in an Intensive Care Unit: The Effects of an Educational Program and Its Relationship to Infection Rates
Conly JM, Hill S, Ross J, Lertzman J, Louie TJ (Univ of Manitoba, Winnipeg)
Am J Infect Control 17:330–339, 1989   7–9

Handwashing is the single most important procedure in the prevention of nosocomial infections, yet it is often neglected. Patients in intensive care units (ICUs) are at greater risk of infection; however, an evaluation of compliance with handwashing procedures revealed that hospital personnel washed after patient contact less than half the time. The correlation between handwashing practices and nosocomial infection rates in the ICU was studied before and after 2 educational programs.

Before and after the first educational program and twice during the second, handwashing practices were observed in 3 cubicles for 4 hours with personnel in the medical ICU being unaware of the observations. Chlorhexidine gluconate solution was provided at all sinks for handwashing. In the medical ICU site surveillance cultures were obtained twice weekly from endotracheal tubes, tracheostomies, and urinary catheters. Patients suspected of having nosocomial infections were reexamined, and cultures were repeated as necessary. In the education program, personnel were provided with data obtained from observations of poor compliance with handwashing; infection-control posters that emphasized handwashing were placed in the medical ICU, and visitors were required to wash their hands before entering the unit. During the first time period, no attempts were made to reinforce the handwashing program, but during the second, infection control personnel emphasized the importance of handwashing, and results of the 2 previous handwashing surveys were stressed. Also, ICU directors actively encouraged handwashing.

In 1978, before the educational program, the nosocomial infection rate was more than 30%. After the first educational program the rate fell to 12%, but by the latter half of 1982 the rate had risen progressively and was approaching 30%. After the second educational program the nosocomial infection rate was approximately 10%, which was maintained throughout 1983.

Good handwashing practices are associated with a low nosocomial infection rate, whereas poor practices are associated with a high rate. An educational program that includes enforcement can significantly reduce nosocomial infection rates, but these programs must be maintained and monitored to have a sustained effect. Motivational techniques to encourage infection-control practices have yet to be determined.

▶ This study of handwashing practices in a medical ICCU extends the observations of others regarding the benefit of handwashing in the prevention of nosocomial infections. Defined in this study are some of the key factors that go into maintaining favorable handwashing practices by health care givers. These include the following: (1) an educational program administered at frequent levels, (2) surveillance of nosocomial infection attack rates, (3) periodic audits of handwashing practices, (4) feedback of audits and surveillance, and (5) active participation by ICU directors and nursing supervisors. This study emphasizes the responsibility that all health care givers share in reducing the morbidity, mortality, and costs incurred by nosocomial infection through the simple but effective use of proper handwashing habits.—A.L. VanDervort, M.D., and R.L. Danner, M.D.

Electrodiagnostic Features of the Guillain-Barré Syndrome: The Relative Sensitivity of Different Techniques
Olney RK, Aminoff MJ (Univ of California, San Francisco)
Neurology 40:471–475, 1990   7–10

As many as 20% of patients with Guillain-Barré syndrome (GBS) have normal findings on peripheral nerve conduction studies early in the course of illness. The sensitivity of peripheral nerve conduction, F-wave, and somatosensory evoked potential (SEP) studies were examined in 15 patients meeting the criteria for GBS, all of whom were acutely ill. All had neuropathy of grade 3 or higher on the modified Hughes scale. Percutaneous supramaximal stimulation and surface recording were carried out.

Three fourths of the nerves examined had abnormal motor conduction, either a reduction in conduction velocity or increased distal motor latency. In all but 3 of the 15 patients abnormalities were detected. Sensory nerve conduction was abnormal in 60% of the patients and F-wave studies in 87%. Only about half of the patients had abnormal SEP recordings. In all, significant electrodiagnostic abnormalities were recorded in 42 of 44 nerves and in all 15 patients. The F-wave studies were significantly more sensitive than SEP recordings.

Electrophysiologic abnormalities are consistently present in patients with GBS, even early in the course of clinical illness. Abnormal F-wave recordings may be obtained even if nerve conduction studies are normal. Recording of SEPs is indicated only if both peripheral nerve conduction and F-wave studies are normal.

▶ The diagnosis of GBS involves peripheral nerve conduction studies, but the sensitivity of these tests is not high. This paper compares the relative diagnostic sensitivity of peripheral nerve conduction, F-wave, and SEP studies in patients with GBS. Based on this report, SEP studies are not indicated in these patients unless results of peripheral nerve conduction and F-wave studies are normal.—M.C. Rogers, M.D.

Acute Relapsing Guillain-Barré Syndrome After Long Asymptomatic Intervals
Wijdicks EFM, Ropper AH (Massachusetts Gen Hosp, Boston)
Arch Neurol 47:82–84, 1990   7–11

Guillain-Barré syndrome (GBS) characteristically is a monophasic illness, but a few patients relapse acutely some time after recovering from the acute disorder. Five patients who recovered from an initial episode of GBS and had acute relapses after 4, 10, 15, 17, and 36 years, respectively, were studied. Two patients had more than 1 relapse. In 3 patients relapses were less lengthy than the initial episode, but in other respects the episodes were clinically similar. One patient had asymptomatic sarcoidosis. Patients frequently had oculomotor involvement and required ventilatory support. Eventually, they did recover with no more than mild residual deficit. Nerve conduction velocities were not substantially abnormal.

These cases were clinically distinct from typical chronic inflammatory demyelinating neuropathy. Some patients may be susceptible to acquiring GBS, possibly from persistent clones of B cells that reemerge to produce a pathogenetic antibody or, alternatively, from the initial neural damage that permits subsequent lymphocyte access to nerve fibers.

▶ Relapsing of an episode of GBS is not unknown. This generally happens, however, when a patient is only partially recovered from an episode, and this is viewed as a setback rather than a chronic problem. These authors report that acute relapses can occur after long asymptomatic periods. These asymptomatic periods range from 4 to 36 years later, and some of the patients had multiple relapses. This is a phase of the disease with which I am not familiar, and I think it would be of interest to all intensivists to review this paper.—M.C. Rogers, M.D.

The Natural History of the Guillain-Barré Syndrome in 18 Children and 50 Adults
Kleyweg RP, van der Meché FGA, Loonen MCB, de Jonge J, Knip B (Univ Hosp Dijkzigt, Rotterdam; St Elisabeth Ziekenhuis, Tilburg, The Netherlands)
J Neurol Neurosurg Psychiatry 52:853–856, 1989   7–12

Plasma exchange is generally accepted as effective in the treatment of severe Guillain Barré syndrome (GBS) in adults, but the indications for plasma exchange in children with GBS are not clear. Although GBS runs a milder course in children, its natural history in the pediatric age group has not been studied formally. A retrospective study was done to compare disease severity and outcome in children and adults with GBS and to assess the need for specific treatment in children.

The study population consisted of 18 children aged 1–14 years and 50 adults aged 16–74 years, all with GBS. All patients were treated before plasma exchange was introduced as a therapeutic modality for this disorder. None of the patients had been treated with immunoglobulin. Functional status was assessed after 1 year and 2 years, using a slightly modified version of the grading system used for the North American trial of 1985 (Table 1). The need for artificial ventilation, length of hospitalization, and functional outcome after 1 year and 2 years were used as parameters to indicate disease severity.

The mean duration of hospitalization was 84 days for children and 86

TABLE 1.—Functional Grading System

0 = healthy
1 = minor symptoms and signs, fully capable of manual work
2 = able to walk > 10 m without any assistance
3 = able to walk > 10 m with a walker or support
4 = bed or chair-bound (unable to walk > 10 m with a walker or support)
5 = assisted ventilation required for at least part of the day
6 = dead

(Courtesy of Kleyweg RP, van der Meché FGA, Loonen MCB, et al: *J Neurol Neurosurg Psychiatry* 52:853–856, 1989.)

TABLE 2.—Severity of the Disease

	Children (n = 18)	Adults (n = 50)
Mean time, 2 SE until nadir in days	9·6, 3·2	11·0, 1·6*
Artificial ventilation; percentage of patients, between brackets 95% confidence limits	22% (7–45%)	30% (18–45%)†
Duration of artificial ventilation (days) mean:	21·5	32*
range:	16–48	1–126
Duration of hospitalisation (incl. rehabilitation centre) (days) mean:	84	86*
range:	7–449	7–551

*Not significant: Mann Whitney U-test.
†Not significant: Fisher exact test.
(Courtesy of Kleyweg RP, van der Meché FGA, Loonen MCB, et al: *J Neurol Neurosurg Psychiatry* 52:853–856, 1989.)

TABLE 3.—Outcome

Functional grade	One Year		Two Years	
	Children	Adults	Children	Adults
0/1	14 (77%)	43 (86%)	15 (83%)	46 (92%)
2	1 (6%)	4 (8%)	1 (6%)	3 (6%)
3	1 (6%)	1 (2%)	—	—
4	—	2 (4%)	—	1 (2%)
5	—	—	—	—
6	2 (11%)	—	2 (11%)	—

(Courtesy of Kleyweg RP, van der Meché FGA, Loonen MCB, et al: *J Neurol Neurosurg Psychiatry* 52:853–856, 1989.)

days for adults. Four children (22%) and 15 adults (30%) required artificial ventilation. The median duration of artificial ventilation was 21.5 days in children and 32 days in adults. None of these differences was statistically significant (Table 2). Two children died of cardiac arrest, 1 in the acute phase and 1 early in the plateau phase. Fourteen children (77%) and 43 adults (86%) were healthy or had only minor symptoms and signs after 1 year, and 15 children and 46 adults had fully or nearly fully recovered at the 2 year follow-up examination (Table 3). One child (6%) and 4 adults (8%) had not fully recovered after 2 years of follow-up.

Because the course of GBS was similar in children and adults, specific treatment for GBS, (e.g., immunoglobulin infusion and plasma exchange) should also be considered in children. A multicenter trial to compare the effect of plasma exchange with that of immunoglobulin infusion is ongoing and includes both children and adults.

▶ The similarity of GBS between children and adults is shown in this study. Because the study reports patients treated before the use of plasma exchange, it is unclear whether the response of children is similar to that of adults.— R.W. McPherson, M.D.

Glucocorticoid Treatment Does Not Improve Neurological Recovery Following Cardiac Arrest
Jastremski M, Sutton-Tyrrell K, Vaagenes P, Abramson N, Heiselman D, Safar P, and the Brain Resuscitation Clinical Trial I Study Group (Univ of Pittsburgh)
JAMA 262:3427–3430, 1989   7–13

Glucocorticoids are commonly used after global brain ischemia in the hope of improving outcome, but their efficacy for this indication has not been confirmed. The multicenter Brain Resuscitation Clinical Trial I was designed to evaluate the effect of high-dose thiopental sodium therapy on neurologic outcome after global brain ischemia. The database of this trial was used to review retrospectively the effect of glucocorticoids on mortality and neurologic outcome after global brain ischemia.

The study population consisted of 262 initially comatose cardiac arrest survivors who made no purposeful response to pain 10–50 minutes after restoration of spontaneous circulation. The brain-oriented intensive care treatment protocol left the use of glucocorticoids to the discretion of the hospital investigators. A total of 192 patients received steroids within the first 8 hours of restoration of spontaneous circulation. One patient was subsequently excluded from the analysis. Of the 191 steroid-treated patients, 67 received a low dose, 58 a medium dose, and 66 a high dose.

Of 191 patients treated with early-rescue steroid therapy, 171 were still alive at 24 hours. Of these, 140 (82%) had received multiple doses of steroids during the first day after resuscitation. There were no statistically significant differences in mortality or neurologic outcomes among patients who never received steroids, those who received only a single early dose, and those who received multiple doses within the first 24 hours after global brain ischemia. Because the use of glucocorticoids has the potential for causing serious toxicity, and because none of the steroid regimens statistically improved survival or neurologic recovery when compared with no steroid use, the routine clinical practice of giving glucocorticoids after global brain ischemia is not justified.

▶ Glucocorticoids have frequently been advocated as potential therapeutic agents for a variety of insults resulting in brain injury. Most clinicians caring for patients with brain tumors rely on the ability of glucocorticoids to decrease vasogenic brain edema and prevent or treat elevated intracranial pressure. High-dose methylprednisolone treatment has also recently been demonstrated to improve recovery from spinal cord trauma. In a retrospective analysis of data obtained from the Brain Resuscitation Clinical Trial I, Jastremski et al. have concluded that glucocorticoids lack therapeutic efficacy in the setting of cytotoxic edema, such as that occurring with severe transient cerebral ischemia. Their data and conclusions are consistent with other studies in the literature.

The major concerns of this study are its retrospective design, inclusion of only severely damaged patients, not clearly separating patients who received thiopental from those who were given standard therapy, and the small sample size of some subgroups. The authors also suggest that glucocorticoid treatment may be dangerous because it may lead to an increased incidence of infection and nitrogen wasting, although this is not borne out by analysis of their data. The recent demonstration of therapeutic efficacy for methylprednisolone following spinal cord injury will undoubtedly lead other investigators to reevaluate the efficacy of glucocorticoids to decrease brain injury after transient cerebral ischemia in a randomized and prospective fashion. Likewise, other nonglucocorticoid steroids (e.g., the 21-aminosteroids) may be evaluated for therapeutic efficacy because they appear to lack many of the undesired side effects of glucocorticoid steroids.—J.R. Kirsch, M.D.

Nimodipine in Acute Ischemic Stroke: A Double-Blind Controlled Study
Paci A, Ottaviano P, Trenta A, Iannone G, De Santis L, Lancia G, Moschini E, Carosi M, Amigoni S, Caresia L (S Maria Hosp, Terni, Italy; Bayer Italia S.p.A, Milan)
Acta Neurol Scand 80:282–286, 1989   7–14

Nimodipine is a new dihydropyridine derivative that provides protection against calcium-induced ischemic cell damage. This calcium antagonist reduces neurologic outcome deficits and mortality induced by acute cerebral ischemia in experimental studies. The effect of nimodipine in patients with acute ischemic stroke was evaluated in a randomized, placebo-controlled, double-blind, parallel-designed trial.

Among the 54 patients screened during the 3-year study, a focal neurologic deficit occurred suddenly in 41 as a result of an acute ischemic event in the carotic area diagnosed after a complete neurologic work-up. Nineteen patients received nimodipine, 40 mg orally 3 times a day for 28 days, and 22 received placebo. Treatment began within 12 hours after onset of symptoms. Neurologic status and functional recovery were evaluated with the Mathew scale.

All but 1 patient, who had a skin rash after taking nimodipine, completed the study. Comparison of neurologic outcomes showed a significant difference in favor of nimodipine. On the basis of the Mathew scores, a higher rate of improvement was observed in the nimodipine-treated group (14 of 18) compared with the placebo-treated group (12 of 22). Nimodipine was well tolerated and no serious cardiovascular adverse effects were noted.

▶ This study is one of several that has demonstrated therapeutic efficacy for oral nimodipine after ischemic stroke. In this study investigators were able to administer nimodipine within 12 hours of the onset of symptoms, which may be difficult for clinicians to accomplish in practice. Other studies suggest that higher dosages and more frequent administration of nimodipine may make the drug efficacious even when administered at a later time after the onset of ischemic symptoms. However, it is probably premature from this and other studies to support the routine use of nimodipine in all patients with ischemic stroke. Additional studies should be completed to better determine the best patient population to benefit from therapy, dose response information, and the incidence of complications at the best dose and administration frequency.—J.R. Kirsch, M.D.

The Effect of Blood Glucose Concentration on Postasphyxia Cerebral Hemodynamics in Newborn Lambs
Rosenberg AA, Murdaugh E (Univ of Colorado)
Pediatr Res 27:454–459, 1990   7–15

One of the variables that may affect the outcome in perinatal asphyxia is preasphyxia blood concentration of glucose. The newborn lamb postasphyxia model was used to examine the effects of the preasphyxia concentration of glucose on cerebral hemodynamics of post asphyxia. Twenty-one newborn lambs were assigned to 1 of 3 experimental groups. The concentration of glucose was not regulated in the control group and was controlled by glucose clamp in the hyperglycemic and hypoglycemic groups. Cerebral blood flow (CBF) and arterial and sagittal sinus oxygen content were measured at control, 5 minutes and 1, 2, and 4 hours after resuscitation from an asphyxial insult.

The 5-minute postasphyxia CBF was increased significantly and cerebral oxygen consumption ($CMRO_2$) was decreased significantly in all 3 groups. In the late period after asphyxia, cerebral hypoperfusion was present in the unregulated group and $CMRO_2$ remained decreased at 1 hour and 4 hours post asphyxia. Hyperglycemia was associated with a return of CBF, $CMRO_2$, and fractional O_2 extraction to control levels during the late period after asphyxia, whereas hypoglycemia led to a late postasphyxia decrease in $CMRO_2$ despite cerebral perfusion at or above control levels.

These data show that CBF and $CMRO_2$ are improved after asphyxia in the hyperglycemic newborn lamb. Because improved CBF and $CMRO_2$ during the late period after asphyxia are beneficial, these data may have implications in the clinical management of the high-risk pregnancy and the asphyxiated newborn.

▶ Although the effect of hyperglycemia and hypoglycemia following ischemia and hypoxia have been studied extensively in adult animals, few studies have examined newborn animals. In adult animals even mild degrees of hyperglycemia before ischemia or at the time of reperfusion may impair neurologic recovery after transient cerebral ischemia. The mechanism for an impaired neurologic outcome has been hypothesized to possibly involve accumulation of lactic acid or lipid peroxidation within the brain studies have previously evaluated the importance of blood glucose levels on recovery of neurologic function after asphyxia. In the current study, using newborn lambs, recovery of CBF and $CMRO_2$ was actually improved by hyperglycemia. The authors suggest that glucose does not impair recovery of blood flow and oxygen consumption because glucose transport mechanisms are limited in the newborn brain and, therefore, asphyxia would not be anticipated to produce cerebral lactic acidosis. Although the authors suggest that the mechanism for improved recovery of CBF and metabolism is decreased production or improved removal of oxygen-free radicals, there is currently no support in the literature for their hypothesis.—J.R. Kirsch, M.D.

Effect of Indomethacin on the Regulation of Cerebral Blood Flow During Respiratory Alkalosis in Newborn Piglets

DeGiulio PA, Roth RA, Mishra OP, Delivoria-Papadopoulos M, Wagerle LC (Univ of Pennsylvania)
Pediatr Res 26:593–597, 1989   7–16

The effect of cyclooxygenase inhibition by indomethacin on regional cerebral blood flow (CBF) was assessed during hypocapnia induced by hyperventilation and during hypercapnia induced by carbon dioxide (CO_2) inhalation. The study was performed with 27 newborn Yorkshire piglets. Cerebral blood flow was measured by the tracer microsphere technique. Baseline measurements were made during normoxic normocapnia in control animals.

After hyperventilation, the CBF decreased significantly to all regions of the brain in the control group, with a 32% decrease in the cerebral cortex. In piglets treated with indomethacin, blood flow decreased significantly by 35% to 49% in all regions of the brain, except for the cerebral white matter, during normocapnia. There was no additional decrease in flow during subsequent hypocapnia.

Although CBF increased significantly after indomethacin treatment during hypercapnia, the response was considerably limited with blood flow to the cerebral gray matter, hippocampus, and pons. Increases were 42%, 25%, and 42%, respectively, in contrast to 108%, 75%, and 225%, respectively, in controls. In 5 animals, unilateral sympathetic nerve stimulation at 15 Hz was used to test the specificity of indomethacin on hypocapnic vasoconstriction. After hyperventilation with indomethacin, unilateral sympathetic nerve stimulation caused a further statistically significant decrease in CBF on the stimulated side, comparable to that occurring during normocapnia.

Thus indomethacin appears to attenuate the cerebrovascular sensitivity to both increases and decreases in CO_2/H^+. This suggests a possible role for vasoactive prostanoids in mediating the response of CBF to fluctuations in CO_2 in newborn piglets.

▶ The purpose of this study was to determine the ability of indomethacin to block the increase in CBF that occurs with hypercapnia and the decrease in CBF with hypocapnia. In newborn piglets, indomethacin attenuated the increase in blood flow with hypercapnia and ablated the decrease in blood flow that normally occurs with hypocapnia. Because indomethacin treatment did not affect the decrease in CBF that occurs with electrical stimulation of sympathetic nerves, the authors conclude that the attenuated blood flow response with alterations in CO_2 results from an effect on a prostanoid mechanism rather than from some nonspecific effect of indomethacin limiting all blood flow changes in the brain. In interpreting these data it is important to be aware that, although prostanoid mechanisms are clearly important in the regulation of CBF in newborn piglets, they do not appear to be important in regulation of CBF in the cat, goat, rabbit, or dog. The importance of prostanoid mechanisms in regulation of CBF in adult or newborn humans is unclear.—J.R. Kirsch, M.D.

Long-Term Neurophysiologic Outcome After Neonatal Extracorporeal Membrane Oxygenation

Lott IT, McPherson D, Towne B, Johnson D, Starr A (Univ of California, Irvine; Children's Hosp of Orange County, Orange, Calif)
J Pediatr 116:343–349, 1990   7–17

Neonates who undergo extracorporeal membrane oxygenation (ECMO) for treatment of temporary heart and lung failure are at risk for neurologic sequelae. The technique often involves surgical alteration of the major carotid and jugular supplies to the right hemisphere. Ten survivors of ECMO aged 4–9 years who had undergone such surgical techniques were assessed clinically. They were part of a previously studied group of 18 ECMO survivors, 13 of whom had normal growth and development and 5 who remained handicapped. To provide data on carotid blood flow and cerebral evoked potentials (EPs), the children underwent electroencephalography, ultrasound imaging, and EP studies.

Electroencephalographic findings did not correlate with neurodevelopmental status or other neurophysiologic measures of interhemispheric asymmetry. Ultrasound showed that in this patient group, the right internal carotid artery velocity was approximately 62% of that on the left, and the right internal carotid flow was reduced by 74%. A number of EP findings did not differ between patients and controls, but significant differences were seen in patients from both long-latency auditory EPs and somatosensory EPs from median nerve stimulation. Compared with controls, patients had a decrease in the amplitude of the potentials recorded over the right hemisphere relative to those recorded over the left hemisphere (Fig 7–2).

The significance of the EP findings is uncertain, but they may indicate an abnormality not detected by current clinical methods. This, and the changes in carotid flow, may reflect redirected cerebral blood flow patterns after ECMO.

▶ In this study, Lott et al. present clinical and neurophysiologic data on 10 children aged 4–9 years after neonatal ECMO. Following ligation of the right common carotid artery, there was decreased flow in the right internal carotid artery and reduction in the amplitude of the right hemispheric long-latency EP. Electroencephalograms, however, did not correlate with these other measures of interhemispheric asymmetry. Although decreased EP amplitude may be a re-

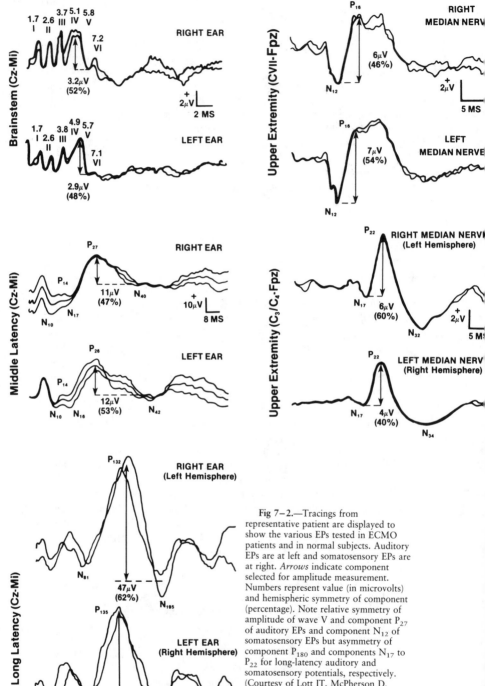

Fig 7–2.—Tracings from representative patient are displayed to show the various EPs tested in ECMO patients and in normal subjects. Auditory EPs are at left and somatosensory EPs are at right. *Arrows* indicate component selected for amplitude measurement. Numbers represent value (in microvolts) and hemispheric symmetry of component (percentage). Note relative symmetry of amplitude of wave V and component P_{27} of auditory EPs and component N_{12} of somatosensory EPs but asymmetry of component P_{180} and components N_{17} to P_{22} for long-latency auditory and somatosensory potentials, respectively. (Courtesy of Lott IT, McPherson D, Towne B, et al: *J Pediatr* 116:343–349, 1990.)

sult of impaired cerebral circulation, decreased cerebral blood flow itself did not predict a poor neurologic outcome. The most interesting finding of this study is that all patients had a patent internal and external right carotid artery despite previous ligation of the right common carotid artery. In each patient, flow through the right internal carotid artery was supplied by retrograde flow from the external carotid circulation.—J.R. Kirsch, M.D.

Cerebral Blood Flow During the Acute Therapy of Severe Hypertension With Oral Clonidine
Greene CS, Gretler DD, Cervenka K, McCoy CE, Brown FD, Murphy MB (Univ of Chicago)
Am J Emerg Med 8:293–296, 1990   7–18

The acute treatment of severe hypertension is associated with the risk of reduction in cerebral blood flow (CBF) with ischemic injury to the CNS. Serial determinations of CBF were made before and after the acute treatment of severe hypertension with clonidine in 13 patients whose diastolic blood pressures were above 115 mm Hg. The goal blood pressure to be reached was a diastolic blood pressure of 105 mm Hg, or a reduction from baseline of 30 mm Hg.

One patient did not reach this goal after treatment with clonidine alone. In the remaining patients, orally administered clonidine decreased the supine blood pressure from a mean 201.7/126.3 mm Hg to 149.4/96.8 mm Hg over an average of 85 minutes. The mean CBF in the group did not change, but there was a significant change in 9 of the 12 responders. The magnitude and direction of the change depended on the initial

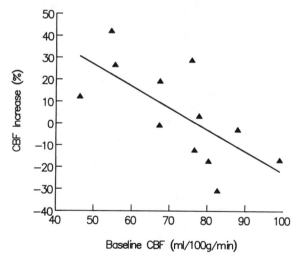

Fig 7–3.—Change in CBF after oral clonidine adminsitration, plotted against baseline CBF (no. = 12, *r* = −.65; *P* < .05). (Courtesy of Greene CS, Gretler DD, Cervenka K, et al: *Am J Emerg Med* 8:293–296, 1990.)

CBF. Patients with a low pretreatment CBF had an increase, and those with high initial flow had a decrease. There were no significant adverse effects (Fig 7–3).

The findings confirm the efficacy and safety of orally administered clonidine in the acute treatment of severe hypertension. The desired decrease in blood pressure was attained in 12 of the 13 patients studied.

▶ Pharmacologic control of blood pressure may have effects on the CBF that may lead to neurologic injury. Many case reports have been published describing an increase in intracranial pressure and decreased CBF leading to ischemia when blood pressure is controlled with direct acting vasodilators. The purpose of the study by Greene et al. was to determine the effect of the α_2 agonist, clonidine, on CBF when used to gain acute control of hypertension. Although the overall effect of clonidine was to produce no change in CBF despite good control of blood pressure, interestingly, those patients with a higher baseline CBF responded to clonidine with a decrease in CBF. Those patients with a lower baseline CBF responded to clonidine with an increase in CBF.

Although the results from this study are very interesting, they leave unanswered how to predict which patients will respond to clonidine with an increase or decrease in CBF, and whether the alteration in level of consciousness and the changes in CBF would be different in patients with preexisting neurologic dysfunction. Because sympathetic stimulation was hypothesized previously to protect the blood-brain barrier integrity by limiting the increase in CBF that occurs with acute hypertension, clonidine may inhibit adrenergically mediated vasoconstriction and accentuate cerebral edema with acute hypertension.—J.R. Kirsch, M.D.

Extensive Dural Sinus Thrombosis Treated by Surgical Removal and Local Streptokinase Infusion
Persson L, Lilja A (Univ Hosp, Uppsala, Sweden)
Neurosurgery 26:117–121, 1990   7–19

Widespread dural sinus thrombosis is a rare condition associated with a high mortality rate. A patient with this condition recovered after surgical treatment and a local infusion of streptokinase in the sagittal sinus.

Woman, 27, was admitted with headache and disorientation. She had recently undergone termination of a pregnancy, was taking oral contraceptives, and had no history of serious illness. Dural sinus thrombosis was suggested at CT, which showed unusually high density in the transverse and sagittal sinuses. The intracranial pressure (ICP) was raised. Within hours of admission, the patient's condition deteriorated and she became deeply comatose. When a cortical vein was accidentally damaged during insertion of a ventricular catheter for ICP measurement, forceful bleeding started. The ICP continued to be dangerously high and death seemed inevitable. Surgery was undertaken to remove thrombotic material from the venous sinuses. The ICP dropped dramatically but increased again 3 days after surgery. This finding, together with CT evidence of bilateral hemorrhages, indicated that venous flow was once again obstructed. A second operation combined surgical removal of thrombotic material with a local infusion of streptokinase. The ICP became normal and radiologic examination showed increased flow in the sinuses. The patient slowly regained consciousness. Although she was at first tetraplegic and mute, the patient was living at home and able to walk 9 months after surgery.

The patient's recovery illustrates that the brain is more resistant to venous obstruction than to cerebral arterial occlusion. The aggressive treatment described should be undertaken in similar cases.

▶ Heroic surgical measures to remove thrombotic material from the dural sinuses appears to have produced a satisfactory outcome in the mother of 2 young children. As our country's health care system comes under intense economic pressure, however, it is unlikely that such extraordinary measures will be preapproved by HMOs or reimbursed by third-party payers such as Blue Cross/Blue Shield.— R.W. McPherson, M.D.

Stroke in Infective Endocarditis
Hart RG, Foster JW, Luther MF, Kanter MC (Univ of Texas, San Antonio; Audie L Murphy VA Hosp, San Antonio)
Stroke 21:695–700, 1990   7–20

Although stroke has long been recognized as a frequent feature of infective endocarditis, its current prevalence is not known. The past 25 years have seen changes in characteristics of the patient population and improvements in therapies and diagnostic techniques. A multicenter retrospective analysis of recent patients with infective endocarditis was un-

TABLE 1.—Stroke and Non-CNS Emboli by Valve

Valve	No.	Mean age* (yr)	Ischemic stroke/TIA	Non-CNS emboli	Brain hemorrhage	Mortality
Native (left-sided)	133	48	19%	11%	7%	20%
Mitral	59	46	19%	10%	3%	14%
Aortic	61	49	16%	11%	8%	21%
Both	13	53	31%	15%	15%	38%
Tricuspid	33	32	6%	0%	0%	9%
Bioprosthetic	17	47	12%	6%	12%	35%
Mechanical	21	51	29%	14%	10%	33%
Congenital	8	29	0%	0%	0%	0%
Total	212	45	17%	9%	6%	20%

Note: *Non-CNS,* not involving the central nervous system; *TIA,* transient ischemic attack. Mortality, for all 212 episodes.
*Standard deviations of age ranges were 16–20 years for each group and do not differ significantly.
(Courtesy of Hart RG, Foster JW, Luther MF, et al: *Stroke* 21:695–700, 1990).

dertaken to reassess the occurrence and implications of stroke and systemic embolism.

The 6 study institutions included 3 university-affiliated teaching hospitals, 2 private nonprofit urban hospitals, and 1 university-affiliated Veterans Administration hospital. Study criteria were met by 203 patients who sustained 212 episodes of endocarditis. Stroke occurred in 21% of these episodes.

Stroke and non–CNS emboli were analyzed by affected valve (Table

TABLE 2.—Stroke Prevalence by Valve and Organism

Valve	No.	Mean age* (yr)	Ischemic stroke	Ischemic stroke or non-CNS emboli	Brain hemorrhage	Mortality
Staphylococcus aureus						
Mitral	18	46	28%	33%	6%	22%
Aortic	12	54	17%	25%	33%	50%
Streptococci						
Mitral	31	47	16%	23%	3%	6%
Aortic	33	48	12%	21%	3%	9%

Note: Mortality, for all 94 episodes. Excludes cases with simultaneous mitral and aortic valve infective endocarditis. Streptococci includes all *Streptococcus* species except virulent β-hemolytic streptococci.
*Standard deviations of age ranges were 18–20 years in all groups.
(Courtesy of Hart RG, Foster JW, Luther MF, et al: *Stroke* 21:695–700, 1990.)

1). Of 133 episodes involving native mitral and/or aortic valves, brain ischemia occurred in 19%, brain hemorrhage in 7%, and non–CNS emboli in 11%. Most (74%) ischemic strokes associated with native valve endocarditis had occurred at the time of presentation. Stroke recurrence often indicated relapse/uncontrolled infection and occurred at a rate of .5% per day. Large ischemic infarcts were uncommon (9%), and all occurred in patients with *Staphylococcus aureus* infection. No important differences in the rates of stroke or systemic embolism were observed when comparing valve sites with the same infecting organism (Table 2).

Characteristics of endocarditis-associated stroke include the clustering of events during uncontrolled infection, a relatively low risk of recurrent and late embolism when infection is controlled, and an infrequency of symptomatic mycotic aneurysms. The use of anticoagulation for primary or secondary prevention of stroke complicating endocarditis is not supported. Embolism occurring before control of infection does not appear, by itself, to warrant valve replacement.

▶ Stroke is a common presenting symptom of infective endocarditis, and it will be difficult to address that incidence of stroke short of preventing endocarditis. However, a significant number of strokes occur after diagnosis. This study shows that recurrent emboli are uncommon, so that anticoagulation based on previous cerebral embolic events may be inappropriate. Perhaps all patients with endocarditis should receive anticoagulation to decrease the risk of cerebral emboli.— R.W. McPherson, M.D.

Myasthenia Gravis Presenting as Isolated Respiratory Failure
Dushay KM, Zibrak JD, Jensen WA (New England Deaconess Hosp, Boston)
Chest 97:232–234, 1990   7–21

Neuromuscular disease is part of the differential diagnosis of progressive respiratory insufficiency.

Man, 64, was thought to have obesity-hypoventilation syndrome with recurrent cor pulmonale 3 months after presenting with peripheral edema and weight gain. Increasing lethargy, weakness, exertional dyspnea, cyanosis, and weight gain ensued, and blood gases indicated worsening carbon dioxide retention and hypoxemia. Dyspnea progressed despite diuretics and intravenously administered aminophylline. Nocturnal apneic spells were described, and the patient also reported difficulty in swallowing. Respiratory distress developed fairly rapidly. There was paradoxical abdominal movement without muscle weakness elsewhere. An edrophonium test did not alter lung function. A trial of neostigmine therapy led to the resolution of diplopia and, after some time, improved respiratory mechanics. Antibody titers confirmed the presence of myasthenia gravis. Neostigmine and prednisone were given, and plasmapheresis allowed extubation.

There are no well-documented reports of myasthenia limited to the ventilatory muscles. Myasthenia gravis is a consideration when acute respiratory failure occurs. Treatment with acetylcholinesterase inhibitors and steroids was not adequate in the described patient.

▶ When a patient presents with respiratory failure and that failure is thought to be caused by neuromuscular involvement, many disease entities are considered. If there is no peripheral neuromuscular involvement, it is difficult to believe that the patient has myasthenia gravis. Despite this, these authors document such a case and point out that the diagnosis should be pursued aggressively because it can be confused in this setting.— M.C. Rogers, M.D.

Electroencephalograph in Tetanus
Luisto M, Seppäläinen A-M (Kivelä Hosp; Univ of Helsinki, Finland)
Acta Neurol Scand 80:157–161, 1989   7–22

The frequency and extent of brain damage caused by tetanus are not known. To define these parameters, 39 patients aged 21–79 years who recovered from tetanus and 39 age- and sex-matched controls underwent electroencephalographic (EEG) examination. Clinically, 26 patients with tetanus had severe, generalized convulsions, including 18 who required mechanical ventilation; 13 had only local symptoms or trismus. The median interval between first symptoms of tetanus and EEG examination was 7 years, 6 months (range, 11 months to 13 years).

Patients, after recovery from tetanus, had significantly more frequent and more severe EEG abnormalities than controls. Graded diffuse EEG abnormality was found only in patients, not in controls, and there was a trend toward higher scores for focal and paroxysmal abnormalities among patients. Twenty patients had normal EEG examination. Of 14 patients who had EEG examinations during the acute phase of tetanus, generalized EEG abnormalities were noted in 13. All 3 patients who had repeated EEGs improved with time.

This is the first controlled EEG study of posttetanus patients. After tetanus, patients may have frequent and severe EEG abnormalities, consisting mainly of diffuse slow-wave abnormalities. The EEG is helpful in revealing brain involvement in patients after tetanus.

▶ This article is provocative. Clearly, there are long-lasting changes in brain electrical function. Because most of the data are retrospective, the mechanism of injury is unclear. Unless oxygen availability is limited, short seizures do not produce cerebral oxygen deprivation. Prolonged seizures in patients who have unsecured airways may produce systemic hypoxia and cerebral oxygen deprivation.— R.W. McPherson, M.D.

Epileptic Seizures in Acute Stroke
Kilpatrick CJ, Davis SM, Tress BM, Rossiter SC, Hopper JL, Vandendriesen ML (Royal Melbourne Hosp; Univ of Melbourne, Victoria, Australia)
Arch Neurol 47:157–160, 1990   7–23

A prospective study was conducted to assess the incidence of early seizures in patients hospitalized with stroke and transient ischemic attacks (TIAs) and to determine whether seizure occurrence correlates with stroke type, pathogenesis, and outcome. Early seizures (within 2 weeks of stroke onset) occurred in 44 of 1,000 consecutive patients with stroke and TIAs, including 10 of 65 patients with lobar or extensive hemorrhage, 6 of 71 with subarachnoid hemorrhage, 24 of 370 with cortical infarctions, and 4 of 109 with hemispheric TIAs. Most seizures were single, partial, and readily controlled. Most occurred within 48 hours of stroke onset, and all seizures with subarachnoid hemorrhage occurred at stroke onset.

Early seizures occurred significantly more often in patients with cortical stroke than in those without cortical involvement, and in those with lobar hemorrhages more often than in those with cortical infarcts. Intracerebral hemorrhages secondary to a ruptured arteriovenous malformation were frequently associated with early seizures. Lacunar infarcts and deep hemorrhages were not associated with seizures. There was no significant association between infarct pathogenesis and seizure occurrence in cortical infarcts. Early seizures were not associated with higher mortality or worse functional outcome. At a mean follow-up of 7 months, 4 of 35 survivors reported recurrent seizures.

▶ This is a very nice study that clearly documents factors influencing seizures associated with stroke. These data may contribute to selective administration of antiseizure medications in patients who have had a stroke.— R.W. McPherson, M.D.

Ibuprofen-Induced Meningitis: Detection of Intrathecal IgG Synthesis and Immune Complexes

Chez M, Sila CA, Ransohoff RM, Longworth DL, Weida C (Cleveland Clinic Found; M.S. Hershey Med School, Hershey, Pa)
Neurology 39:1578–1580, 1989   7–24

Several reports have implicated ibuprofen and other arylalkanoic nonsteroidal anti-inflammatory drugs in the production of meningitis.

Man, 43, had signs of lumbar radiculopathy after a work-related injury, and myelography showed herniation of the L4-5 disk. Ibuprofen was given after the patient refused operation. Within 12 hours, headache, chills, photophobia, and increased radicular leg pain developed. Aseptic meningitis had occurred several years earlier, apparently after the patient had taken an anti-inflammatory drug. He had a severe headache after ingesting ibuprofen on several occasions. There was no indication of collagen-vascular disease. The patient was febrile and lethargic, and Kernig's and Brudzinski's signs were noted. The CSF exhibited neutrophilic pleocytosis but no bacteria. After ibuprofen was withdrawn and penicillin G given, the patient improved within 24 hours. After 4 days, an 800-mg dose of ibuprofen was given, followed within an hour by severe headache, fever, nuchal rigidity, and markedly increased radicular pain. A striking increase in CSF C1q-binding activity was seen, and calculated intrathecal IgG synthesis was markedly elevated. Improvement occurred with high-dose steroid treatment. The CSF was normal 6 weeks later.

This is the first documentation of elevated intrathecal IgG synthesis in ibuprofen-induced meningitis, which apparently involves reactivity to a specific antigen. The tendency for this form of meningitis to occur in patients with autoimmune disorders might indicate a disposition to autoreactivity or the frequent administration of nonsteroidal anti-inflammatory drugs.

▶ The increasing use of ibuprofen or other nonsteroidal anti-inflammatory drugs has resulted in the observation that these agents can produce meningitis. What is interesting about this report is that it documents the intrathecal IgG immune complex formation as the basis for this disorder. As such, it is important to recognize this as an unusual cause of immunologically mediated meningitis in the intensive care unit.—M.C. Rogers, M.D.

Carbamate and Organophosphate Poisoning in Early Childhood
Sofer S, Tal A, Shahak E (Soroka Med Ctr; Ben-Gurion Univ of the Negev, Beer-Sheba, Israel)
Pediatr Emerg Care 5:222–225, 1989   7–25

Organophosphate compound and carbamate insecticides are widely used around the world, but only a few reports of organophosphate compound poisoning in infants and young children have been published. Twenty-five infants and young children were treated for carbamate and organophosphorus compound intoxication.

The presenting signs and symptoms, different from those described in adults, were related mainly to severe CNS depression, coma and stupor, dyspnea, and flaccidity. Other signs (e.g., miosis, excessive salivation and tearing, sweaty cold skin, and gastrointestinal symptoms) were less common. Fasciculations and bradycardia were unusual on arrival. Only 2 children had all of the typical signs of organophosphate poisoning as described in adults. The signs of carbamate poisoning were indistinguishable from those of organophosphate poisoning. They included signs of myoneural and CNS cholinergic receptor involvement in addition to parasympathetic muscarinic dysfunction. Atropine sulfate had a clear beneficial effect on the CNS, as well as a peripheral antimuscarinic effect. The patients' response to treatment differs from that of older patients. Seven patients recovered completely within a day after receiving atropine, and an eighth child recovered within 2 days.

▶ This report focuses on 25 children who were treated for carbamate and organophosphorus compound intoxication. It is important because the presentation in the pediatric age group appears to be different from that in adults or older children. In children, the symptoms involve severe CNS depression including coma and flaccidity, whereas gastrointestinal symptoms and bradycardia were uncommon.—M.C. Rogers, M.D.

Correlation of Interleukin-1β and Cachectin Concentrations in Cerebrospinal Fluid and Outcome From Bacterial Meningitis
Mustafa MM, Lebel MH, Ramilo O, Olsen KD, Reisch JS, Beutler B, McCracken GH Jr (Univ of Texas, Dallas)
J Pediatr 115:208–213, 1989   7–26

Interleukin-1β (IL-1β) and cachectin (tumor necrosis factor, TNF) play a major role in the body's response to infection. In vitro studies suggest that brain cells release these cytokines after endotoxin stimulation. This is further supported by the detection of TNF in the CSF, but not in sera, of animals with meningitis induced by intracisternal inoculation of *Hemophilus* colonies or its endotoxin. Prompted by these findings, IL-1β and TNF were measured in paired CSF samples obtained from 106 infants and children with bacterial meningitis. The samples were obtained on admission to the hospital (CSF1) and 18–30 hours later (CSF2).

Both IL-1β and TNF were present in the CSF of most patients at the time of admission and again 18–30 hours later. In CSF1, IL-1β was present in 95% of patients at a mean concentration of 944 pg/mL and TNF was present in 75% at a mean concentration of 787 pg/mL. In CSF2, IL-1β was detected in 66% of patients at a mean concentration of 135 pg/mL and TNF was detected in 50% at a mean concentration of 21 pg/mL. Patients with CSF1 IL-1β concentrations ≥500 pg/mL were more likely to have neurologic sequelae, whereas CSF2 IL-1β concentrations correlated significantly with the CSF2 leukocyte count, glucose, lactate, protein, and TNF concentrations, and with neurologic sequelae. Forty-seven patients were treated with dexamethasone and 59 received placebo at diagnosis. Patients treated with dexamethasone had significantly lower mean CSF2 IL-1β concentrations and shorter duration of fever than patients treated with placebo.

There may be a role for IL-1β and TNF as mediators of meningeal inflammation in patients with bacterial meningitis. The significant inverse correlation between IL-1β concentrations and improvement in the indices of meningeal inflammation and outcome may explain, in part, the beneficial effects of dexamethasone as adjuvant therapy in bacterial meningitis.

▶ This paper reviews the levels of IL-1β and cachectin (TNF) in patients with meningitis of bacterial origin. The authors suggest that there is a possible role for IL-1β and TNF as mediators of meningeal inflammation in patients with bacterial meningitis. They use this suggestion to explain the potential beneficial role of dexamethasone as part of the treatment of this disease.—M.C. Rogers, M.D.

Diseases That Mimic Herpes Simplex Encephalitis: Diagnosis, Presentation, and Outcome

Whitley RJ, Cobbs CG, Alford CA Jr, Soong S-J, Hirsch MS, Connor JD, Corey L, Hanley DF, Levin M, Powell DA, and the NIAID Collaborative Antiviral Study Group (Univ of Alabama, Birmingham)

JAMA 262:234–239, 1989   7–27

Herpes simplex encephalitis (HSE) is a difficult disease to diagnose. The National Institute of Allergy and Infectious Diseases Collaborative Antiviral Study Group has evaluated patients with focal encephalitis presumed to be caused by herpes simplex virus (HSV). A total of 432 patients underwent brain biopsy.

Three groups of patients were identified. The first consisted of 195 patients (45%) who had HSE confirmed by isolation of HSV from brain tissue at biopsy or autopsy. The second included 95 patients (22%) with diseases that were not caused by HS. Three subgroups were identified: 38 patients (9%) had treatable diseases such as bacterial infection or cancer; 40 patients (9%) had a diagnosed viral infection for which there was no established therapy (togavirus and Epstein-Barr virus infections accounted for 24 of these 40 diagnoses); and 17 patients (4%) had identified diseases that were neither of viral etiology nor treatable. The third group included 142 patients (33%) without a diagnosis.

The historical, clinical, and neurodiagnostic assessments of patients with diseases that mimic HSE (group 2) were similar to those of patients with HSE and those without a diagnosis. Overall, morbidity was similar among patients with identified non–HSV diseases and those with HSE. Antiviral therapy appeared to be of no value to patients without HSE. Patients with nontreatable but diagnosed viral infections were most likely to return to normal.

Identification of patients with other diagnoses is relevant in treatment of a focal encephalopathic process. Brain biopsy appears to enhance the ability to diagnose HSE and to recognize other treatable conditions as well as nontreatable conditions for which antiviral therapy is of no value.

▶ The presentation of patients with symptoms that appear to be HSE is now a cause for administering antiviral therapy. Because this therapy is now so easily available, it is most important to ensure that herpes simplex is the disease being treated. Previously, brain biopsy was used, but that is no longer the clinical standard. This review, which describes 432 patients who did undergo brain biopsy, and found that only 45% of them had herpes simplex. A third of the patients had diseases that could not be clearly identified. Of the 22% who had identifiable diseases, 9% had bacterial infections or cancer. This distribution of patients indicates that herpes simplex is a diagnosis that is made in error in more than half of the patients, and that antiviral therapy may be inappropriate in patients who present with symptoms that mimic herpes but in fact have other conditions such as meningitis or cancer.—M.C. Rogers, M.D.

Placebo-Controlled Trial of Nimodipine in the Treatment of Acute Ischemic Cerebral Infarction

Martínez-Vila E, Guillén F, Villanueva JA, Matías-Guiu J, Bigorra J, Gil P, Carbonell A, Martínez-Lage JM (Clinica Universitaria de Navarra, Pamplona; Hosp Gen de la Cruz Roja, Madrid; Hosp Provincial de Navarra, Pamplona; Hosp del Insalud Virgen de los Lirios, Alcoy-Alicante, Spain)
Stroke 21:1023–1028, 1990   7–28

Nimodipine, a 1,4-dihydropyridine derivative, has preferential cerebrovascular activity in experimental animals. Clinical data suggest that this agent may have a beneficial effect on the neurologic outcome of victims of acute ischemic stroke. A double-blind, placebo-controlled, multicenter trial was initiated to assess the effects or oral nimodipine on the death rate and neurologic outcomes of 164 patients with an acute ischemic stroke.

The patients were randomly assigned to receive nimodipine tablets, 30 mg 4 times a day, or identical placebo tablets for 28 days. Treatment was

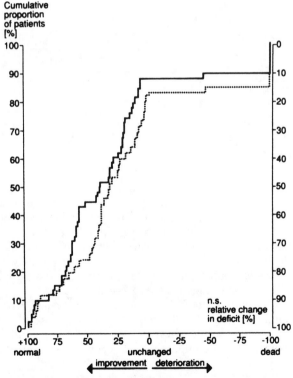

Fig 7–4.—Cumulative frequency diagram of relative change in neurologic deficit for 123 stroke patients valid for efficacy analysis. Nimodipine group *(solid line)*, no. = 58; placebo group *(broken line)*, no. = 65. (Courtesy of Martínez-Vila E, Guillén F, Villanueva JA, et al: *Stroke* 21:1023–1028, 1990.)

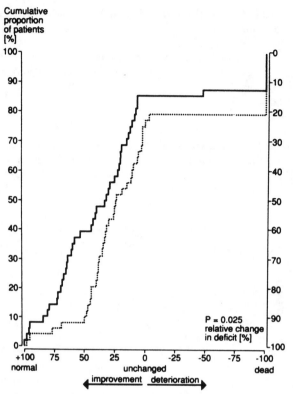

Fig 7−5.—Cumulative frequency diagram of relative change in neurologic deficit for 96 stroke patients valid for efficacy analysis with Mathew Scale sum score at baseline of 65. Nimodipine group *(solid line)*, no. = 48; placebo group *(broken line)*, no. = 48. (Courtesy of Martínez-Vila E, Guillén F, Villanueva JA, et al: *Stroke* 21:1023–1028, 1990.)

always begun 48 hours or less after the acute event. A slightly modified Mathew Scale was used to assess neurologic conditions. In all, 123 patients were assessable. Death rates did not differ between the treatment and control groups. Neurologic outcome after 28 days of treatment also did not differ between groups. However, when only patients most likely to benefit from any intervention were analyzed separately in post hoc subgroups, the subgroup treated with nimodipine had a significantly better neurologic outcome (Figs 7−4 and 7−5).

Some patients with acute ischemic stroke may benefit from treatment with nimodipine tablets. A subgroup of patients most likely to benefit from any intervention and given nimodipine had significantly better neurologic outcomes than a comparable subgroup in the control group.

▶ This study was done to test the hypothesis that neurologic outcome is improved by treatment with nimodipine within 48 hours after onset of symptoms of an acute ischemic event. Although the patients were treated with nimodipine or placebo in a randomized fashion, it is not clear whether the investigators were blinded to treatment. The nimodipine dose was submaximal at 30 mg every 6 hours. Nonetheless, patients with a Mathew Scale sum score of 65 or less who received nimodipine had a better neurologic outcome than patients receiving placebo. Perhaps the differences between groups may have even been more different if more nimodipine was administered. It is surprising that there was no difference between groups in number of cardiovascular complications.—J.R. Kirsch, M.D.

Effects of Sodium Dichloroacetate Dose: Brain Metabolites Associated With Cerebral Ischemia

Dimlich RVW, Timerding BL, Kaplan J, Cammenga R, Van Ligten PF (Univ of Cincinnati)
Ann Emerg Med 18:1172–1180, 1989   7–29

Excess brain lactate is an important cause of irreversible cell damage in cerebral ischemia. In studies of bilateral carotid ligation combined with systemic hypotension, sodium dichloroacetate (DCA), 25 mg/kg, has effectively lowered brain lactate levels. The efficacy of higher doses was examined in adult rats subjected to real or sham ischemia and sacrificed after 30 minutes of reperfusion.

Lactate levels were higher in the cerebral cortex than in the hippocampus after induction of ischemia, and DCA was most effective in lowering cortical levels. No rise in lactate occurred in the cerebellum. A dose-related effect on lactate was evident in the animals that responded. Administration of DCA did not alter adenosine triphosphate levels at any brain site. Levels of phosphocreatine in the cortex were higher in responding animals given DCA, 200 or 300 mg/kg, than on nonresponders. Glucose and glycogen levels did not change significantly with DCA.

Sodium dichloroacetate is of value in lowering brain lactate levels in animals with cerebral ischemia. Doses higher than 25 mg/kg may be optimally effective.

▶ The role of brain lactate in cerebral ischemia has been under active investigation. This is particularly true since there is increasng evidence that hyperglycemia contributes to poor brain recovery from ischemia because of the development of lactate. This remains an ambiguous area, however, with basic physiologic mechanisms not well understood. This study shows that sodium DCA can lower high levels of brain lactate, particularly when 25 mg/kg are given. Nevertheless, the real clinical utility of these measures remains to be demonstrated.— M.C. Rogers, M.D.

Cerebral Vasoreactivity to Carbon Dioxide During Cardiopulmonary Perfusion at Normothermia and Hypothermia

Johnsson P, Messeter K, Ryding E, Kugelberg J, Ståhl E (Univ of Lund, Sweden)
Ann Thorac Surg 48:769–775, 1989   7–30

The pH-stat acid-base strategy for hypothermic cardiopulmonary bypass (CPB) entails administration of carbon dioxide (CO_2) to maintain the partial pressure of CO_2 higher than with the alpha-stat method. If CO_2 vasoreactivity is preserved, the induction of "respiratory acidosis" can lead to a much higher cerebral blood flow than occurs metabolically. In 18 men undergoing coronary bypass surgery, cerebral blood flow was measured by the radioxenon washout technique before, during, and after CPB at varying CO_2 levels. Patients were operated on under both normothermic and hypothermic conditions.

Overall CO_2 reactivity was 1.2 mL/100 g/min/mm Hg, and values were not influenced by temperature of CPB. Induced hemodilution led to greater cerebral blood flow, but this was counteracted by a temperature-related reduction in the hypothermia group. Flow increased transiently after CPB in this group. The cerebral delivery rate of oxygen increased transiently in the hypothermia group but remained constant in the normothermia group.

Cerebral vasoreactivity to altered partial pressure of arterial CO_2 ($PaCO_2$) is preserved during both normothermic and hypothermic CPB. As a result, the respiratory acidosis occurring during hypothermic CPB with pH-stat management leads to cerebral hyperemia that endangers autoregulation. Alpha-stat management is the preferred approach in hypothermic CPB. This implies that a non–temperature-corrected $PaCO_2$ of about 40 mm Hg is maintained during the entire period of CPB.

▶ This study was done to test the hypothesis that alpha-stat management of arterial blood gases during CPB results in preserved cerebral blood flow reactivity to CO_2. The findings confirm data from other studies and suggest that alpha-stat management results in preserved cerebral blood flow reactivity to CO_2 during hypothermia with either CPB or spontaneous circulation. The authors appropriately speculate from their data and from the data of other laboratories that alpha-stat management of arterial blood gases is preferred because it leads to preserved autoregulation and flow-metabolism coupling. Based on data from this and other studies, there currently appears to be no good reason for the use of pH-stat management of arterial blood gases during CPB.—J.R. Kirsch, M.D.

Pericardial Effusion After Cardiac Surgery in Children and Effects of Aspirin for Prevention
Béland MJ, Paquet M, Gibbons JE, Tchervenkov CI, Dobell ARC (Montreal Children's Hosp; McGill Univ)
Am J Cardiol 65:1238–1241, 1990   7–31

To determine the incidence of pericardial effusion in children who have undergone cardiac surgery and the value of the prophylactic use of aspirin in these patients data on 74 open-heart cases were examined. An attempt was also made to identify patients at risk for effusion.

Children older than 3 months of age were eligible for the study. The median age of the group was 4 years. All had undergone palliative or corrective procedures for a variety of congenital heart diseases. Thirty-two children were randomly assigned to receive a 7-day course of aspirin (60 mg/kg/day) starting on the third postoperative day. Echocardiograms were obtained on postoperative days 4, 7, 14, and 28.

Pericardial effusions were seen in 48 patients (65%) on at least 1 of the 4 echocardiographic studies. The effusions were classified as grade 0 in 56% of the studies, grade 1 in 21%, grade 2 in 18%, grade 3 in 3%, and grade 4 in 2%. No grade 5 effusions were seen. Most effusions disappeared spontaneously without therapy. Three patients, however, required pericardiocentesis, and a fourth died of tamponade on postoperative day 20 because of delayed recognition of her condition.

Patients without an effusion in the first days after surgery were at low risk for later having a grade 4 effusion. Those with a grade 4 effusion in the first month after surgery appear to be at greater risk for cardiovascular compromise. Closure of the pericardium at the end of the surgical procedure had no effect on the rate of grade 4 effusions. Children younger than age 2 years had the same risk as older children for a significant effusion developing. Aspirin, in this small series of patients, did not significantly affect outcome.

▶ Béland et al. have provided several important insights. Although pericardial effusion is relatively common in children after cardiac surgery, only 5% will have clinically significant effusions. The risk of hemodynamic compromise is present when the size of the effusion is approximately equal to the aortic root. The mechanism of postoperative pericardial effusions remains unclear. However, these data are consistent with the concept that late effusions develop as a reaction to blood remaining in the pericardial space, because the absence of pericardial fluid (blood) on the second and third postoperative days was associated with a significantly reduced risk of late development of large pericardial effusions. The patients in this study were not closely investigated for all the features of the postpericardiotomy syndrome, so it is unclear whether effusions were related to this syndrome. Yet, the prophylactic administration of aspirin to all pediatric postoperative heart patients does not affect the incidence of effusion.—D.G. Nichols, M.D.

Myosin: A Highly Sensitive Indicator of Myocardial Necrosis After Cardiac Operations
Séguin JR, Saussine M, Ferrière M, Léger JJ, Léger J, Larue C, Calzolari C, Grolleau R, Chaptal PA (Hôp Saint Eloi; Centre de Recherche Clin-Midy, Montpellier, France)
J Thorac Cardiovasc Surg 98:397–401, 1989　　　　　　　　　7–32

Myocardial infarction remains one of the most serious complications of heart surgery. Because plasma levels of ventricular myosin fragments reportedly increase 4–5 days after infarction, levels were estimated in 27 patients having cardiac operations. Seventeen patients received 3 or more bypass grafts, and 10 had double valve replacements. Six patients having thoracic surgery via sternotomy with the same anesthesia also were assessed. Surgery was performed under hypothermic bypass with moderate hemodilution and cold crystalloid cardioplegia.

None of the patients required inotropic support, and none had arrhythmia postoperatively. Myosin levels, determined by immunoradiometric assay, were normal until the third postoperative day and peaked on day 7. Among patients having bypass graft surgery, those with perioperative infarction had higher myosin levels on postoperative days 7–12 than those without infarction. Plasma ventricular myosin levels were higher on days 4–7 after valve replacement than in patients having bypass surgery or thoracic noncardiac operations.

High plasma levels of ventricular myosin after cardiac surgery are indicative of perioperative myocardial necrosis. Myosin levels are a more reliable marker of such necrosis than either ECG changes or increased creatine kinase-MB levels.

▶ Following cardiac surgery, the detection of myocardial infarction is particularly challenging. Traditional markers of myocardial infarction such as ECG changes or determination of cardiac enzymes may be difficult to evaluate in the setting of heart surgery, for obvious reasons. These investigators conclude that the plasma level of ventricular myosin fragments is a specific and accurate marker of perioperative myocardial necrosis that is much more effective in detecting myocardial infarction than is the ECG or creatine kinase-MB level.—M.C. Rogers, M.D.

Effects of Bilateral Transvenous Diaphragm Pacing on Hemodynamic Function in Patients After Cardiac Operations: Experimental and Clinical Study
Ishii K, Kurosawa H, Koyanagi H, Nakano K, Sakakibara N, Sato I, Noshiro M, Ohsawa M (Tokyo Women's Med College; Saga Med School, Saga; Sato Clinic, Yamaguchi; Tokyo Med and Dental Univ; Seirei Hamamatsu Hosp, Shizuoka, Japan)
J Thorac Cardiovasc Surg 100:108–114, 1990   7–33

In contrast to positive-pressure breathing, diaphragmatic pacing has favorable effects on the circulation and the pacer is implantable. The safety of bilateral transvenous electrical stimulation of the phrenic nerve was examined in adult dogs. The stimulator delivered 1-msec capacitor-discharged biphasic pulses at a rate of 25 pulses per second. No arrhythmia occurred with the catheter tip more than 30 mm from the sinus node and with an applied voltage of 3.1 V or less. Aortic, pulmonary artery, and right and left atrial pressures all increased on diaphragm pacing, as did aortic flow. Similar changes occurred in animals with induced tricuspid insufficiency.

The same pacing catheter was used in 14 patients undergoing cardiac surgery. Pacing produced tidal volumes of 7.2–12 mL/kg, which sufficed to maintain normal blood gas levels. All patients recovered spontaneous breathing without weaning problems after 2–6 hours of diaphragm pacing. The average time required for recovery was 3.2 hours.

The hemodynamic sequelae of diaphragm pacing are superior to those of intermittent positive-pressure ventilation. It will be especially useful when a decrease in loading of the right heart is desired.

▶ The use of transvenous diaphragmatic pacing is now at clinical potential and has several major advantages over positive pressure respiration. Foremost among these advantages is the fact that the hemodynamic effects of diaphragmatic pacing may be superior to positive pressure ventilation. These authors clearly demonstrate, in patients, that the hemodynamic consequences of diaphragmatic pacing are better than the consequences of intermittent positive pressure ventilation. This study, which includes animal and human data, is worthy of review because of the discussion and background it gives in this interesting and developing field.—M.C. Rogers, M.D.

Internal Mammary Artery Bypass After the Arterial Switch Operation
Rheuban KS, Kron IL, Bulatovic A (Univ of Virginia)
Ann Thorac Surg 50:125–126, 1990   7–34

A right internal mammary artery to right coronary artery anastomosis was successfully performed during an arterial switch operation in a neonate with transposition.

Male infant, 3.2 kg, had findings characteristic of d-transposition with a 7-mm perimembraneous ventricular septal defect and a patent ductus on day 1 of life. A balloon atrial septostomy was performed shortly after admission, and an arterial switch procedure was performed on day 9 with closure of the ventricular and atrial septal defects and ligation of the patent ductus. When the right coronary artery was excised, little aortic tissue remained for anastomosis with the neoaorta, and the inferior cardiac wall became cyanotic on rewarming. The right internal mammary artery then was joined end-to-side to the right coronary artery and myocardial perfusion improved markedly. Normal left coronary flow was present at age 5 months, and a widely patent anastomosis was present between the internal mammary and coronary vessels. There was no anterograde flow from the aortic root through the proximal right coronary artery.

This procedure allows improved coronary perfusion and myocardial function when traditional coronary artery translocation fails or is not feasible. Further growth of the vessel is expected.

Preservation of Pancreatic Beta Cell Function With Pulsatile Cardiopulmonary Bypass
Nagaoka H, Innami R, Watanabe M, Satoh M, Murayama F, Funakoshi N
(Tsuchiura Kyodo Gen Hosp, Ibaraki, Japan)
Ann Thorac Surg 48:798–802, 1989   7–35

The effects of pulsatile cardiopulmonary bypass on insulin-glucagon relationships were examined in 38 consecutive patients, not diabetic, who underwent elective cardiac surgery. Twenty-one patients had coronary bypass grafting, and 17 had valve operations. Twenty patients had pulsatile bypass, and 18 were maintained by nonpulsatile cardiopulmonary bypass.

Blood glucose and immunoreactive insulin levels were significantly elevated during pulsatile bypass. Levels of C-peptide were elevated in both groups. Immunoreactive glucagon levels did not change significantly in either group. Lactate was increased in patients on nonpulsatile bypass. Hyperglycemia was present shortly after surgery in both groups. Patients on pulsatile bypass had higher insulin and C-peptide levels and a higher insulin/glucagon ratio an hour postoperatively. The blood lactate level was lower than in the patients on nonpulsatile bypass at this stage. Pulsatile cardiopulmonary bypass preserves pancreatic β cell function and tissue metabolism well during open-heart surgery and in the early postoperative period.

▶ The effective cardiopulmonary bypass is being studied in a wide range of organ systems that go well beyond the heart. These include the brain and, more recently, key elements of gastrointestinal, endocrinologic, and metabolic systems. This interesting paper discusses the preservation of pancreatic β cell function with the use of cardiopulmonary bypass. It concludes that pulsatile cardiopulmonary bypass is effective in preserving pancreatic β cell function and is an indicator that there may be specific settings in which pulsatile cardiopulmonary bypass may be preferred over more conventional methods.—M.C. Rogers, M.D.

Management of Extensive Right Ventricular Injury or Rupture
Slater AD, Gott JP, Tobin GR II, Gray LA Jr (Univ of Louisville; Jewish Hosp Heart and Lung Inst, Louisville)
Ann Thorac Surg 49:810–813, 1990   7–36

It may not be possible to repair extensive tears or rupture of the right ventricle with sutures, with death occurring as the result. Two patients, were successfully treated by repair with a tissue patch.

Case 1.—Man, 73, experienced cardiac arrest during balloon angioplasty. When efforts at defibrillation were unsuccessful, the patient was transferred to the operating room for open cardiac massage. During massage the assistant's thumb perforated the right ventricular outflow tract. Bypass was started, and an attempt was made to repair the defect with felt-pledgetted sutures. Because bleeding persisted, a patch of anterior pericardium was obtained and secured to the myocardium around the tear with interrupted Prolene sutures reinforced with Teflon felt.

Case 2.—Man, 53, had undergone 3-vessel coronary bypass grafting for unstable angina pectoris. When his wound failed to heal, he was returned to the operating room for débridement. Two days later, massive bleeding developed. The patient was found at surgery to have a 7-cm tear in the anterior wall of the right ventricle adjacent to the interventricular septum. Because the tear could not be closed completely with sutures reinforced with Teflon felt pledgets, surgeons obtained a 10 × 10 patch of fascia from the left anterior rectus sheath to cover the defect.

Both patients recovered. The first remains asymptomatic of cardiac disease after 3 years, and the second left the hospital on postoperative day 21 with a well-healed incision and no cardiac symptoms. The area to be treated should be compressed and early cardiopulmonary bypass should be instituted. Coverage with a tissue patch results in hemostatic control of the defect without compromise of ventricular function.

▶ Because the right ventricle sits under the interior chest wall, it is particularly susceptible to problems with trauma or laceration. These authors report their experience in right ventricular injury and rupture, and the concepts of their approach will be of interest to intensivists who care for patients in the trauma setting.—M.C. Rogers, M.D.

Alterations in Serum Creatine Kinase and Lactate Dehydrogenase: Association With Abdominal Aortic Surgery, Myocardial Infarction, and Bowel Necrosis
Graeber GM, Clagett GP, Wolf RE, Cafferty PJ, Harmon JW, Rich NM (Walter Reed Army Med Ctr, Washington, DC; Uniformed Services Univ of the Health Sciences, Bethesda, Md)
Chest 97:521–527, 1990   7–37

There is experimental evidence that serum creatine kinase (CK) and lactate dehydrogenase (LD) change after bowel infarction. A prospective study was undertaken to monitor these parameters in 15 patients with ECG evidence of acute transmural myocardial infarction, 13 undergoing aortobifemoral bypass grafting for occlusive or aneurysmal disease, and 8 with suspected bowel infarction.

All 3 groups had elevated serum levels of total CK. The elevation occurred most rapidly in those with myocardial infarction. Patients with infarction and those with bowel necrosis had increased serum CK-MB levels. Only patients with necrotic bowel had CK-BB detected in the serum in the first 24 hours. All 3 groups had elevated serum total LD levels. Patients with bowel necrosis and those having major aortic reconstruction had LD_1/LD_2 ratios below unity, whereas patients with myocardial infarction had ratios above unity. Estimates of CK and LD isoenzymes can help to distinguish between acute myocardial infarction, bowel necrosis, and the changes attending major abdominal aortic surgery.

▶ This clinical study extends experimental work from the laboratory that peripheral serum CK levels become elevated with acute bowel infarction. This is an important distinction in patients with abdominal surgery or abdominal trauma in whom serum levels of either CK-MB or CK-BB are elevated. In the absence of ECG changes, the origin of these enzymes appears to be mesenteric rather than myocardial. The authors caution, however, that this approach needs to be further evaluated through analysis of serum LB_1-LB_2 ratios.—M.C. Rogers, M.D.

Gastrointestinal Complications After Cardiac Transplantation: Potential Benefit of Early Diagnoses and Prompt Surgical Intervention
Kirklin JK, Holm A, Aldrete JS, White C, Bourge RC (Univ of Alabama, Birmingham)
Ann Surg 211:538–542, 1990   7–38

Although acute gastrointestinal (GI) illnesses after cardiac transplantation are rare, the mortality rate is high when surgery is required. In a retrospective review of 169 cardiac transplant operations, the frequency, etiology, and severity of GI complications and the value of early diagnosis and prompt surgical intervention were determined.

Between 1981 and July 1988, 31 major GI complications occurred in 26 patients at a median of 58 days after cardiac transplantation. The median age was 44 years; all 26 patients had received cyclosporine and prednisone, with or without azathioprine. The GI complications were most common within the first 30 days after transplantation and were associated with a rejection episode.

Five patients died after a GI complication, for an overall mortality rate of 16%. Two of these patients were being treated medically. Death in the other 3 patients, who underwent emergent surgical therapy, was associated with multisystem failure. All but 2 of the surviving patients received prompt surgical intervention within 48 hours after the development of symptoms, whereas 2 of 3 nonsurvivors had a delay of more than 10 days before surgery.

The immunosuppressive regimen required for transplantation may make patients vulnerable to serious GI complications. Such complications may occur in association with other morbid events that make diagnosis difficult. Early detection and prompt treatment should lower mortality rates. Surgery, when necessary, should be undertaken even in the presence of acute cardiac or multisystem dysfunction.

▶ The increasing frequency of cardiac transplant patients means that many intensivists get to see these patients on a rather routine basis. For those of us who care for these patients, the potential for GI complications is quite significant. This paper reviews the etiology and frequency of specific GI complications of cardiac transplantation that required surgical intervention and is a useful review of the subject for intensive care specialists.—M.C. Rogers, M.D.

Increased Risk of Pneumococcal Infections in Cardiac Transplant Recipients

Amber IJ, Gilbert EM, Schiffman G, Jacobson JA (Univ of Utah; VA Med Ctr, Salt Lake City; LDS Hosp, Salt Lake City; State Univ of New York, Brooklyn)
Transplantation 49:122–125, 1990   7–39

Infectious complications remain a major cause of morbidity and mortality in cardiac transplant patients. Prompted by the preliminary observation of an increased incidence of pneumococcal infection in heart transplant recipients, as compared with the general population, a prospective surveillance and retrospective chart review was conducted to determine whether cardiac transplant patients are at increased risk of pneumococcal infection.

The study included 129 patients who underwent cardiac transplantation from March 1985 through December 1987. Five patients had pneumococcal infection, yielding an estimated incidence of 36 cases per 1,000 patient-years. All 5 patients were male (mean age, 44 years), and none had previous pneumococcal vaccination. Pneumococcal infections occurred within a mean 58 days after transplantation. Three patients had pneumococcal pneumonia, 1 had bacteremia with empyema, and another had bacteremia alone. All 5 patients had an adequate number of neutrophils, but both patients with bacteremia had extremely low lymphocyte counts at the time of infection. The occurrence of pneumococcal infection did not correlate with age, sex, immunosuppression, or rejection episodes. All 5 patients recovered from their infection.

Serum antibody levels to 12 pneumococcal antigens were measured in 6 unvaccinated, uninfected patients before and after cardiac transplantation. Protective levels of antibody, defined as ≥300 ng of anticapsular antibody nitrogen per millimeter of serum, were to a mean of 8.7 pneumococcal serotypes before and a mean of 6.5 after transplantation. In 1 of these 6 patients pneumococcal pneumonia subsequently developed.

Cardiac transplant patients apparently are at increased risk of serious pneumococcal infections. Vaccinating transplant candidates before transplantation may provide protection against pneumococcal infection.

▶ This interesting paper documents that cardiac transplant recipients are at a higher risk for the development of pneumococcal infections than was previously believed. Of the 129 cardiac transplant patients followed in this study, 5 episodes of significant pneumococcal infection were documented. Interestingly, infections occurred rather late (58 days after transplantation), but they were significant, although all patients recovered. The authors conclude that cardiac transplant patients may require vaccination before transplantation, and I would add that the potential for the late onset of pneumococcal infections must be kept in mind.—M.C. Rogers, M.D.

Amrinone in Neonates and Infants After Cardiac Surgery

Lawless S, Burckart G, Diven W, Thompson A, Siewers R (Children's Hosp of Pittsburgh; Univ of Pittsburgh)
Crit Care Med 17:751–754, 1989   7–40

Amrinone is an inotropic agent that is used as adjunctive therapy for pulmonary hypertension, congestive heart failure, and postoperative low cardiac output. Despite its frequent use in critically ill pediatric patients, few data are available concerning its pharmacokinetics, proper dosage, and adverse effects. To address these issues, studies were made in 18 critically ill patients less than 1 year of age who had undergone surgery for congenital heart disease with cardiopulmonary bypass.

After surgery, patients received an intravenous bolus of amrinone at doses of up to 2.3 mg/kg, followed by a continuous intravenous infusion of 5–10 μg/kg/min. Plasma samples were obtained every 12 hours during infusion and within 24 hours after it was discontinued. Elimination half-life (T-½), total body clearance, and volume of distribution were calculated from the plasma amrinone concentrations.

The amrinone concentration at the time the infusion was discontinued ranged from 1 μg/mL to 13.7 μg/mL. Both mean elimination T-½ (22.2 hours vs. 6.8 hours) and mean total body clearance (1.1 mL/min/kg vs. 2.6 mL/min/kg) differed significantly in patients <4 weeks old compared with patients >4 weeks of age. There was a negative correlation between age and T-½ after 4 weeks of age. The frequency of platelet transfusion did not differ significantly between study patients and another sample of patients who did not receive amrinone. Except for transient hypotension during the initial bolus, which resolved with a decrease in infusion rate, no other adverse reactions, particularly arrhythmias, were observed.

These data demonstrate that, to obtain the plasma amrinone concentration that is therapeutic in adults (2–7 μg/mL), current dosage recommendations are inadequate for neonates and infants. In infants the initial intravenous bolus of amrinone should be 3–4.5 mg/kg in divided doses followed by a continuous infusion of 10 μg/kg/min. Neonates should receive a similar initial bolus followed by a continuous infusion of 3–5 μg/kg/min.

▶ There is some concern that the lack of information on the use of amrinone in neonates and infants severely limits the administration of this drug to children. Because many cardiac drugs must be modified specifically in their use in infants, these investigators looked carefully at 18 critically ill patients given amrinone in the first year of life. They concluded that to achieve the plasma concentrations of amrinone defined as therapeutic in adults, significantly higher doses of the drug are required in infants. Their conclusions, described in detail in the abstract above, are in keeping with the need to modify inotropic drugs in infants and children in a way similar to the observations made on digitalis many years ago.— M.C. Rogers, M.D.

8 Pulmonary Pathophysiology

Improved Survival in ARDS Patients Associated With a Reduction in Pulmonary Capillary Wedge Pressure
Humphrey H, Hall J, Sznajder I, Silverstein M, Wood L (Univ of Chicago Hosps and Clinics)
Chest 97:1176–1180, 1990

8–1

Adult respiratory distress syndrome (ARDS) continues to result in high mortality, even with aggressive supportive therapy. The acute lung injury that initiates ARDS leads to alveolar flooding and mechanical and gas exchange abnormalities in the lung. Animal studies have shown that a reduction of hydrostatic pressures in the pulmonary circulation, as judged by the measured pulmonary capillary wedge pressure (Ppw), reduces lung edema and improves gas exchange.

In a retrospective study the association between lowered Ppw and increased survival or a decreased stay in the intensive care unit (ICU) was studied in 20 men and 20 women (mean age, 46 years). At entry into the study the mean Ppw for all patients was 12 mm Hg. Patients were divided into 2 groups: group 1, 16 patients in whom a Ppw reduction of at least 25% was achieved, and group 2, 24 who did not have such a reduction.

Survival was significantly different in the 2 groups, even after stratification by age and severity of illness. Twelve patients from group 1 (75%) survived, but only 7 (29%) from group 2 survived. The stay in the ICU was shorter for patients in group 1 but not significantly so.

During the first 5 days after lung injury, ARDS can be considered a reversible condition. However, in patients who still require mechanical ventilatory support after 1 or 2 weeks, extensive pulmonary fibrosis and distortion of lung architecture often develop. Thus reducing lung edema in the early stages may shorten the duration and intensity of supportive therapy and improve outcome. Intervention directed at the reduction of Ppw should increase survival in these patients.

▶ Controversy continues to surround the management of patients with ARDS. One of the focal points of disagreement is fluid management. There are staunch proponents for increased fluids and maintaining a normal Ppw, or even lowering it as much as can be tolerated. Although the results of this study are interesting, their present clinical application is questionable.

This retrospective study compares patients who tolerated maneuvers to reduce the Ppw by 25% with patients who did not tolerate such maneuvers.

Even though efforts were made to correct for the severity of illness between the 2 groups, it is likely that the very nature of the study selected a group that was destined to have a better prognosis. At present, whether there is improvement in survival from ARDS associated with decreasing the amount of lung water is controversial. It is also worth noting that the ability to insure adequate perfusion of the various systems appears to be a critical determinant in the production of multisystem organ failure and potentially recurrent sepsis. The practice of lowering the Ppw, even to the point of embarrassing organ system perfusion could have disastrous consequences. The concept of lowering the wedge in ARDS should not be clinically accepted until this principle has support from a prospectively performed, randomized study with a control group.— R.A. Balk, M.D., and J.E. Parrillo, M.D.

Assessment of Routine Chest Roentgenograms and the Physical Examination to Confirm Endotracheal Tube Position
Brunel W, Coleman DL, Schwartz DE, Peper E, Cohen NH (Univ of California, San Francisco)
Chest 96:1043–1045, 1989   8–2

Malpositioning of the endotracheal tube is a serious complication of intubation. The Amerian Heart Association has recommended auscultation of the bilateral breath sounds to confirm proper positioning, but recent studies suggest that this may not be an accurate approach. The reliability of physical findings in determining the position of the endotracheal tube (ETT) was studied in 219 patients intubated for surgery or respiratory failure.

Only 7 patients were thought to have an improperly positioned ETT on physical grounds, but a review of postintubation chest films showed that 30 of the patients (14%) required repositioning. Ten had main-stem intubations, all of them after oral intubation. Among 58 patients who had no other indications for chest films, 12 required repositioning of the ETT. Use of the centimeter markings on the tube did not always prevent endobronchial placement.

Physical examination cannot be relied upon to confirm correct ETT positioning. Postintubation chest films are indicated for this purpose, particularly after emergency intubation. The lighted stylet may prove reliable in determining ETT position.

▶ Insuring proper ETT position is an important component in the process of establishing an artificial airway. Conrardy et al. (1) have previously emphasized the importance of proper positioning of the ETT and its range of motion with changes in head position. The standard practice of determining the adequacy of ETT position using clinical criteria (bilateral and equal breath sounds, bilateral and equal chest wall expansion, and ETT cuff ballotment in the suprasternal notch) were found to be unreliable in 21% of the patients in this study. Not unexpected was the finding that emergent intubations were more likely to result in mainstem bronchus intubation. This study helps to support the practice of obtaining a postintubation chest x-ray view to confirm the proper position of the ETT.—R.A. Balk, M.D., and J.E. Parrillo, M.D.

Reference

1. Conrardy PA, et al: *Crit Care Med* 4:8, 1976.

Nifedipine for High Altitude Pulmonary Oedema
Oelz O, Maggiorini M, Ritter M, Waber U, Jenni R, Vock P, Bärtsch P (Univ Hosp, Zurich; Inselspital Bern, Switzerland)
Lancet 2:1241–1244, 1989   8–3

A simple drug treatment for high-altitude pulmonary edema (HAPE) is desirable for use when descent is not feasible for any reason. High-altitude pulmonary edema is a permeability edema, and hypoxic pulmonary hypertension, probably a critical factor, is reversed in rats by calcium antagonists. The value of nifedipine, therefore, was studied in 6 men who participated in a prospective study at an altitude of 4,559 m. Five had experienced HAPE in the previous 4 years.

No unpleasant side effects occurred from treatment with 10 mg of sublingual nifedipine and 20 mg of slow-release drug. If necessary, a dose of 20 mg was given at 6-hour intervals throughout the stay at high altitude. Shortness of breath and chest pressure were relieved within an hour of treatment. Symptoms of acute mountain sickness also responded but less consistently. Hypoxemia resolved but not completely. The alveolar-arterial oxygen gradient decreased in all subjects in the first 12 hours of treatment. The pulmonary artery pressure fell to the still elevated level seen in controls and remained there.

Nifedipine is worthwhile for persons with HAPE when descent is not possible and supplementary oxygen is unavailable. Improvement, however, should not lead to continued activity at high altitude.

▶ High-altitude pulmonary edema is typically prevented by gradual ascent up the mountain, or treated by descent to lower altitude and supplemental oxygen. This study describes the potential role for calcium channel blockers, such as nifedipine, to acutely reduce pulmonary hypertension and thereby improve oxygenation in this disorder. There was also rapid improvement in the clinical symptoms of shortness of breath and chest pressure, in addition, to improvement in chest radiograph appearances. These findings may be important additions to the emergent treatment of patients with HAPE, especially when weather or other factors prohibit rapid descent. It also emphasizes the importance of pulmonary hypertension in the early symptomatology of these patients.—R.A. Balk, M.D., and J.E. Parrillo, M.D.

Clinical Validity of a Normal Perfusion Lung Scan in Patients With Suspected Pulmonary Embolism

Hull RD, Raskob GE, Coates G, Panju AA (Univ of Calgary, Alta; Chedoke-McMaster Hosps, Hamilton, Ont)
Chest 97:23–26, 1990   8–4

The safety of withholding anticoagulant treatment from patients with clinically suspected pulmonary embolism but normal perfusion lung scans was tested in 515 consecutive patients. Anticoagulant therapy was withheld or withdrawn from all but those in whom deep-vein thrombosis was detected.

At follow-up only 3 patients had symptomatic venous thromboembolism and 1 had symptomatic pulmonary embolism. With knowledge of the normal findings by perfusion scanning an alternative diagnosis could be established in 367 patients. The cause of symptoms was uncertain in 148.

Withholding anticoagulant therapy from patients with suspected pulmonary embolism and normal perfusion scans proved to be safe, regardless of the clinical manifestations. A normal perfusion scan excludes the presence of clinically important pulmonary embolism and obviates the need for pulmonary angiography.

▶ The value of a normal perfusion lung scan was assessed in this prospective study of 515 patients who presented with clinically suspected pulmonary emboli. Conventional wisdom has held that a normal ventilation/perfusion (V̇/Q̇) scan virtually eliminates the clinical possibility of significant pulmonary emboli. In this study only 1 (.2%) pulmonary embolism occurred subsequently during the 3-month follow-up period. The authors concluded that if findings on noninvasive assessment of the deep veins of the thigh and the V̇/Q̇ scan are normal, it is safe to withhold anticoagulant therapy. The potential risks and complications associated with the use of anticoagulants makes this information of tremendous importance in the initial management of patients suspected of having a pulmonary embolus. The PIOPED study (see Abstract 8–5) also confirms the low likelihood of a pulmonary embolus in the face of a normal V̇/Q̇ scan.—R.A. Balk, M.D., and J.E. Parrillo, M.D.

Value of the Ventilation/Perfusion Scan in Acute Pulmonary Embolism: Results of the Prospective Investigation of Pulmonary Embolism Diagnosis (PIOPED)

Vreim C, et al (Natl Heart, Lung, and Blood Inst, Bethesda, Md)
JAMA 263:2753–2759, 1990   8–5

A sample of 933 patients undergoing ventilation-perfusion lung scanning was studied prospectively. Pulmonary angiography was performed in 755 patients, 33% of whom had a pulmonary embolism. The patients were aged 18 years and older and were seen at 6 clinical centers in a 20-

TABLE 1.—Comparison of Scan Category With Angiogram Findings, Sensitivity and Specificity

Scan Category	Sensitivity, %	Specificity, %
High probability	41	97
High or intermediate probability	82	52
High, intermediate, or low probability	98	10

(Courtesy of Vreim C, et al.: *JAMA* 263:2753–2759, 1990.)

month period. Lung scans were done using radioxenon and ^{99m}Tc-macroaggregated albumin.

Lung scans were 98% sensitive overall in detecting pulmonary embolism but only 10% specific (Table 1). All but 14 of 116 patients with high-probability scans and definitive angiograms had pulmonary embolism, but only some of those with pulmonary embolism had high-probability scans. Embolism was present in one third of the patients with intermediate-probability scans and definitive angiograms. The angiographic and follow-up findings suggested that pulmonary embolism occurred in 12% of patients having low-probability lung scans (Table 2).

Whereas a high-probability lung scan usually indicates pulmonary embolism, only some of the affected patients have such scans. A low-probability scan makes pulmonary embolism unlikely if supported by the clinical picture. A normal or nearly normal scan makes acute pulmonary embolism very unlikely.

▶ This large prospective investigation of the value of ventilation/perfusion lung scans in assessment of patients with suspected pulmonary embolism continues to keep the uncertainty in this diagnostic entity. This condition continues to be one of the most difficult diagnoses to establish with assurance, short of performing invasive pulmonary angiography. The results of the PIOPED study confirm the low diagnostic value of the intermediate and low probability ventilation/ perfusion scan in either ruling in or ruling out the diagnosis of pulmonary embolism. As can be seen in Table 1, a high probability scan was fairly sensitive for the presence of a pulmonary embolus, and the normal or near-normal scan was

TABLE 2.—Comparison of Scan Category With Angiogram Findings

Scan Category	Pulmonary Embolism Present	Pulmonary Embolism Absent	Pulmonary Embolism Uncertain	No Angiogram	Total No.
High probability	102	14	1	7	**124**
Intermediate probability	105	217	9	33	**364**
Low probability	39	199	12	62	**312**
Near normal/normal	5	50	2	74	**131**
Total	**251**	**480**	**24**	**176**	**931**

(Courtesy of Vreim C, et al.: *JAMA* 263:2753–2759, 1990.)

helpful in excluding the diagnosis of pulmonary embolus. Of interest in this study was that pulmonary embolism was found on pulmonary angiography in 5 of 131 patients with a normal or near-normal ventilation/perfusion lung scan (see Abstract 8–4). This study sheds important light on our ability to diagnose pulmonary emboli noninvasively, and emphasizes the importance of the clinician's judgment in defining the extent of the diagnostic work-up.— R.A. Balk, M.D., and J.E. Parrillo, M.D.

Effects of Volume Loading During Experimental Acute Pulmonary Embolism

Belenkie I, Dani R, Smith ER, Tyberg JV (Univ of Calgary, Alta)

Circulation 80:178–188, 1989   8–6

Volume loading has been proposed in acute pulmonary embolism to raise the right ventricular (RV) end-diastolic volume and thereby the cardiac output. However, a leftward shift in the ventricular septum could decrease left ventricular (LV) end-diastolic volume and stroke work. The effects of volume loading were examined in anesthetized, closed-chest, ventilated dogs with increased RV afterload caused by pulmonary embolization from injected clot fragments.

The LV area index, which reflects LV volume, increased during baseline volume loading and decreased after repeated embolizations. Left ventricular stroke work increased on volume loading and decreased markedly after repeated embolizations. The decrease in the LV area index correlated with an increased septum-to-RV free wall diameter and a decreased septum-to-LV free wall diameter. Left ventricular transmural pressure decreased in response to volume loading after repeated embolizations, indicating a marked increase in pericardial pressure.

Volume loading can cause hemodynamic deterioration after pulmonary embolism in this model through both a leftward septal shift and increased pericardial pressure. In addition, LV transmural pressure (preload) is reduced. Stroke work declines by the Frank-Starling mechanism. It should not be assumed that volume loading will help patients who are hemodynamically impaired after acute pulmonary embolism. If it is attempted, it might be worthwhile to monitor the estimated transmural LV end-diastolic pressure.

▶ This elaborate and well-done study evaluated the effect of volume loading as part of the acute resuscitative efforts in the treatment of hemodynamically unstable pulmonary embolism. Initially, LV function improved with volume loading. However, after repeated embolization there was a decrease in LV systolic function. The mechanism for the decrease in ventricular function in this anesthetized canine model of repeated embolization appears to be related to the decrease in LV end-diastolic volume that is mediated by increased pericardial constraint and a leftward shift of the intraventricular septum. Volume loading produces an increase in right heart volume and pressure and results in increased pericardial pressure. The increased pulmonary artery resistance results in a greater increase in right-sided pressures compared to LV end-diastolic pressure and leads to the bulging of the intraventricular septum into the left ventricle.

This study raises some valid concerns for caution when using volume loading without the guidance of hemodynamic monitors in the acute management of hemodynamically unstable patients with pulmonary emboli. These observations warrant further evaluation in patients with massive pulmonary emboli.—R.A. Balk, M.D., and J.E. Parrillo, M.D.

Mechanisms of Pulsus Paradoxus in Airway Obstruction
Viola AR, Puy RJM, Goldman E (Hosp Nacional María Ferrer, Buenos Aires; Ohio State Univ Hosp)
J Appl Physiol 68:1927–1931, 1990   8–7

Pulsus paradoxus refers to an inspiratory decrease of 10 mm Hg or more in systolic blood pressure. It is a common finding in patients with severe airway obstruction. Transmission of the increased swings in pleural pressure to the intrathoracic vasculature could explain this phenomenon. Alternatively, a decrease in left ventricular stroke volume during inspiration may be responsible.

Twelve patients with chronic airflow obstruction before and during breathing through an external resistance that provided loads during inspiration and expiration were studied to assess the mechanisms of pulsus paradoxus. Esophageal pressure (Ppl) and brachial artery pressure, relative to atmospheric (Pa) or esophageal pressure (Pa_{tm}), were measured in each patient during normal and loaded breathing.

There were no significant differences between systolic fluctuation (ΔPa) and pleural pressure swings (ΔPpl) during the control period. Inspiratory and expiratory Pa_{tm} were almost identical. Under maximally loaded conditions, however, higher magnitudes of ΔPpl than ΔPa were noted. The Pa_{tm} consequently rose with inspiration. The plot of ΔPa against ΔPpl demonstrated that the slopes for ΔPpl of 15 mm Hg of less and ΔPpl of more than 15 mm Hg were significantly different. Under all experimental conditions there was a rise in diastolic Pa_{tm} during inspiration that was consistent with an increase in left ventricular afterload.

Direct transmission of intrapleural pressure to the vascular tree is the primary explanation for the nearly equal ΔPpl and ΔPa. With increasing ΔPpl, smaller pressure fluctuation in the artery than in the thorax further supports direct transmission and suggests the presence of certain mechanisms attenuating the inspiratory drop in blood pressure in severe airway obstruction.

▶ The magnitude of the pulsus paradoxus has been considered an index of the severity of airflow obstruction in patients with obstructive lung disease. There has been controversy over the mechanism responsible for the paradoxical pulse in this group of patients. This study evaluated 12 patients with airflow obstruction and concluded that direct transmission of the intrathoracic pressure to the vascular tree was the primary determinant of the pulsus paradoxus in patients with airway obstruction. It is important to remember, however, that there are reports of poor correlation of the paradoxical pulse and the degree of airflow obstruction. In these circumstances, pulsus paradoxus may be related to pulmonary hyperinflation, pulmonary flow rates, and changes in the breathing pattern.— R.A. Balk, M.D., and J.E. Parrillo, M.D.

Effects of Intravenous Fat Emulsion on Respiratory Failure
Hwang T-L, Huang S-L, Chen M-F (Chang Gung Mem Hosp; Chang Gung Med College, Taipei, Taiwan)
Chest 97:934–938, 1990   8–8

A high glucose intake during administration of total parenteral nutrition can increase carbon dioxide (CO_2) production. High CO_2 production may precipitate respiratory distress in patients whose pulmonary function is compromised. Fat emulsions may serve as a source of nonprotein calories and have been associated with less CO_2 production than glucose. Intravenous infusion of a fat emulsion is widely used in critically ill patients as a source of calories for parenteral nutritional support. The effects of intravenous fat emulsion on ventilated normal, diseased, or distressed lungs were investigated in 48 patients with different types of respiratory failure.

The patients were divided into 4 groups: normal lung condition, infectious pulmonary condition and respiratory failure, chronic obstructive pulmonary disease and repiratory failure, and adult respiratory distress syndrome (ARDS). Ten percent fat emulsion, 500 mL, was infused in 4 hours as partial parenteral nutritional support. Intravenous fat infusion reduced the partial pressure of oxygen in arterial blood/fraction of oxygen in inspired air (PaO_2/FIO_2) and increased the alveolar-arterial oxygen ($P(A-a)O_2$) difference and intrapulmonary shunt in the patients with ARDS. It had little effect on patients with infectious pulmonary disease or chronic obstructive pulmonary disease. The fat emulsion infusion had positive effects on the patients with normal lungs, with increased PaO_2/FIO_2 and reduced $P(A-a)O_2$ and shunt.

There appear to be no advantages or disadvantages to giving a fat emulsion to patients with infectious lung conditions and chronic obstructive pulmonary disease. Patients with disrupted alveolar capillary membrane had reduced PaO_2/FIO_2, increased $P(A-a)O_2$, and intrapulmonary shunting. Because fat emulsion can change ventilation-perfusion inequalities, the apparent reduction in diffusion capacity might actually represent an increased ventilation-perfusion inequality for CO rather than a decreased diffusion capacity.

▶ There are still many unresolved issues in the nutritional management of the critically ill. There is widespread acceptance that nutritional support has many benefits in critically ill patients; however, there are a growing number of reports and anecdotes emphasizing that this therapeutic modality must be individualized to a given patient's needs. The finding that lipid solutions may spare the excess CO_2 production associated with carbohydrate metabolism in patients with limited ventilatory reserves has led to their widespread use in clinical practice. This article details the potential detrimental effects on oxygenation associated with the infusion of intralipid in patients with capillary permeability defects as seen in ARDS. These findings are very important and will likely have much clinical utility, because lipid infusions have become a major component of parenteral nutrition. The observation that the oxygenation abnormalities could be helped by slowing the infusion to an 8-hour rate instead of a 4-hour rate may be what is needed to continue to utilize this form of therapy in this cohort of patients. As with many therapeutic endeavors, it appears that nutritional management may also involve balancing potential risks and benefits and therefore require individualized decisions, rather than simply looking up a formula in one's "cookbook."—R.A. Balk, M.D., and J.E. Parrillo, M.D.

Isoflurane for Refractory Status Epilepiticus: A Clinical Series
Kofke WA, Young RSK, Davis P, Woelfel SK, Gray L, Johnson D, Gelb A, Meeke R, Warner DS, Pearson KS, Gibson JR Jr, Koncelik J, Wessel HB (Univ of Pittsburgh; Yale Univ; Wright State Univ, Dayton, OH; Univ of Western Ontario, London, Ont; Cork Regional Hosp, Wilton, Cork, Ireland; et al)
Anesthesiology 71:653–659, 1989   8–9

Isoflurane may be preferable to halothane in controlling seizures because it can produce electroencephalographic (EEG) suppression at concentrations not usually associated with adverse hemodynamic effects and because it lacks known organ toxicity. Isoflurane was evaluated 11 times in 9 patients with convulsive generalized status epilepticus or subtle status epilepticus.

Isoflurane substantially attenuated EEG and convulsive seizure activity or stopped activity in all instances. Fluid administration and/or pressor support was consistently necessary. Seizures recurred in 8 of 11 instances when isoflurane was withdrawn. All 3 surviving patients had cognitive deficits. Two patients had multiorgan failure after isoflurane administration.

Isoflurane effectively controls intractable seizures but, until more definitive results are available, it cannot be recommended as a first-line anesthetic to control convulsive status epilepticus. Isoflurane may be used when intravenous agents such as barbiturates and benzodiazepines fail to control seizure activity or produce physical dependence. Isoflurane also is useful if intravenous anesthetics produce unacceptable hemodynamic sequelae.

▶ This article is a collection of case reports clearly showing that isoflurane temporarily suppresses seizure activity. The extremely poor outcome of this group suggests that seizures refractory to conventional medications may be stopped temporarily with isoflurane but the outcome is not improved.— R.W. McPherson, M.D.

Early Administration of Corticosteroids in Emergency Room Treatment of Acute Asthma

Stein LM, Cole RP (Columbia Univ)
Ann Intern Med 112:822–827, 1990   8–10

Corticosteroids are effective in asthma refractory to other therapies, but their effectiveness in treating acute exacerbations is less clear. Early administration of high-dose intravenous corticosteroids and the effect on duration of emergency room treatment and hospital admission were investigated in a double-blind, randomized, placebo-controlled trial in a large urban hospital. Eighty-one patients aged 18–45 years with acute bronchial asthma and without pneumonitis or other serious underlying illnesses were studied during 91 patient visits to the emergency room.

Initially, all patients received aerosolized metaproterenol, followed by 125 mg of methylprednisolone intravenously or normal saline (control). Additional treatment included aerosolized metaproterenol and oral theophylline. Six hours after entry into the study, those who still required treatment received 40 mg of methylprednisolone intravenously at 6-hour intervals until hospital discharge or admission. Hospitalization was mandatory when total treatment time was longer than 12 hours.

Age, sex, peak expiratory flow at entry, and prevalence of recent use of corticosteroids were similar in both the steroid-treated and control groups. The duration of emergency room treatment, percentage of patients requiring hospitalization, and frequency of return visits because of acute asthma 2 days after emergency room discharge did not differ significantly between the treatment groups. The peak expiratory flow (PEF) after 2 hours of intensive bronchodilator therapy was significantly reduced in patients who required hospital admission. Administration of oral corticosteroids at discharge did not influence the frequency of return visits.

The overall outcome for patients with acute exacerbations of asthma is not improved by early administration of high-dose corticosteroids intravenously. It appears that routine administration of corticosteroids to these patients at initial presentation may not be warranted.

▶ Steroids are effective in the treatment of asthmatic episodes that are refractory to standard therapies. However, their role in the early management of asthmatic attacks is controversial. This study by Stein and Cole indicates that early administration of steroids does not lead to improved resolution of asthma within the first 6 hours in the emergency room. Similarly, steroid administration on arrival at the emergency room did not affect the number of patients requiring hospital admission at 12 hours. These results suggest that steroids should not be given routinely to asthmatics presenting with acute exacerbation. Of note, however, patients eventually requiring admission had substantially lower peak expiratory flow rates 2.5 hours after arrival in the emergency room. Evaluating the efficacy of treatment at this point using these flow rate measurements may provide a means of identifying patients who are unlikely to improve. These data can then be used as a basis on which to administer steroids early to this subset of patients.—M.J. Breslow, M.D.

Effect of Increased Intracranial Pressure on Regional Hypoxic Pulmonary Vasoconstriction
Domino KB, Hlastala MP, Cheney FW (Univ of Washington)
Anesthesiology 72:490–495, 1990   8–11

Many patients with injury to the CNS have hypoxemia in the absence of clinical or physiologic evidence of lung abnormalities. When intracranial pressure (ICP) is increased, the sympathetic nervous system is activated and cardiac output, mixed venous oxygen tension, pulmonary artery pressure, and pulmonary venous pressure are all increased. These changes may inhibit regional hypoxic pulmonary vasoconstriction (HPV) and the result is reduced diversion of flow from hypoxic to normoxic lung regions. The effects of increased ICP and cardiac output on the pulmonary vascular response to regional alveolar hypoxia were investigated in 6 phenobarbital-anesthetized dogs with closed chests.

After a bronchial divider was inserted, the right lung was continuously ventilated with 100% oxygen while the left lung was ventilated with either 100% oxygen or a hypoxic gas mixture. The response to left lung alveolar hypoxia was studied before, during, and after the ICP was increased by infusion of mock CSF into a lateral ventricle to yield a cerebral perfusion pressure of 25 mm Hg. During both control periods cardiac output was randomly altered by opening or closing 2 arteriovenous fistulas.

Increasing the ICP significantly increased cardiac output, pulmonary artery pressure, and mixed venous oxygen tension, compared with normal cardiac output in controls. Similar increases were obtained by opening the arteriovenous fistula. During hyperoxic conditions the mean percentage of blood flow to the left lung was 43.9% and did not vary with manipulation of cardiac output or ICP. In contrast, during hypoxia the mean percentage of blood flow to the left lung was significantly increased by both increased ICP and high cardiac output. Therefore, flow diversion with HPV was reduced equally by both increasing ICP and cardiac output. Ventilation-perfusion matching did not change with increased ICP. These data suggest that impaired oxygenation with increased ICP may be partly the result of attenuation of regional HPV, which is caused by increased cardiac output.

▶ This animal study shows that decreasing cerebral perfusion pressure to 25 mm Hg moderately diminishes hypoxic pulmonary vasoconstriction. It is unlikely that this degree of pulmonary abnormality will result in hypoxemia if a high inspired oxygen concentration is used.—R.W. McPherson, M.D.

Respiratory and Hemodynamic Effects of Halothane in Status Asthmaticus

Saulnier FF, Durocher AV, Deturck RA, Lefèbvre MC, Wattel FE (Hôp Albert Calmette, Lille, France)
Intensive Care Med 16:104–107, 1990   8–12

Inhalational anesthetics (e.g., halothane) are often used for anesthesia in asthmatic patients. The effects of halothane were studied in 12 patients with status asthmaticus who required mechanical ventilation. A flow-generated ventilator was used to administer 1% halothane for 30 minutes.

The peak inspiratory pressure fell significantly after halothane administration. The dead space-tidal volume ratio decreased significantly. The $PaCO_2$ was decreased by 10 mm Hg 30 minutes after halothane administration and the pH rose significantly. Intravascular pressures decreased after halothane, whereas cardiac index, vascular resistances, and the left ventricular stroke work index remained normal. The mean systemic blood pressure decreased but remained at acceptable levels. Arrhythmias did not develop during halothane exposure.

Halothane rapidly controls bronchospasm in patients with status asthmaticus and improves respiratory efficiency. Adverse hemodynamics are not observed. Administration of 1% halothane appears to be effective.

▶ The salutary effects of halothane in status asthmaticus are clearly demonstrated in the absence of surgical stimulation. This study supports previous anesthesia literature concerning bronchospasm resolution attributable to halothane.— R.W. McPherson, M.D.

Barotrauma Related to Inhalational Drug Abuse

Seaman ME (Valley Med Ctr, Fresno, Calif)
J Emerg Med 8:141–149, 1990   8–13

Twenty-five cases of barotrauma after inhalation of cocaine were reported in the last decade. Other drugs (e.g., marijuana and nitrous oxide) have also caused pneumomediastinum. In the 3 case reports, the inhalation of cocaine and an amphetamine resulted in barotrauma. One patient had a "clicking pneumothorax" and the others had pneumomediastinum.

Man, 19, had pleuritic chest pain after inhaling amphetamine. Subcutaneous emphysema was evident on examination of the neck, and a Hamman's sign was noted during cardiac auscultation. Radiographs showed elevation of the pleura along the left mediastinal border, a collection of retrosternal air, air posterior to the cardiac silhouette, and air outlining the aorta. By the second hospital day the patient had no symptoms and was released. Although the pneumomediastinum persisted, there was no increase in the mediastinal air.

The other 2 patients, also young men, had smoked cocaine. Both went to the emergency department with sharp, pleuritic chest pain. One patient was discharged after 2 days, but the third patient was found to have a pneumothorax and required tube thoracostomy.

Subcutaneous emphysema and the presence of Hamman's crunch are the principal signs of pneumomediastinum in cocaine abusers. The diagnosis is supported by radiographic evidence of gas collections within mediastinal structures and air in the neck that has escaped from the mediastinum.

Cocaine and amphetamines both have potent vasoconstrictive properties that may lead to increased pressure gradients between the alveolus and interstitium. Use of the Valsalva maneuver during inhalation of cocaine may lower the interstitial pressure. Patients with barotrauma after inhalational drug abuse often require analgesics and oxygen therapy. They should avoid strenuous activities for several weeks so as not to promote further dissection of air from the lungs to the mediastinum.

▶ Another interesting complication of cocaine abuse is presented that should be considered in the evaluation of patients admitted for cocaine toxicity.—R.W. McPherson, M.D.

Hydrochlorothiazide-Induced Acute Pulmonary Edema
Kavaru MS, Ahmad M, Amirthalingam KN (Cleveland Clinic Found; Trumbull Meml Hosp, Warren, Oh)
Cleve Clin J Med 57:181–184, 1990   8–14

Acute noncardiogenic pulmonary edema is a rare life-threatening complication of hydrochlorothiazide therapy. In 1 new case and 16 previously reported cases the mean age of the patients was 54 years. Of the 17 patients, 16 were women.

Hydrochlorothiazide-induced pulmonary edema appeared to have a sudden onset, with an average of 50 minutes from drug ingestion to onset of symptoms. Patients were acutely ill with hypotension and hypoxemia. Dyspnea was present in 16 of 17 cases, and there were systemic manifestations such as fever, chills, and gastrointestinal symptoms. Chest films showed bilateral diffuse pulmonary infiltrates, usually without cardiomegaly. Hemodynamic studies in 7 patients supported a noncardiogenic etiology.

Most patients recovered rapidly. Chest film appearances and oxygen saturation normalized within a mean of 5 days. Therapy was usually supportive; 5 patients required mechanical ventilation for a mean of 2 days. There were no fatalities.

Hydrochlorothiazide-induced pulmonary edema appears to be specific for hydrochlorothiazide alone and does not occur with other thiazide preparations. It has occurred with or without previous exposure to the drug. This syndrome has developed in patients receiving intermittent therapy with hydrochlorothiazide but not in those receiving chronic daily therapy with the drug.

Despite the widespread use of hydrochlorothiazide and the potential seriousness of this reaction, little information about hydrochlorothiazide-induced pulmonary edema has appeared in the literature. Acute noncardiogenic pulmonary edema should be considered in the differential diagnosis in patients with bilateral pulmonary infiltrates and exposure to hydrochlorothiazide.

▶ This case report and review of 16 previously reported cases is interesting for the discussion it develops on noncardiogenic pulmonary edema. Apparently, this condition can occur with or without previous exposure to the agent. Although rare, this is exactly the kind of complication from the use of a common drug that intensivists need to know in order to function in the intensive care unit.—M.C. Rogers, M.D.

Comparison of Bronchial and Per Oral Provocation With Aspirin in Aspirin-Sensitive Asthmatics
Dahlén B, Zetterström O (Karolinska Inst, Stockholm)
Eur Respir J 3:527–534, 1990   8–15

For reasons that are not clear, very severe reactions develop in some asthmatics after they ingest aspirin. Most of these patients have severe, chronic asthma of the endogenous type with nasal symptoms. Patients do not always recognize sensitivity to nonsteroidal anti-inflammatory drugs. Oral challenge with acetylsalicylic acid was compared with inhalation of lysine acetylsalicylic acid for diagnosing aspirin idiosyncracy in 17 asthmatics and 5 patients with chiefly nasal symptoms. The patients underwent both oral and bronchial provocation.

Significant bronchoconstriction occurred in 10 patients during either challenge; the 2 tests had the same absolute sensitivity. Reactions occurred about 20 minutes after bronchial provocation and 1 hour after oral administration. Reactions to orally administered aspirin often were more marked and lasted longer, and generalized symptoms occurred more frequently. Asthmatics with comparably severe disease did not have bronchoconstriction in response to lysine acetylsalicylic acid. More medication was needed to reverse the reactions to oral administration.

Bronchial provocation testing with acetylsalicylic acid is easily controlled, even in severe asthmatics, and is readily interpreted. It also may be safer than the oral test. Oral provocation, however, is necessary to diagnose extrapulmonary features of aspirin sensitivity.

▶ Approximately 10% to 20% of adult asthmatics respond to the ingestion of aspirin with severe bronchoconstriction. Historically, it has been recognized that the combination of asthma, rhinorrhea, and nasal polyps is a good marker for aspirin sensitivity that induces bronchoconstriction. This study considered whether or not these patients could be recognized by all challenges or by inhalation with lysine acetylsalicylic acid. The bronchial provocation method appeared best, and this is a useful contribution. More importantly, this is a very good review of the basis of the airway response and an analysis of the provocation and treatment of patients with aspirin-induced bronchoconstriction.— M.C. Rogers, M.D.

High-Frequency Oscillatory Ventilation and Extracorporeal Membrane Oxygenation for the Treatment of Acute Neonatal Respiratory Failure
Carter JM, Gerstmann DR, Clark RH, Snyder G, Cornish JD, Null DM Jr, deLemos RA (Wilford Hall USAF Med Ctr, Lackland AFB, Tex; Southwest Found for Biomedical Research, San Antonio)
Pediatrics 85:159–164, 1990   8–16

For the past 15 years, extracorporeal membrane oxygenation (ECMO) has been used to treat neonates in acute respiratory failure. Although the procedure has had success, its safety has been questioned. Fifty infants admitted for ECMO were first given high-frequency oscillatory ventilation (HFOV) as a rescue therapy before resorting to ECMO support.

All of the infants had severe acute cardiorespiratory failure that did not respond to conventional ventilatory and pharmacologic treatment. Four infants died before either treatment could be initiated. Twenty-one responded to HFOV with improved oxygenation and stabilized cardiovascular status. The remaining 25 infants had persistent, severe hypoxia despite HFOV rescue and were subsequently given ECMO treatment.

Responders to HFOV had a younger gestational age (38 weeks) than the nonresponders (40 weeks). Nonresponders were slightly more hypoxic and hypercarbic at the start of HFOV treatment than those who responded favorably. Eleven of the responders to HFOV, but only 2 of the nonresponders, had pneumonia. None of the infants with congenital diaphragmatic hernia responded to HFOV. Survival to hospital discharge was 100% in infants treated with HFOV and 88% for those receiving EMCO. Complications appeared related to treatment modality, with bleeding abnormalities, seizures, and acute renal failure greater in EMCO-treated HFOV nonresponders.

Because nearly half of the infants required only HFOV, this treatment modality should be considered for certain infants with acute respiratory failure. Determining which patients are likely to respond to HFOV, EMCO, or combined treatments should help to maintain the best possible risk to benefit ratio.

▶ This study looks at the use of HFOV and/or ECMO in the treatment of acute neonatal respiratory failure. The conclusion is that some patients benefit from one therapy and some benefit from the other. The authors tried to understand the reasons for this finding, but failed to reach any meaningful conclusion. I agree with the authors that "It is unlikely that there will be any single therapy that will be 'optimal'. . . ."—M.C. Rogers, M.D.

Vitamin E Deficiency and Lipoperoxidation During Adult Respiratory Distress Syndrome

Richard C, Lemonnier F, Thibault M, Couturier M, Auzepy P (Hôp de Bicêtre, Université Paris-Sud, Paris)
Crit Care Med 18:4–9, 1990   8–17

The mechanism of lung injury in adult respiratory distress syndrome (ARDS) is not yet completely understood. However, vitamin E acts as a chain-breaking antioxidant and thus inhibits lipid peroxidation associated with the loss of functional integrity of the pulmonary endothelial cell barrier. To determine whether ARDS is associated with a decrease in vitamin E plasma levels linked to an increase in lipoperoxide plasma levels as an indication of enhanced lipoperoxidation, vitamin E, lipoperoxides, total lipids, and fatty acid plasma levels were measured in 8 men and 4 women aged 36–82 years with ARDS caused by pulmonary or extrapulmonary sepsis. All patients were on mechanical ventilation. The same tests were performed in a group of healthy controls breathing room air.

At the onset of ARDS, patients had significantly decreased vitamin E plasma levels when compared with normal controls. This decrease in vitamin E was associated with an increase in lipoperoxide plasma levels. Lipoperoxide plasma levels were inversely correlated with vitamin E plasma levels (Fig 8–1). Plasma vitamin E deficiency was associated with a low level of total plasma lipids and plasma cholesterol. Patients with ARDS also had a significant decrease in essential fatty acid, linoleic acid,

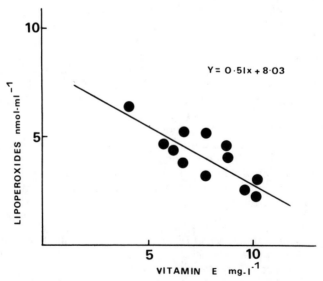

Fig 8–1.—Correlation between vitamin E and lipoperoxide plasma levels at the onset of ARDS, $r = .78$, $P < .01$, df = 10. (Courtesy of Richard C, Lemonnier F, Thibault M, et al: Crit Care Med 18:4–9, 1990.)

and arachidonic acid plasma levels, and a significant increase in the oleic/linoleic acid ratio when compared with control values.

During the first 24 hours after ARDS onset, there was a significant decrease in lipoperoxide plasma levels associated with a decrease in vitamin E plasma levels plotted against time. There was no significant change in the vitamin E/total lipid ratio or the oleic/linoleic acid ratio during the first 24 hours after the onset of ARDS. The low basal vitamin E plasma levels were probably a consequence of malnutrition. The decreases in vitamin E plasma levels observed during the first 24 hours after ARDS onset were probably the result of increased vitamin E utilization or decreased vitamin E absorption.

Adult respiratory distress syndrome is associated with vitamin E deficiency and increased plasma lipoperoxide levels. Vitamin E plasma levels do not correlate with the risk of acute respiratory failure developing, or with the overall course or prognosis of the disease. However, because vitamin E is capable of preventing oxidant-mediated cytotoxicity, critically ill patients should be given parenteral vitamin E supplementation, as this might delay the onset of acute respiratory failure.

▶ This interesting paper documents that the vitamin E plasma level is decreased in the course of ARDS. This observation, in turn, raises the question of whether or not the vitamin E plasma level is decreased as a cause of the disease or as a response to it. Because vitamin E plays such a key role in lipoperoxidation, these observations are worth further investigations. Intensivists should be cautioned, however, that these observations are too preliminary to raise the potential for treating patients with vitamin E in the face of ARDS. Clearly, a lot more work needs to be done before these thoughts can be considered.—M.C. Rogers, M.D.

Clinical Efficacy and Cost Benefit of Pulse Flow Oxygen in Hospitalized Patients
Kerby GR, O'Donohue WJ, Romberger DJ, Hanson FN, Koenig GA (Univ of Kansas; Creighton Univ, Omaha)
Chest 97:369–372, 1990   8–18

Intermittent pulse-flow oxygen delivery devices are promising tools for oxygen conservation. In previous studies in the intensive care unit, pulse-flow oxygen offered equivalent arterial PO_2 values, 55% to 60% oxygen savings, and no reduction of nasal humidity compared with continuous-flow nasal cannula oxygen. The clinical efficacy and cost benefit of pulse-flow and continuous-flow oxygen were compared in 100 patients recently hospitalized for diseases requiring oxygen therapy. Pulse and continuous oxygen were administered alternately during 4 sessions of 5½ hours in an unblinded crossover manner.

Oxygen saturation during pulse flow (mean, 95.6%) was clinically equivalent to oxygen saturation during continuous flow (mean, 95.3%). The mean oxygen saturation between the 30-minute crossover periods was not significantly different. Analysis of potential savings, when the pulse-flow delivery device is used in a 350-bed hospital, suggests a saving of about $55,000 annually, largely because of elimination of oxygen humidifiers.

▶ There is the thought that every new medical technology raises a new expense without any compensatory cost savings. This paper documents that pulse-flow oxygenation may be helpful in saving hospital expense.

This minor adaptation of existing techniques of oxygen delivery can save tens of thousands of dollars a year per hospital and is really worth noting. Unless intensivists can find ways to save money for the hospital, they will not be able to continue to spend money for the hospital.—M.C. Rogers, M.D.

Acute Eosinophilic Pneumonia as a Reversible Cause of Noninfectious Respiratory Failure
Allen JN, Pacht ER, Gadek JE, Davis WB (Ohio State Univ)
N Engl J Med 321:569–574, 1989   8–19

Four patients were seen in the past 2 years with a distinct form of idiopathic lung disease presenting as acute respiratory failure. The patients, all previously healthy, had marked eosinophilia in the bronchoalveolar lavage fluid. Infectious causes of lung disease were excluded, and the patients responded promptly to steroid therapy.

The patients had an acute febrile illness for less than a week when first seen. Severe hypoxemia was present, and there were diffuse lung infiltrates. Lavage fluid contained more than 25% eosinophils, and the average was 42% of effector cells. Erythromycin therapy was ineffective, but the dyspnea, infiltrates, and hypoxemia resolved rapidly when steroid therapy was begun. Symptoms did not recur after prednisone was tapered during follow-up ranging from 5 to 21 months. Lavage fluid at this time contained 1% or fewer eosinophils. Differential cell counts should be done routinely on bronchoalveolar lavage specimens because acute eosinophilic pneumonia may be clinically indistinguishable from acute infectious pneumonia and adult respiratory distress syndrome.

▶ This interesting observation on acute eosinophilic lung disease was of particular interest to me. In the past decade I have met with other individuals who have seen an occasional patient with acute pneumonia characterized by diffused pulmonary infiltrates and an increased number of eosinophils in the bronchoalveolar lavage fluid. These investigators document this as a distinct syndrome, and it is likely, now that it is recognized, that there will be increasing reports of this entity.—M.C. Rogers, M.D.

Functional Loss of Chemotactic Factor Inactivator in the Adult Respiratory Distress Syndrome

Robbins R, Maunder R, Gossman G, Kendall T, Hudson L, Rennard S (Omaha VA Med Ctr; Univ of Nebraska)
Am Rev Respir Dis 141:1463–1468, 1990   8–20

Current concepts suggest that acute respiratory distress syndrome (ARDS) is characterized by neutrophilic alveolitis in the lung that, in part, may be the result of activation of the potent neutrophil chemotactic factor C5a. Because chemotactic factor inactivator (CFI) can reduce C5a-directed neutrohil chemotaxis, loss of CFI activity in the ARDS lung could result in increased ability of C5a to attract neutrophils. To test this hypothesis, the antigenic and functional levels of CFI were measured in bronchoalveolar lavage (BAL) fluid obtained from 29 patients with ARDS and 14 normal nonsmoking controls.

Antigenic levels of CFI were markedly elevated in the patients with ARDS, compared to controls. In contrast, functional levels of CFI were markedly decreased in ARDS BAL fluid, compared with those in normal BAL fluid, and there was no correlation between the antigenic and functional amounts of CFI.

To determine whether CFI was an important inhibitor of C5a-induced chemotaxis in BAL, normal and BAL fluids were fractionated at less than 45%, 45%–65%, and greater than 65% ammonium sulfate saturation. The 45% to 65% fraction containing CFI caused significant inhibition of C5a-induced neutrophil chemotaxis, and depleting this fraction resulted in significantly reduced inhibitory activity. Furthermore, although purified CFI inhibited the C5a-directed neutrophil chemotactic activity, this activity was decreased when ARDS BAL fluid was incubated with CFI.

These findings suggest that patients with ARDS are functionally deficient in CFI, resulting in an increased ability of C5a to attract neutrophils. The loss of CFI activity may play a role in the pathogenesis of ARDS.

▶ Among the interesting observations in ARDS is the fact that there is an accumulation of neutrophils in the ARDS lung. Mechanisms for explaining this phenomenon remain unclear, and these investigators have documented that patients with ARDS are functionally deficient in CFI. In turn, this leads to an increased ability of C5a to attract neutrophils. This interesting and important observation on the interrelationship between chemotactic factor inactivator (CFI) and the accumulation of neutrophils may be related to the underlying ARDS or to the ability of patients with ARDS to respond to immunologic problems. In either event, this is an important observation that is at the heart of explaining the inflammatory response of the lung in ARDS.—M.C. Rogers, M.D.

Prolonged Neuromuscular Blockade After Long-Term Administration of Vecuronium in Two Critically Ill Patients

Segredo V, Matthay MA, Sharma ML, Gruenke LD, Caldwell JE, Miller RD (Univ of California, San Francisco)
Anesthesiology 72:566–570, 1990   8–21

Vecuronium often is used for neuromuscular blockade in critically ill patients because it lacks hemodynamic side effects and is not primarily dependent on the kidneys for its elimination. Two women aged 49 years and 35 years with renal functional impairment were evaluated. Both had neuromuscular blockade lasting for several hours to several days after long-term vecuronium therapy was withdrawn. Renal failure had necessitated hemodialysis in both patients.

The first patient received vecuronium for 19 days followed by a week of paralysis. The second patient had neuromuscular blockade lasting for 40 hours after termination of vecuronium administration. In both cases, vecuronium disappeared relatively rapidly from the plasma after its withdrawal, but 3-desacetylvecuronium persisted in high concentration.

Prolonged neuromuscular blockade in these patients probably reflected the accumulation of an active metabolite of vecuronium, 3-desacetylvecuronium. Elimination of this metabolite appears to be highly dependent on renal function. Neuromuscular function should be closely monitored in critically ill patients with renal dysfunction who are treated with vecuronium.

▶ The choice of neuromuscular blocking agents in renal failure is difficult because these patients require surgery for renal transplantation as well as other associated medical problems. Currently, vecuronium is frequently used because of less dependence on renal excretion than pancuronium. The findings reported here show that neuromuscular blockade should be evaluated carefully in patients with renal failure who have received vecuronium.—R.W. McPherson, M.D.

Impact of C-Reactive Protein (CRP) on Surfactant Function

Li JJ, Sanders RL, McAdam KPWJ, Hales CA, Thompson BT, Gelfand JA, Burke JF (Shriners Burns Inst, Boston; Harvard Med School; Tufts Univ)
J Trauma 29:1690–1697, 1989   8–22

C-reactive protein (CRP), a major marker of acute inflammation in man, binds to phosphorylcholine. Because of the structural homology between phosophorylcholine and dipalmitoyl phosphatidylcholine (DPPC), the major component of lung surfactant, CRP levels were determined in bronchoalveolar fluid specimens obtained from 6 patients with adult respiratory distress syndrome (ARDS) and 7 normal controls.

The mean CRP level in lavage fluid from patients with ARDS was 98 μg/mg of total protein, compared with 4 μg/mg in control specimens. In vitro studies showed that CRP binds to liposomes containing DPPC and phosphatidylglycerol. The surface activity of Surfactant TA, a clinical surfactant replacement, was markedly impaired by CRP in a dose-dependent manner. The human serum albumin level did not inhibit the activity of this material.

C-reactive protein could contribute to abnormal surfactant function in ARDS and thereby to the pathogenesis of pulmonary function in this disorder. In addition to CRP, other plasma proteins of an amphiphilic nature bind to liposomes made of phospholipids and could interefere with surfactant function in the lung.

▶ Along with many other observations on ARDS that are discussed in this issue of the YEAR BOOK, this paper continues the discussion of the immunologic interactions that appear to be intermittently involved in the genesis of the inflammatory response in the lung. In particular, these authors suggest that CRP may contribute to abnormalities of surfactant function in ARDS. Although the authors clearly show that CRP is not an initiating insult in ARDS, it may be a major contributor to the pathogenesis of pulmonary dysfunction seen in this syndrome.—M.C. Rogers, M.D.

The Association of Circulating Endotoxin With the Development of the Adult Respiratory Distress Syndrome
Parsons PE, Worthen GS, Moore EE, Tate RM, Henson PM (Univ of Colorado; Denver Gen Hosp)
Am Rev Respir Dis 140:294–301, 1989   8–23

Despite extensive investigation, the pathogenesis of adult respiratory distress syndrome (ARDS) has not been clearly defined. Complement-mediated neurophil sequestration in pulmonary capillaries can cause pulmonary vascular endothelial injury leading to ARDS, but complement activation alone does not fully account for the development of ARDS. Whether some mechanism involving a synergistic interaction between circulating endotoxin and the presence of complement fragments in plasma might be responsible for the development of ARDS was investigated in 98 patients.

At the time of enrollment, 15 patients already had established ARDS and 83 had at least 1 major predisposing risk factor for ARDS. Blood samples for the measurement of C5 fragments, C3 fragments, and plasma endotoxin levels were obtained at the time of enrollment in the study, and at 24 hours and 1 week thereafter. Illness severity was assessed by calculating APACHE II scores.

Nine of the 83 patients at risk of ARDS developing died before completion of the study, but none had evidence of ARDS at the time of death. Nine other patients with either transferred or discharged from the hospital before all 3 blood samples had been obtained. Of the remaining 65 at-risk patients, 56 completed the study and ARDS did not develop during their hospital stay; the other 9 had ARDS during the study.

There were no significant differences between the C5 fragment levels in the 23 patients with ARDS, the 56 patients who were at risk at enrollment but did not have ARDS during the study period, and the 9 patients who were at risk for ARDS at the time of enrollment and subsequently, in fact, had the disease. Increased plasma C3 fragment levels were found in 89% of the patients with ARDS and in 62% of those at risk for ARDS. Endotoxin was detected in the plasma of 74% of the at-risk patients who subsequently had ARDS, 64% of the patients who already had ARDS, and only 22% of the at-risk patients who did not have ARDS. Thus the combination of endotoxin and complement fragments may be important in the pathogenesis of ARDS.

▶ Although certain clinical events clearly predispose to the development of ARDS, the pathogenesis of lung injury in these patients is unclear. Parsons et al. demonstrate in this article an increased incidence of detectible endotoxin in "at risk" patients in whom ARDS did in fact develop. The authors hypothesize that endotoxin is an important mediator of ARDS that acts to prime white blood cells, and these leukocytes are then activated by complement fragments. However, not all patients with endotoxemia had ARDS and some patients without endotoxemia experienced lung injury, indicating that considerable uncertainty remains concerning the pathogenesis of this often lethal pulmonary injury.—M.J. Breslow, M.D.

Long-Term Survival of Patients With Chronic Obstructive Pulmonary Disease Following Mechanical Ventilation
Shachor Y, Liberman D, Tamir A, Schindler D, Weiler Z, Bruderman I (Tel Aviv Univ; Technion-Israel Inst of Technology, Haifa, Israel)
Isr J Med Sci 25:617–619, 1989   8–24

Initial mechanical ventilation has a worsening prognosis for patients with chronic obstructive lung disease. Fifty patients were followed for 15 years after surviving their first episode of artificial ventilation. All 50 patients had chronic bronchitis or pulmonary emphysema; asthmatics were excluded. None of the patients had used long-term domiciliary oxygen therapy after discharge.

All but 3 patients had died by the time of final follow-up. The 5-year survival rate was 30%, and the median survival time was 23.5 months. The average length of survival was 45 months. Nearly half of the patients died suddenly, most of them at home. Survival correlated positively with the partial pressure of arterial oxygen (PaO_2) value at the time of discharge, the presence of wheezing or rhonchi, and the absence of right heart failure at admission. Males did better than females. Survival correlated negatively with age. The outlook improved with the number of ventilations after the initial episode.

In this series, survival of patients with chronic obstructive lung disease after initial ventilatory therapy correlated best with the PaO_2 at the time of discharge. The positive effect of repeated ventilations on survival may indicate an advantage of home ventilation.

▶ This study provides long-term follow-up of patients with chronic obstructive lung disease who required mechanical ventilation during an acute exacerbation of their disease. Approximately half of the patients survived the initial hospitalization and were followed. Survival was most highly correlated with PaO_2. Most patients died suddenly, suggesting a cardiac event, most likely an arrhythmia.

Given these observations, one can only speculate whether home oxygen therapy, which was not used in these patients, would substantially alter the outcome. Of interest, this study identified a group of patients, presumably with some degree of reversible airway disease, who recovered uneventfully from mechanical ventilation on several occasions.—M.J. Breslow, M.D.

Abnormal Patterns of Pulmonary Neuroendocrine Cells in Victims of Sudden Infant Death Syndrome
Gillan JE, Curran C, O'Reilly E, Cahalane SF, Unwin AR (Trinity College; Rotunda Hosp; Children's Hosp, Dublin)
Pediatrics 84:828–834, 1989   8–25

Ventilatory dysfunction in sudden infant death syndrome (SIDS) has been associated with structural abnormalities in the carotid body and respiratory nuclei of the brain stem. The pulmonary neuroendocrine cells are thought to represent intrapulmonary chemoreceptors, which are affected by the denervating effect of asphyxial brain stem dysfunction. The pulmonary neuroendocrine system was studied in 25 victims of SIDS aged 3 weeks to 7 months and 20 control infants aged 1–12 months. The pulmonary neuroendocrine cells were stained by the Churukian-Schenck method, and the neuroendocrine cell-positive airway values were expressed as the percentage of the total number of airways.

The number of neuroendocrine-positive airways in SIDS victims ranged from 2% to 97% (median, 73%), whereas those from controls ranged from 1% to 44% (median, 25.5%); the difference was significant. Similarly, the number of neuroendocrine cells in the neuroendocrine-positive airways in SIDS victims was significantly increased, as compared with control infants. The neuroendocrine cell cytoplasmic staining in SIDS was distinctive, showing both increased granularity and confluence of granules; however, it was not present in all cases of SIDS. In addition, new neuroendocrine cells were present distal to the terminal bronchiole within the respiratory units in 40% of SIDS victims, but in none of the control infants.

The presence of a pulmonary chemoreceptor reaction to a ventilatory abnormality in SIDS was confirmed. The altered pulmonary neuroendocrine cell pattern could be attributed to either brain stem dysfunction or chronic hypoxia. Brain stem dysfunction may cause failure of neuroendocrine cell degranulation, whereas hypoxia may induce reactive hyperplasia of the pulmonary neuroendocrine cells. These mechanisms are not mutually exclusive of one another but may, in fact, both be operative in SIDS.

▶ The sudden infant death syndrome (SIDS) has been a difficult problem to understand. Many theories have been advanced to explain the unfortunate presentation of "perfectly healthy children" who die in the first several months of life. This paper documents that there is an abnormal pattern in the development of pulmonary neuroendocrine cells, which function as chemoreceptors in these children. It is not clear, however, whether pulmonary neuroendocrine abnormalities are primary changes or are caused by brain stem dysfunction or chronic hypoxia. In fact, both possibilities exist.—M.C. Rogers, M.D.

Clinical Features of Amiodarone-Induced Pulmonary Toxicity

Dusman RE, Stanton MS, Miles WM, Klein LS, Zipes DP, Fineberg NS, Heger JJ (Indiana Univ, Indianapolis; VA Med Ctr, Indianapolis)
Circulation 82:51–59, 1990   8–26

Pulmonary toxicity induced by amiodarone was diagnosed in 33 of 573 patients (5.3%) given the drug for recurrent tachyarrhythmia. The loading dose of amiodarone in later patients was 1,600 mg daily for 1 week, followed by 800 mg daily for 1 month. Daily maintenance doses ranged from 50 mg to 800 mg. The cumulative incidence of pulmonary toxicity at 121 months of treatment was 9.1% (Fig 8–2). Toxicity did not occur when treatment began at age 40 years or younger (Fig 8–3).

The diagnosis of amiodarone pulmonary toxicity was supported by abnormal findings on lung biopsy specimens in 13 patients, abnormal findings on gallium lung scans in 11, and low pulmonary diffusing capacity in 9. A low diffusing capacity predicted the occurrence of toxicity. Affected patients received higher daily maintenance doses of amiodarone, but there was no difference in loading doses. Three of the 33 patients with pulmonary toxicity died of this cause.

Pulmonary toxicity remains a significant complication of amiodarone therapy; it may be fatal. The risk can be minimized by giving the lowest effective maintenance dose and by closely monitoring patients whose pretreatment pulmonary diffusing capacity is low.

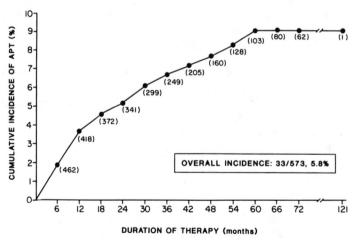

DURATION OF THERAPY (months)

Fig 8–2.—Life-table analysis of amiodarone pulmonary toxicity (APT) and duration of therapy in 373 patients treated with amiodarone. Numbers in parentheses denote number of patients remaining available for analysis. (Courtesy of Dusman RE, Stanton MS, Miles WM, et al: *Circulation* 82:51–59, 1990.)

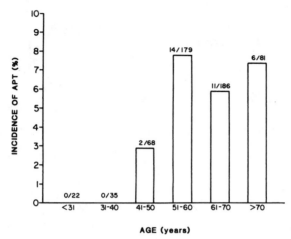

AGE (years)

Fig 8–3.—Incidence of amiodarone pulmonary toxicity (APT) based on age at which therapy was started. (Courtesy of Dusman RE, Stanton MS, Miles WM, et al: *Circulation* 82:51–59, 1990.)

▶ The increasing use of amiodarone for arrhythmias has resulted in the documentation of a clear-cut relationship between amiodarone and pulmonary toxicity. It appears that amiodarone-associated pulmonary toxicity is related to the level of the maintenance dose, the age of the patient, and preexisting lung disease. This is of significance to patients who require this drug for life-threatening arrhythmias because approximately 1 in 20 patients given amiodarone is likely to have major pulmonary complications.—M.C. Rogers, M.D.

Steroids in Croup: Do They Increase the Incidence of Successful Extubation?
Freezer N, Butt W, Phelan P (Royal Children's Hosp, Melbourne)
Anaesth Intensive Care 18:224–228, 1990   8–27

Steroid use in the treatment of croup is controversial. From 1983 to 1988, 2,623 children were admitted to a children's hospital for the treatment of croup. Of these, 416 (16%) were admitted to the intensive care unit. Intubation was required in 176 children; 117 of them were successfully extubated at the first attempt, but 59 needed reintubation. Of the children who needed reintubation, 35 were given steroids before subsequent attempts at extubation. In only 1 child who received steroids did extubation fail. By contrast, 59% of those who did not receive steroids required reintubation (table).

Although this was a retrospective study and patients were not randomly allocated to treatment with corticosteroids, the results supporting the use of steroids seem strong. The use of steroids before extubation significantly increased the incidence of successful extubation in children with croup in whom the first extubation failed.

▶ Although this report suffers from all of the problems (uncontrolled and retrospective) that have plagued the "steroids in croup" controversy, it reinforces a

	SUCCEEDED	FAILED	HOURS INTUBATED Mean (SD)
Use of Steroids Before Subsequent Extubations			
2ND EXTUBATION (n=59)			
Steroids (n=16)	16 (100%)	0	167 (47)
No Steroids (n=43)	17 (40%) ‡	26*	136 (54)
3RD EXTUBATION (n=25)			
Steroids (n=14)	13 (93%)	1 §	225 (76)
No Steroids (n=11)	5 (45%) †	6*	168 (46)
4TH EXTUBATION			
Steroids (n=6)	6 (100%)	0	

*One patient had a tracheostomy.
†P < .001.
‡P < .02.
§In patient who received steroids extubation failed and a second course was given before the next extubation.
(Courtesy of Freezer N, Butt W, Phelan P: *Anaesth Intensive Care* 18:224–228, 1990.)

gradual trend in the management of severe croup. A prospective, randomized, double-blind study by Super et al. (1) showed that a single dose of dexamethasone, .6 mg/kg, was associated with a reduced croup score and a reduced need for racemic epinephrine. The present study suggests that oral prednisolone, 2 mg/kg/day, may improve the chances of successful extubation in croup patients in whom previous extubation attempts have failed. A prospective, controlled study is needed to confirm this conclusion.—D.G. Nichols, M.D.

Reference

1. Super DM, et al: *J Pediatr* 115:323, 1989.

Effects of Aerosolized Artificial Surfactant on Repeated Oleic Acid Injury in Sheep

Zelter M, Escudier BJ, Hoeffel JM, Murray JF (San Francisco Gen Hosp; Univ of California, San Francisco)
Am Rev Respir Dis 141:1014–1019, 1990   8–28

Therapeutic administration of surfactant may mitigate some of the mechanical and gas exchange anomalies found in pulmonary edema accompanying acute lung injury in adults. The effects of giving surfactant as an aerosol to sheep with oleic acid-induced acute lung injury were studied to test this hypothesis.

An artificial surfactant, Exosurf, was administered in aerosol form and its effects on respiratory system compliance (Crs), total respiratory resistance (RT), and gas exchange (PO_2) were determined. Paired experiments were done on 10 sheep, 5 of which received Exosurf in the first experiment and aerosolized .9% NaCl in the second, and 5 of which received these agents in the reverse order. Paired experiments without oleic acid were done in 6 additional sheep that served as controls.

Oleic acid caused significant abnormalities when compared with control and baseline values in Crs, RT, and PO_2. No differences were found between animals that received Exosurf and NaCl. In the second experiment, baseline values for PO_2 and Crs with oleic acid were lower than control values, indicating that the sheep had not fully recovered from their initial injury. After oleic acid, the animals given NaCl had higher PO_2 and Crs values than those given NaCl first and Exosurf second. No differences were found in postmortem lung water content between sheep given Exosurf or NaCl first. Both groups had higher lung water content than the control group had. Peripheral deposition of aerosol was noted in 3 additional sheep.

The results fail to show an acutely beneficial effect of Exosurf administration to oleic acid-injured lungs. Increased surface forces may play a minor role in the gas exchange and mechanical abnormalities that occur in the oleic acid model of acute lung injury. Another possible explanation is that artificial surfactant may be less suitable than natural surfactant in this experimental model. Alternatively, aerosolization may have been unable to deliver enough surface-active material to overcome the effect of inhibitors released into the lungs in oleic acid injury.

▶ The phenomenal success of surfactant replacement therapy in neonatal respiratory distress syndrome has stimulated investigation of this therapy in adult respiratory distress syndrome (ARDS). However, as pointed out by the negative results of this study by Zelter et al., application of surfactant replacement therapy in ARDS will be much more complex.

Depending on the model, increased surface tension in ARDS may be attributable to absolute reduction in alveolar surfactant levels (oxygen toxicity, paraquat intoxication models) or functional inactivation of surfactant in the face of normal or even increased surfactant levels (oleic acid embolism model). Exogenous surfactant administrataion in those animal models of ARDS with reduced surfactant levels has demonstrated improvement in lung mechanics, oxygenation, and survival (1). The failure of surfactant to improve lung function in the oleic acid model used in this study may be because of continued inactivation of the administered surfactant by plasma proteins or membrane lipids in pulmonary edema fluid. Because inactivation of surfactant can be overcome by high surfactant concentration, it is possible that insufficient surfactant was administered in this study.

It is likely that the role of surfactant deficiency/dysfunction in ARDS patients is at least as diverse as in the animal models. Nevertheless, isolated case reports suggest that there may be a subgroup of patients whose lung function will improve after exogenous surfactant administration (2). Future research will have to concentrate on identification of ARDS patients who will benefit from surfactant administration and the ways in which surfactant inhibition may be prevented or overcome.— D.G. Nichols, M.D.

References

1. Matalon S, et al: *J Appl Physiol* 62:756, 1987.
2. Richman PS, et al: *Am Rev Respir Dis* 135:5, 1987.

Depressed Bronchoalveolar Urokinase Activity in Patients With Adult Respiratory Distress Syndrome

Bertozzi P, Astedt B, Zenzius L, Lynch K, LeMaire F, Zapol W, Chapman HA Jr (Brigham and Women's Hosp, Boston; Massachusetts Gen Hosp, Boston; Harvard Med School; Univ of Lund, Sweden; Henri Mondor Hosp, Créteil, France)
N Engl J Med 322:890–897, 1990   8–29

Abundant deposition of bronchoalveolar fibrin and fibronectin occurs during the exudative phase of the adult respiratory distress syndrome (ARDS). The deposition of fibrin and fibronectin promotes hyaline-membrane formation and subsequent alveolar fibrosis. Patients with idiopathic pulmonary fibrosis or sarcoidosis have diminished urokinase activity when compared with normal controls. To identify the mechanisms responsible for the persistence of bronchoalveolar fibrin and fibronectin in ARDS, the urokinase activity in cell-free bronchoalveolar-lavage (BAL) fluid obtained from 8 patients with ARDS was compared with that in 9 patients with pulmonary diseases other than ARDS and 10 normal controls.

Patients with ARDS had almost no measurable urokinase activity in their BAL fluid, whereas patients with other pulmonary diseases and normal controls had easily measurable urokinase activity. Bronchoalveolar-lavage fluid from all ARDS patients also had antiplasmin activity, which promotes the persistence of fibrin.

The true decrease in urokinase activity was confirmed by the failure of the BAL from patients with ARDS to convert [^{125}I]plasminogen to plasmin. Despite low urokinase activity in the BAL fluid of patients with ARDS, immunochemical assays revealed normal BAL fluid urokinase antigen levels that suggested the presence of urokinase inhibitors (Fig 8–4). The fibrin gel-underlay assay technique, which can detect complexes of urokinase with inhibitors, was then used to determine whether the BAL fluid from ARDS patients contained urokinase inhibitors. Inhibitors were demonstrated directly by this technique, with plasminogen-activator inhibitor type 1 being the principal inhibitor identified. Thus antifibrinolytic activity caused by urokinase inhibitors and antiplasmins present in the bronchoalveolar compartment of patients with ARDS contributes

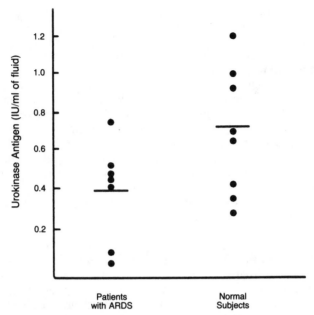

Fig 8–4.—Comparison of urokinase-antigen levels in the BAL fluid from normal subjects and patients with ARDS. Unconcentrated BAL fluid from each group was assayed for urokinase antigen in a sandwich enzyme-linked immunosorbent assay that used monoclonal and polyclonal urokinase antibodies. The results are expressed as IU of urokinase per milliliter of lavage fluid on the basis of a standard curve for purified urokinase done with each assay. Urokinase was detected in complexes with urokinase inhibitor at approximately half its actual concentration in this assay. (Courtesy of Bertozzi P, Astedt B, Zenzius L, et al: *N Engl J Med* 322:890–897, 1990.)

to the formation and persistence of hyaline membranes, a key component of the alveolar histopathology in ARDS.

▶ The adult respiratory distress syndrome (ARDS) can be triggered by many different events. However, once established, ARDS often develops into a progressive lung injury despite resolution of the original precipitant. The self-perpetuating character of ARDS is poorly understood but is of major clinical importance. The study by Bertozzi et al., demonstrating depressed pulmonary urokinase activity in patients with ARDS, may shed some light on why this process fails to resolve. Without urokinase to activate plasminogen, fibrin-containing hyaline membranes cannot be lysed. Persistence of alveolar fibrin can inactivate surfactant and serve as a nidus for collagen deposition. Whether a therapy can be developed that will provide alternate mechanisms for plasminogen activation, and whether these will lead to resolution of ARDS, remain to be determined.—M.J. Breslow, M.D.

Circumstances Surrounding the Deaths of Children Due to Asthma: A Case-Control Study

Miller BD, Strunk RC (Univ of Colorado; Children's Hosp, St Louis)
Am J Dis Child 143:1294–1299, 1989

The circumstances surrounding deaths caused by asthma have been investigated but none of the studies have been case controlled. The life circumstances and course of events in children who died of an acute asthma episode were compared with those in children who also had a life-threatening asthma attack but survived.

The study population consisted of 12 cases aged 10–18 years (mean, 14 years) who died during an asthma attack and 12 controls aged 11–17 years (mean, 13.8 years). Information was obtained in structured interviews with families and physicians and from medical records. The data were used to characterize the patient and his or her family. They were also used to define the severity and treatment of asthma during the 6 months before the attack, as well as the medical circumstances and patient characteristics that occurred on the day of and during the acute episode. The 12 cases were carefully matched with their controls for similar long-term medication use histories and overall disease severity ratings.

Analysis of the variables pertaining to the 6-month period preceding the attack showed that 2 physiologic variables and 3 psychological variables distinguished between cases and controls. The 2 physiologic variables were a history of respiratory failure requiring intubation, and a reduction in steroid dosage by more than 50% in the month before the attack. The psychological variables identified were dysfunction in the family, a history of reactions to separation or loss, and feelings of hopelessness and despair in the month before the attack.

Analysis of the variables pertaining to the medical circumstances and patient charateristics on the day of the attack showed that cases more often had attacks starting during sleep but less frequently experienced vomiting during the course of the attacks. Treatment of the attack by the parents was inadequate in 7 of the 12 children who died but also in 6 of the 12 children who survived. None of the many other variables analyzed for this study discriminated between cases and controls. Although the data suggest that certain characteristics of asthmatic children may place them at greater risk for death from an acute asthma attack, there may be as yet unidentified inherent differences in the mechanisms that precipitate acute asthma attacks that result in death or in survival.

▶ Although subject to the limitations of a retrospective, case-control study with a small number of participants, the study by Miller and Strunk suggests that a life-threatening asthma attack was more likely to lead to death if (1) the patient had a history of respiratory failure requiring ventilation within the past 6 months; (2) the steroid dosage had been decreased by more than 50% in the month before the attack; (3) there was family dysfunction; (4) a severe psychological reaction to separation or loss, or (5) a sense of hopelessness and despair had been experienced; (6) the attack began during sleep; (7) the patient did not vomit during the attack.

These data suggest approaches to reducing the mortality in acute asthma and understanding the mechanisms that lead to a severe asthma attack. In the at-risk population (history of respiratory failure), steroids are important in limiting airway inflammation, which may provide the substrate for a life-threatening attack. Furthermore, other recent studies have highlighted the importance of the prompt addition of high-dose intravenous steroids in the emergency room if the patient does not respond to inhaled β agonists alone within 1 hour. During sleep there is a cholinergic predominance of the nervous system, which may explain the propensity for fatal attacks to begin during sleep. Finally, this report highlights the timeliness of the NIH Asthma Education Project recommendations, which are anticipated in 1991. Parents need to be taught to recognize severe asthma attacks, preferably by objective measurement such as a reduction in peak airflow of more than 50%. Paramedics should administer nebulized β agonists and oxygen in the field. Greater efforts are needed to train paramedics in intravenous access and in intubation techniques for children. Families must understand the important psychological aspects of this disease and receive appropriate counseling and support.—D.G. Nichols, M.D.

Elevated Production of Neutrophil Leukotriene B_4 Precedes Pulmonary Failure in Critically Ill Surgical Patients

Davis JM, Meyer JD, Barie PS, Yurt RW, Duhaney R, Dineen P, Shires GT (Cornell Univ; Beth Israel Hosp, Boston)
Surg Gynecol Obstet 170:495–500, 1990   8–31

Leukotriene B_4 (LTB_4) is a potent neutrophil chemotactic factor that is also produced by neutrophils. The relationship between LTB_4 production and adult respiratory distress syndrome (ARDS) has not been defined. Neutrophil function was examined in 12 patients at risk for the development of ARDS. Peripheral blood neutrophils were tested for chemotaxis to f-met-leu-phe and LTB_4 and for production of LTB_4. Plasma was assessed for C3a desArg levels.

Five of the 12 patients had ARDS within 3 days of hospital admission. Neutrophil production of LTB_4 was significantly enhanced on day 1 in these patients, as compared to those that did not have ARDS. Chemotaxis to f-met-leu-phe and LTB_4 was significantly reduced in all 12 patients. Neutrophil chemotaxis improved in patients who did not have pulmonary failure and worsened in those who did. Plasma C3a desArg levels were significantly elevated on day 1 in those patients in whom ARDS developed subsequently.

Leukotriene production by neutrophils increases simultaneously with complement activation in patients who subsequently have ARDS. Leukotriene may play a role in the development of pulmonary failure in patients who have ARDS.

▶ This is yet another paper in a series dealing with the area of complement activation in the development of ARDS. This particular paper indicates that LTB_4 is elevated before clinical onset of pulmonary failure in critically ill patients. This paper, when read in concert with other papers in this section dealing with related issues in ARDS, provides increasing evidence that we are moving from physiologic to biochemical and neurohormonal understanding of the pathogenesis of ARDS. Any one of these papers cannot fully explain the phenomenon of ARDS. On the other hand, I am increasingly convinced that we are moving closer to an understanding of how this disease process is triggered and the cascade of events that result in continuation of this process. All of these papers are worth reading in their entirety as a "package" because they provide updated information on the latest developments in this field.—M.C. Rogers, M.D.

Surfactant Therapy for Pulmonary Edema Due to Intratracheally Injected Bile Acid

Kaneko T, Sato T, Katsuya H, Miyauchi Y (Kumamoto Univ, Kumamoto, Japan)
Crit Care Med 18:77–82, 1990   8–32

Human bile injected into the trachea of rabbits causes pulmonary edema and severe lung hemorrhage. In a clinical setting, a patient who had aspirated stomach contents, including bile, after operation for esophageal cancer died about 9 hours after aspiration. Autopsy revealed massive bleeding and the presence of hyaline membrane in the lung. Because conventional mechanical ventilation was not sufficient in treating pulmonary edema caused by bile aspiration, the therapeutic effect of an exogenous surfactant on bile aspiration-induced pulmonary damage was assessed.

Thirty anesthetized New Zealand white rabbits were injected intratracheally with taurocholic acid, 1 mL/kg, diluted to .6% with normal saline solution. The animals were then divided into 3 groups. Ten rabbits were left untreated, 10 were treated by intratracheal instillation of 3 mL of surfactant solution 15 minutes after injection of bile acid, and 10 were given surfactant solution at 15 minutes and 90 minutes after bile acid injection. All animals were observed for 6 hours and killed. The thorax was opened, the lung was photographed macroscopically, pressure-volume curves were recorded at the time of death, and portions of lung tissue were examined histologically.

Between 20 and 40 minutes after bile acid injection, all animals in the control group had moist rales in both lungs, and pink, foamy sputa appeared in the endotracheal tube. All 10 untreated rabbits died within 2.5–4.5 hours. The mean survival time was 3.3 hours. None of the treated rabbits died before the end of the 6-hour study period, and none had rales or sputa. After surfactant injection, the animals improved, but pulmonary edema recurred after 1 hour. After additional surfactant injection, the improved condition was sustained for the full 6 hours of observation.

Macroscopic examination showed that all lobes in the control animals were dark red, swollen, and liver-like in appearance. In contrast, the only irregularity in the once-treated animals was localized atelectasis in both lower lobes. The appearance of the lungs in the twice-treated animals

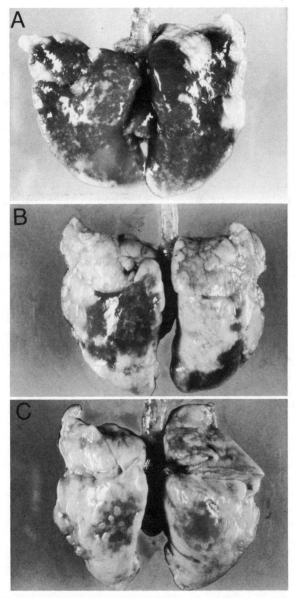

Fig 8–5.—Macroscopic findings from rabbits: **A,** 3 hours after intratracheal administration of bile acid (group 1); the dark congested appearance is apparent in all positions. **B,** 6 hours after intratracheal administration of bile acid (group 2); there is localized atelectasis in both lower lung fields. **C,** 6 hours after intratracheal administration of bile acid (group 3); almost normal findings are present. (Courtesy of Kaneko T, Sato T, Katsuya H, et al: *Crit Care Med* 18:77–82, 1990.)

was almost normal (Fig 8–5). Microscopic examination revealed no pulmonary edema in the twice-treated animals.

▶ The approval of surfactant therapy for use in respiratory distress syndrome of the newborn has raised the possibility that this clinically approved agent might be useful in other settings as well. This study examined in a rabbit model, the potential for surfactant therapy for pulmonary edema after aspiration of bile. These investigators show that, in this model, surfactant therapy is useful. It is my expectation that surfactant use will proliferate from the original neonatal respiratory distress setting to other settings, and this is just one example.—M.C. Rogers, M.D.

Seasonal Trends in US Asthma Hospitalizations and Mortality
Weiss KB (George Washington Univ)
JAMA 263:2323–2328, 1990   8–33

Asthma morbidity exhibits seasonal periodicity, but little is known of the seasonal trends in asthma mortality. By using 2 population-based information systems, the United States Vital Records and the National Hospital Discharge Survey, the seasonal trends in asthma hospitalizations and mortality in the United States population was compared.

From 1982 through 1986 there were 1.92 hospital discharges for asthma per 1,000 population. During the same period the average annual mortality associated with asthma was 1.52/100,000 population. Both hospitalizations and mortality exhibited periodic seasonal trends that were age specific and similar for sex, race, or region. In persons aged 5 through 34 years hospitalizations peaked in September through November, whereas mortality peaked in June through August. However, in those aged 65 years and older hospitalizations and mortality both increased from December through February. This seasonal trend in asthma hospitalizations and mortality in older adults is similar to that reported for pneumonia and influenza.

There appear to be age-specific variations in hospitalization rates and mortality associated with asthma. Further understanding of these trends may perhaps improve the treatment and prevention of asthma morbidity and mortality.

▶ There are many factors involved in changes in mortality associated with asthma. Recent concerns have focused on the fact that the mortality rate is rising. This study evaluates seasonal trends and concludes that there are age-specific variations in hospital and mortality rates for asthma. Although these authors do not explain those trends, this information is important in understanding the increasing rate of mortality for asthma.—M.C. Rogers, M.D.

Respiratory Distress Syndrome and Tracheoesophageal Fistula: Management With High-Frequency Ventilation

Bloom BT, Delmore P, Park VI, Nelson RA (HCA Wesley Med Ctr, Wichita, Kan)
Crit Care Med 18:447–448, 1990   8–34

Innovative airway management, such as endotracheal tube positioning, unilateral main stem intubation, and bronchoscopic placement of a balloon catheter, have been successful in the respiratory management of infants with tracheoesophageal fistula (TEF) and respiratory distress syndrome (RDS). One infant with very low birth weight and RDS and TEF was managed by high-frequency ventilation.

Male infant, born at 29 weeks' gestation, weighed 1,180 g and had esophageal atresia, TEF, and life-threatening RDS. Conventional mechanical ventilation resulted in gastric perforation and pneumoperitoneum, and repositioning of the endotracheal tube did not improve the infant's condition. High-frequency ventilation stabilized the infant, allowing distal occlusion of the esophagus with a Silastic band. Subsequently, fistula ligation was performed under more optimal physiologic conditions.

This is believed to be the first report of an infant with TEF and RDS who was managed successfully with high-frequency ventilation. The latter appears to improve carbon dioxide removal and oxygenation by minimizing peak to baseline airway pressure fluctuation and reducing loss of ventilation through a low compliance fistula. Infants with RDS and TEF who do not respond to mechanical ventilation may respond to high-frequency ventilation.

▶ This brief report of high-frequency ventilation use in a patient who had both RDS and TEF is useful for the specifics it gives in the techniques used.—M.C. Rogers, M.D.

Effect of Endothelin-1 on Pulmonary Resistance in Rats
Matsuse T, Fukuchi Y, Suruda T, Nagase T, Ouchi Y, Orimo H (Univ of Tokyo)
J Appl Physiol 68:2391–2393, 1990   8–35

Intravenous administration of the peptide endothelin-1 (ET-1) reportedly provokes a sustained increase in blood pressure in rats. The possibility that ET-1 may play a role in the development of respiratory disease was investigated by examining the peptide's effect on pulmonary resistance (RL) in Wistar rats.

Lung volume, tracheal flow, and transpulmonary pressure were measured in tracheotomized and paralyzed animals by means of a fluid-filled esophageal catheter and a pressure-sensitive body plethysmograph. The femoral artery was cannulated to measure the mean arterial blood pressure.

In the first experiment, RL increased at once after the injection of ET-1. This increase was sustained for at least 10 minutes, with the maximal response obtained 5 minutes after the injection. No such effect was seen in

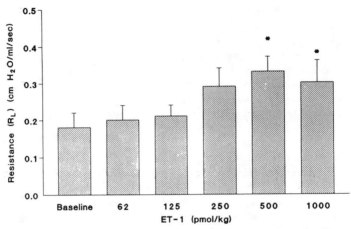

Fig 8–6.—Responses of pulmonary resistance with increasing doses of endothelin-1 (ET-1). Data 10 minutes after bolus injection of each dose of ET-1. Values are means ± 1 SE of 6 animals. *$P < .05$ compared with baseline (study 2). (Courtesy of Matsuse T, Fukuchi Y, Suruda T, et al: *J Appl Physiol* 68:2391–2393, 1990.)

control rats. In a second experiment, serially increasing doses of ET-1 were administered, followed by histamine, 1 μmol/kg, 60 minutes after the final injection of ET-1, 1,000 pmol/kg. After an initial small and transient fall in systemic blood pressure, ET-1 provoked a sustained increase in mean arterial blood pressure. Endothelin-1 provoked a dose-dependent increase in mean arterial blood pressure up to the maximum dose administered. An increase in R_L was observed within 5 minutes that was dose dependent (Fig 8–6). The response to ET-1, 1,000 pmol/kg, was comparable to the respnse to histamine, 1 μmol/kg, and the latter did not produce an additional change in R_L.

Endothelin-1 acted as a bronchoconstrictor on the airways in this animal model. The potential role of this peptide in the development of respiratory disease remains to be determined.

▶ Physiologists have been increasingly interested in endothelin, and this report looks at the effect of ET-1 on pulmonary resistance in a rat model. Although there is no confirmed role for endothelin in respiratory disease, the potency of this agent as a bronchoconstrictor and the fact that it occurs naturally mean that there is likely to be such a clinical condition identified in the not too distant future.—M.C. Rogers, M.D.

Respiratory Mechanics in Adult Rats Hypercapnic in the Neonatal Period
Rezzonico R, Gleed RD, Mortola JP (McGill Univ)
J Appl Physiol 68:2274–2279, 1990   8–36

When rats are exposed to chronic hypoxia during the neonatal period, they exhibit changes in the mechanical properties of the respiratory system as adults. Whether similar effects would occur after neonatal exposure to hypercapnia was investigated in 3 groups of Sprague-Dawley rats. The first group was exposed to 7% CO_2 in normoxia during the first week after birth, then returned to normocapnia (NB-CO_2). Animals in the second group were exposed to the same level and duration of hypercapnia from days 36 to 42 after birth (AD-CO_2). A control group was raised in normoxia and normocapnia. When the rats were approximately 7 weeks of age, the mechanical properties of the respiratory system, lung, and chest were measured during artificial ventilation in the anesthetized and paralyzed animals.

Similar results were found in the AD-CO_2 group and controls. The NB-CO_2 group, however, had higher compliance of the lung and respiratory system than the other 2 groups. Consistently lower average values of resistance of the total respiratory system, lung, and chest wall were noted in the NB-CO_2 animals. Lung compliance, measured during spontaneous breathing in a separate group of NB-CO_2 animals, averaged 34% more than in controls. Also significantly higher in NB-CO_2 animals was the exponential constant of the deflation quasistatic pressure-volume curve of the liquid-filled lungs.

In the rat, hypercapnia in the neonatal period produces long-term effects on passive respiratory system mechanics that are not apparent when the exposure occurs at later stages of the animal's development. It appears that it is not hyperventilation per se but, rather, its occurrence in the neonatal period that brings about these changes.

▶ The developmental effects of exposure to hypoxia hypercapnia and the potential for the effects to be long lasting is of interest to the pediatric intensivists. This animal model demonstrates clearly that hypercapnia in the neonatal period can result in significant changes in respiratory system mechanics. Furthermore, when a similar level of hypercapnia occurs at a later stage of the animal's development, these changes are not observed. As a result, the dynamics of respiratory development and the potential for significant susceptibility of the neonate to respiratory changes in response to hypercapnia needs to be borne in mind by neonatologists and pediatric intensivists.—M.C. Rogers, M.D.

Respiratory Muscle Insufficiency in Acute Respiratory Failure of Subjects With Severe COPD: Treatment With Intermittent Negative Pressure Ventilation

Corrado A, Bruscoli G, De Paola E, Ciardi-Dupre GF, Baccini A, Taddei M (Dept of Pneumology-Villa D'Ognissanti, Florence, Italy)
Eur Respir J 3:644–648, 1990   8–37

Inspiratory muscle weakness in patients with chronic obstructive lung disease leads to malfunction of the respiratory pump and progressive carbon dioxide retention. Nine patients with severe obstructive lung disease in acute respiratory failure who had marked respiratory muscle weakness underwent intermittent negative-pressure ventilation in an iron lung for 8 hours a day for 1 week. Seven control patients in stable chronic respiratory failure did not receive ventilator therapy, but their care otherwise was the same.

The study patients had increases in maximum inspiratory and expiratory pressures, vital capacity, oxygen pressure, and pH, and decreases in residual volume, total lung capacity, and carbon dioxide pressure. No comparable functional improvement occurred in the control patients.

These findings indicate that the expiratory muscles have a determining role in acute respriatory failure. The iron lung is helpful by lessening muscle fatigue and restoring an adequate level of respiratory compensation in patients with severe chronic obstructive lung disease in whom acute respiratory failure develops. As the expiratory muscles recover contractile force, they move the chest-lung system toward a point of elastic equilibrium. The energy cost of breathing declines as a result.

▶ This paper concludes that the iron lung is a useful therapeutic defense in relieving muscular fatigue in patients with acute respiratory failure who have underlying severe chronic obstructive pulmonary disease. This is really not a new thought, simply the resurfacing of an old one. It is likely that we will have increasing use for intermittent negative pressure ventilation in a wide variety of settings that go beyond the use described by these authors. I expect that negative pressure ventilation will be used to supplement ventilation in infants with unstable chest walls, and that there will be other similar specific conditions in which it will replace the problems associated with intubation and positive pressure ventilation.— M.C. Rogers, M.D.

Inhaled or Intravenous Pentamidine Therapy for *Pneumocystis carinii* Pneumonia in AIDS: A Randomized Trial
Soo Hoo GW, Mohsenifar Z, Meyer RD (Cedars-Sinai Med Ctr, Los Angeles; Univ of California, Los Angeles)
Ann Intern Med 113:195–202, 1990   8–38

The standard treatments for *Pneumocystis carinii* pneumonia— trimethoprim-sulfamethoxazole or pentamidine parenterally—frequently cause adverse reactions. Inhaled pentamidine has had some success as an alternative therapy for patients with AIDS and *Pneumocystis* pneumonia, but results of these trials have been mixed. The inhaled and intravenous forms of pentamidine therapy were compared.

Eligible patients were stratified into groups according to room-air PaO_2 (< 8 kPa or ≥ 8 kPa) and the episode of *Pneumocystis* pneumonia (initial or recurrent). They were then randomly assigned to treatment with inhaled pentamidine (11 patients) or intravenously administered pentamidine (10 patients), given daily for 21 days. Follow-up continued for at least 3 months.

Intravenously administered pentamidine resulted in a 100% response. In contrast, only 6 patients (55%) responded to the inhaled form of the drug. Three of the 5 patients who failed to respond were successfully treated with trimethoprim-sulfamethoxazole. The death of the other 2 patients resulted in an 18% mortality rate in the inhaled pentamidine

Toxicity Associated With Pentamidine Therapy

Toxicity	Intravenous Pentamidine ($n = 10$)	Inhaled Pentamidine ($n = 11$)	P Value*
	n (%)		
Clinical			
Hypotension	4 (40)	0 (0)	0.04
Nausea or emesis	6 (60)	2 (18)	0.06
Rash	1 (10)	0 (0)	0.48
Drug fever	2 (20)	0 (0)	0.21
Dysgeusia	5 (50)	0 (0)	0.01
Cough or wheezing	0 (0)	9 (82)	0.002
Laboratory			
Neutropenia	5 (50)	0 (0)	0.01
Thrombocytopenia	1 (10)	0 (0)	0.48
Azotemia	3 (30)	0 (0)	0.09
Dysglycemia	5 (50)	3 (27)	0.27
Hypoglycemia	3 (30)	3 (27)	0.63
Hyperglycemia	2 (20)	0 (0)	0.21

*P value from the Fisher exact test.
(Courtesy of Soo Hoo GW, Mohsenifar Z, Meyer RD: *Ann Intern Med* 113:195–202, 1990.)

group. Because of this adverse response rate, the study was terminated before its scheduled completion.

Patients who failed to respond to inhaled pentamidine appeared to have a greater severity of illness at study entry. Compared with responders, nonresponders had a lower mean PaO_2 and a higher arterial PO_2 difference. Those with milder disease clearly improved with inhaled pentamidine, but this form of therapy should not be used in patients with moderate or severe disease. Although intravenous therapy resulted in a higher response rate, it also caused substantially more adverse systemic effects (table).

▶ This is an important prospective randomized trial on the use of inhaled pentamidine for treatment of *P. carinii* pneumonia in AIDS patients. Although previous results had not indicated clear-cut success with this treatment, this study clearly demonstrates that inhaled pentamidine is probably as effective as intravenous pentamidine when the patient has mild *Pneumocystis* pneumonia. It is not clear, however, that this relationship holds when moderate or severe infections are encountered.—M.C. Rogers, M.D.

Effect of Naloxone on Spectral Shifts of the Diaphragm EMG During Inspiratory Loading

Petrozzino JJ, Scardella AT, Li JK-J, Krawciw N, Edelman NH, Santiago TV (Univ of Medicine and Dentistry of New Jersey, New Brunswick; Rutgers Univ, Piscataway, NJ)
J Appl Physiol 68:1376–1385, 1990

A shift in the power spectrum of the diaphragmatic electromyogram to lower frequencies may accompany fatiguing inspiratory flow-resistive loading (IRL). A similar shift might follow a reduction in end-inspiratory high-frequency power. Studies were performed in unanesthetized goats to determine whether activation of endogenous opioids by IRL can differentially lower central respiratory output, thereby reducing the centroid frequency. Respiratory studies were done in 5 animals. Naloxone was given in a dose of .1 mg/kg after imposing IRL for 1½ hours.

Inspiratory flow-resistive loading lowered the centroid frequency from 148 Hz to 141 Hz within 1½ hours. Naloxone administration increased the frequency to 149 Hz. The decline in centroid frequency during IRL resulted from a decrease in high-frequency power, that occurred mainly toward the end of inspiration. Reversal of the frequency shift after naloxone suggests a central mechanism involving the elaboration of endogenous opioids.

There may be a role for central respiratory drive in the altered diaphragmatic power spectrum that accompanies inspiratory loading. Endogenous opioid formation, rather than a muscular event secondary to fatigue, is implicated.

▶ The causes for diaphragmatic fatigue during inspiratory loading are quite complex. This interesting paper reviews this subject and investigates the potential role for narcotic reversal (naloxone) to alter the central respiratory drive that accompanies inspiratory loading. The fact that naloxone was effective suggests that endogenous opioid formation may play a role in the diaphragmatic fatigue associated with inspiratory loading, and that such fatigue may not be a simple peripheral muscular problem.—M.C. Rogers, M.D.

Unilateral Lung Hyperinflation and Herniation as a Manifestation of Intrinsic PEEP
Eveloff SE, Rounds S, Braman SS (Rhode Island Hosp, Providence; VA Med Ctr, Providence, RI; Brown Univ)
Chest 98:228–229, 1990   8–40

Occult or "intrinsic" positive end-expiratory pressure (PEEP) can occur. Patients with a prolonged expiratory time constant caused by increased airway resistance or reduced elastic recoil are at high risk. Manifestations of intrinsic PEEP range from overt hemodynamic compromise to unexplained hypoxemia, hypercarbia, tachycardia, and oliguria.

Man, 64, with chronic obstructive pulmonary disease became febrile after being stable for 5 years on mechanical ventilation. A right upper lobe infiltrate, a left upper lobe bulla, and generalized hyperinflation were noted on chest radiographs. Culture of endotracheal secretions showed *Pseudomonas aeruginosa*. Despite appropriate antibiotic treatment, the infiltrate cavitated and progressed radiographically to involve the right lower lobe. Intrinsic PEEP was 10 cm H_2O. An on-line suction catheter was placed to facilitate suctioning. On subsequent

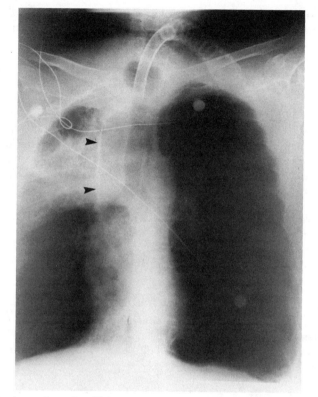

Fig 8–7.—*Arrows* show edge of left upper lobe bulla herniated across midline. Note contralateral shift of mediastinum. (Courtesy of Eveloff SE, Rounds S, Braman SS: *Chest* 98:228–229, 1990.)

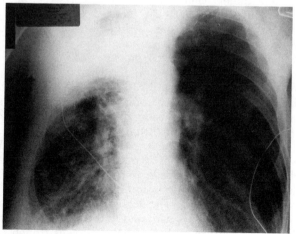

Fig 8–8.—On-line suction catheter removal resulted in reduced intrinsic PEEP and reversal of left lung herniation and mediastinal shift. (Courtesy of Eveloff SE, Rounds S, Braman SS: *Chest* 98:228–229, 1990.)

days, routine chest radiographs showed hyperinflation of the left lung with herniation of the upper lobe bulla across the midline (Fig 8–7). At this time, intrinsic PEEP measurements were 20 cm H_2O. Although little improvement was noted in the patient's pneumonia, later radiographs showed improvement in the hyperinflation of the left lung and a reduction in the size of the left upper lobe bullous lesion (Fig 8–8).

Intrinsic PEEP became evident when the chest radiograph showed unilateral lung hyperinflation and herniation of a large bulla to the contralateral hemithorax. The use of the on-line suction catheter on the ventilator apparatus may have contributed to the development of intrinsic PEEP. Radiographic and clinical improvement occurred when the catheter was removed.

▶ This case report was included because it reviews the potential for occult or "intrinsic PEEP" to develop in patients with a prolonged expiratory time constant caused by airway resistance or reduced elastic recoil. The case description is interesting, and the discussion of the subject is informative for the intensive care audience.—M.C. Rogers, M.D.

Pulmonary Gas Exchange During Dialysis in Patients With Obstructive Lung Disease
Pitcher WD, Diamond SM, Henrich WL (Dallas VA Med Ctr; Univ of Texas, Dallas)
Chest 96:1136–1141, 1989   8–41

Hypoxemia occurs in virtually all hemodialysis procedures and may contribute to the associated morbidity. Gas exchange was measured in 12 stable men undergoing hemodialysis 3 times per week. Six patients had chronic obstructive pulmonary disease and 6 had normal pulmonary function. Measurements were obtained before dialysis, after 1 hour, and after dialysis. Both acetate and bicarbonate dialysates were used.

Acetate dialysis lowered oxygen pressure in both groups of patients. Respiratory carbon dioxide excretion decreased and hypoventilation was noted, but the carbon dioxide pressure was unchanged. Hypoxemia occurred only after dialysis with bicarbonate dialysate. With both dialysates the arterial-alveolar oxygen tension difference increased after dialysis, particularly in the patients with chronic lung disease.

Dialysis hypoxemia is related in part to the use of acetate dialysate buffer, which produces alveolar hypoventilation chiefly because of reduced delivery of carbon dioxide secondary to acetate metabolism. In addition, abnormal ventilation-perfusion relationships within the lung contribute to dialysis hypoxemia. The degree of reduction in arterial oxygen pressure is similar in patients with and without chronic obstructive lung disease, but those with lung disease have a lower trough oxygen pressure.

▶ The observation that hypoxemia occurs during hemodialysis was investigated in this study by evaluating 12 stable patients undergoing standard hemodialysis 3 times weekly. The authors conclude that 2 mechanisms contribute to dialysis hypoxemia. One cause is related to the type of dialysis, and it is clear that acetate dialysate can produce alveolar hypoventilation from CO_2 unloading as a result of acetate metabolism. Regardless of the dialysate, however, abnormalities in ventilation/perfusion contribute to postdialysate hypoxemia. This interesting paper provides insight into the relationship between kidney disease, dialysis, and lung failure.—M.C. Rogers, M.D.

9 Other (Nutritional, Gastrointestinal, Metabolic, and Renal) Concerns

---

Effects of Metabolic Alkalosis on Pulmonary Gas Exchange
Brimioulle S, Kahn RJ (Erasme Univ Hosp, Brussels)
Am Rev Respir Dis 141:1185–1189, 1990

9–1

Metabolic alkalosis is a frequent acid-base disorder in hospitalized patients and generally is associated with an increased alveolar-arterial oxygen tension difference secondary to hypoventilatory atelectasis. Changes in arterial oxygen pressure were monitored in 8 critically ill patients who had respiratory failure, most often a result of chronic obstructive lung disease or bronchopneumonia. The patients were maintained by mechanical ventilation and were restudied after the selective correction of metabolic alkalosis by infusing 1N HCl.

The most frequent causes of metabolic alkalosis in these patients were previous hypercapnia and acute renal failure. Alkalosis was corrected by infusing a mean of 6 mmol of HCl per kg; no clinical complications resulted. The arterial pH decreased from 7.55 to 7.38 and the bicarbonate

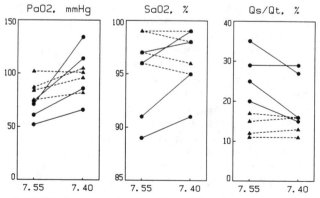

Fig 9–1.—Arterial blood oxygen tension (Pao$_2$), hemoglobin saturation (Sao$_2$), and venous admixture (QS/QT) at pH 7.55 and 7.4, respectively, before and at 12 hours after the HCl infusion. In patients with initial QS/QT < 20% *(dotted lines)*, Pao$_2$ tended to increase, whereas Sao$_2$ decreased and QS/QT did not change. Patients with initial QS/QT > 20% *(solid lines)* showed a significant improvement in Pao$_2$, Sao$_2$, and QS/QT. (Courtesy of Brimioulle S, Kahn RJ: *Am Rev Respir Dis* 141:1185–1189, 1990.)

decreased from 36 mmol/L to 23 mmol/L. Pulmonary artery pressure was increased 2 hours after the infusion. Oxygen pressure increased from 76 mm Hg to 114 mm Hg. Patients whose respiratory failure was more marked had a greater increase in oxygen pressure as well as significant improvement in arterial oxygen saturation (Fig 9–1).

The improved arterial blood oxygenation seen when metabolic alkalosis is corrected in patients in respiratory failure can be ascribed to both a shift in the oxyhemoglobin dissociation curve and a lessening of ventilation-perfusion mismatching. The latter effect probably is caused by enhanced hypoxic pulmonary vasoconstriction.

▶ This is a very interesting study detailing the use of 1N HCl in the correction of metabolic alkalosis in patients on mechanical ventilatory support. The study involved only 8 patients, who had a variety of etiologies for their metabolic alkalosis. The use of 1N HCl was said to be safe, although there was a significant drop in platelet count and an increase in the blood urea nitrogen with treatment. There was improvement in oxygenation, which presumably (as the authors argue) reflects improvement in the ventilation/perfusion relationships. This observation warrants further evaluation and should be tested in a prospective, randomized, controlled trial using a larger number of patients who are better matched for the etiology of their metabolic alkalosis.—R.A. Balk, M.D., and J.E. Parrillo, M.D.

Bolus or Intravenous Infusion of Ranitidine: Effects on Gastric pH and Acid Secretion: A Comparison of Relative Efficacy and Cost

Ballesteros MA, Hogan DL, Koss MA, Isenberg JI (Univ of California, San Diego)

Ann Intern Med 112:334–339, 1990   9–2

The parenteral administration of histamine H_2-receptor antagonists is a common procedure in the intensive care unit (ICU) to prevent acute hemorrhagic gastritis. To compare the effects of intravenous bolus injection and continuous intravenous infusion on gastric pH and acid secretion, 6 different ranitidine treatment regimens were evaluated. Also, 8 hospitals were polled for information on the use of histamine H_2-receptor antagonists in their ICUs.

Twelve men with inactive duodenal ulcer disease participated in the double-blind, Latin-square randomized, prospective study. Gastric acid secretion, pH, and the plasma level of ranitidine were monitored for 24 hours on 6 separate days in response to placebo, intravenous bolus injection of ranitidine 50 mg every 8 hours and 75 mg every 12 hours, and continuous intravenous infusion of ranitidine 75 mg, 150 mg, and 300 mg every 24 hours.

Continuous intravenous ranitidine infusion was significantly more effective than intermittent bolus injections. The total 24-hour gastric acid output during continuous intravenous infusion of 150 mg over 24 hours was approximately half the output seen with 2 divided bolus doses of 75

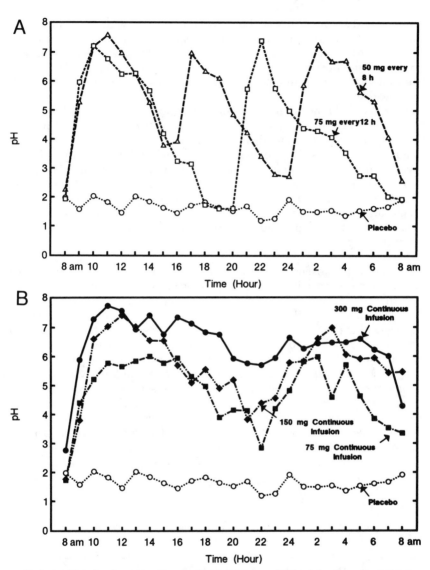

Fig 9–2.—Mean hourly gastric pH in 12 subjects with inactive duodenal ulcer disease studied during 6 seperate 24-hour periods. **A,** effects of ranitidine, 150 mg over 24 hours, given as an intravenous bolus injection of either 50 mg every 8 hours *(open triangles)* or 75 mg every 12 hours *(open squares)* on the 24-hour gastric pH. *Open circles* indicate pH levels in those patients given placebo. **B,** effects of raniti-dine given as a continuous intravenous infusion, 75 mg over 24 hours *(single-dotted line)*, 150 mg over 24 hours *(double-dotted line)*, or 300 mg over 24 hours *(solid line)* on the 24-hour gastric pH. (Courtesy of Ballesteros MA, Hogan DL, Koss MA, et al: *Ann Intern Med* 112:334–339, 1990.)

mg every 12 hours, and a third the output seen with 3 divided bolus doses of 50 mg every 8 hours. Hourly gastric pH values fluctuated widely from 7.6 to 1.6 after bolus injection, whereas the gastric pH remained at 3.8 or higher during continuous intravenous infusion (Fig 9–2). Fluctuations in plasma ranitidine levels corresponded with changes in gastric pH and acid secretion.

Results of the hospital survey indicated that parenteral histamine H_2-receptor antagonists were prescribed for approximately 74% of patients in ICUs. Intravenous administration of ranitidine was prescribed for 77% and cimetidine for 20% of patients. Administration by bolus injection was 4 times more common than continuous intravenous infusion, but the cost of infusion was approximately $40 less than that of bolus injection. Intravenous ranitidine infusion at doses of 150 mg or 300 mg daily is clinically more effective and more cost effective than bolus injection for use in hospitalized patients requiring treatment with histamine H_2-receptor antagonists.

▶ Upper gastrointestinal bleeding remains a serious problem in ICUs. Although prophylaxis with sucralfate is probably preferable to the use of H_2 blockers because of the lower risk of nosocomial pneumonia (1), not all patients can tolerate sucralfate. The study summarized above demonstrates convincingly the superiority of the intravenous infusion of ranitidine over intermittent injections of the drug with respect to gastric pH. Although one might hope that this finding could be extended to the prevention of gastrointestinal bleeding, the study was not designed to address this question. Furthermore, the study was not performed in critically ill patients, whom we would assume to be under somewhat greater stress than the inactive duodenal ulcer patients who served as subjects for this study. Until the findings are confirmed in critically ill patients, it would be imprudent to assume that the continuous infusion of 300 mg of ranitidine each day will keep the gastric pH of a sick, intubated patient above 3.5. However, this study is a necessary and useful first step.— T.P. Bleck, M.D., and J.E. Parrillo, M.D.

Reference

1. Leggner, et al, et al: *Am J Med* 86:81, 1989.

Misoprostol Versus Antacid Titration for Preventing Stress Ulcers in Postoperative Surgical ICU Patients

Zinner MJ, Rypins EB, Martin LR, Jonasson O, Hoover EL, Swab EA, Fakouhi TD (Johns Hopkins Med Inst; Univ of California, Irvine; Long Beach VA Med Ctr, Calif; Hershey Med Ctr, Hershey, Pa; Cook County Hosp, Chicago; et al)
Ann Surg 210:590–595, 1989   9–3

Misoprostol is an alternative to H_2 blockers, sucralfate, and antacids for preventing stress ulceration. It has cytoprotective properties and lowers gastric acid secretion. In a prospective, double-blind study, misoprostol was compared with antacid titration of the gastric pH in 371 patients scheduled for major surgery at 16 centers. Patients were assigned to receive either misoprostol 200 μg every 4 hours plus a placebo liquid every 2 hours, or placebo tablets every 4 hours plus magnesium-aluminum hydroxide liquid antacid every 2 hours. Outcomes were assessed on the basis of deterioration from the initial endoscopic appearance (strict criteria), development of erosions or ulcer craters, and evidence of significant clinical bleeding.

From 26% to 31% of both groups met strict criteria for therapeutic success. Using looser criteria based the development of erosions or ulcer craters, about 70% of both groups had success. No patient in either group had significant clinical bleeding, and follow-up lesion scores were comparable. Although levels of pH remained consistently greater in the antacid-treated patients, mean pH levels in the misoprostol group remained at or above 4. Diarrhea occurred in about 25% of each group.

Misoprostol in fixed dosage and antacid titration are similarly effective in preventing upper gastrointestinal tract bleeding and stress lesions in patients undergoing major surgery. Although misoprostol probably will be more expensive, is is easier to administer and should substantially reduce nursing time.

▶ Although this study effectively demonstrates that misoprostol is as effective as antacids in the prevention of postoperative stress-induced gastroduodenitis, it does not demonstrate any convincing benefit over other agents that do not require routine intragastric pH monitoring, e.g., long-acting H_2 blockers and sucralfate. The study supports adding misoprostol to the list of acceptable agents for stress ulcer prophylaxis, but in the absence of convincing data favoring any one agent, total costs of use should determine drug selection. Studies that can show a difference in efficacy (even if that difference exists) may be difficult in the future because of a probable decline in incidence of clinically relevant stress ulceration in response to improvement in overall perioperative and intensive care unit care management (1).—A. Kumar, M.D., and J.E. Parrillo, M.D.

Reference

1. Schuster DP, et al: *Am J Med* 76:623, 1984.

Open Versus Closed Peritoneal Lavage With Particular Attention to Time, Accuracy, and Cost
Howdieshell TR, Osler TM, Demarest GB (Med College of Georgia, Augusta; Univ of New Mexico, Albuquerque)
Am J Emerg Med 7:367–371, 1989   9–4

Diagnostic peritoneal lavage for the evaluation of blunt and penetrating thoracoabdominal trauma can be performed via an open, surgical technique or a closed, percutaneous technique. With the open approach, the dialysis catheter is inserted into the peritoneal cavity under direct vision. The percutaneous approach requires blind insertion of the catheter. The open surgical technique has been recommended as safer and more accurate than the percutaneous technique. During a 3-month period, the accuracy and safety of the 2 techniques were compared in 100 patients aged 9–75 years who sustained blunt abdominal trauma, thoracoabdominal stab wounds, or anterior abdominal stab wounds with fascial penetration requiring diagnostic peritoneal lavage. Fifty patients were randomly allocated to the open technique and 50 to the closed technique.

Twenty-four lavages were positive, 11 grossly so. Six grossly positive lavages were done with the open technique and 5 with the closed technique. Wound infection developed in 5 patients in the surgical group but in none of the percutaneous group. Wound one patient who had percutaneous lavage sustained an arterial puncture that did not require blood transfusion or surgical treatment. A false negative result was obtained in a patient who had open lavage. This patient was later found to have a bleeding splenic capsular laceration that required suturing. Most of the bleeding apparently occurred after completion of peritoneal lavage. The costs associated with the 2 procedures were approximately the same. However, the closed lavage technique consistently took less time to perform than the open technique.

Percutaneous diagnostic peritoneal lavage is now used almost exclusively at the present institution. Only pregnant women and patients with previous abdominal surgery are still investigated with open peritoneal lavage.

▶ This study documents the superiority of closed peritoneal lavage, performed by surgical residents instructed in the technique (but probably not supervised) in detecting a traumatic hemoperitoneum. This study appears to have been well designed and executed, and the results are clear: The closed technique is faster, less expensive, and at least as accurate as the open technique. There were fewer complications in the closed lavage group as well, although none of the complications in either group was particularly severe. Closed peritoneal lavage was performed with a Seldinger technique, rather than by blind penetration of the abdominal cavity with a peritoneal dialysis catheter. This probably accounts for the safety of the technique.—T.P. Bleck, M.D., and J.E. Parrillo, M.D.

Emergency Surgery for Severe Acute Cholangitis: The High-Risk Patients
Lai ECS, Tam P-C, Paterson IA, Ng MMT, Fan S-T, Choi T-K, Wong J (Univ of Hong Kong; Queen Mary Hosp, Hong Kong)
Ann Surg 211:55–59, 1990   9–5

Emergency biliary decompression in patients with severe acute cholangitis (SAC) is associated with formidable morbidity and mortality risks. Data were reviewed on 41 men and 45 women aged 28–97 years who had SAC secondary to choledocholithiasis. All 86 patients underwent emergency ductal exploration under general anesthesia. Additional procedures included cholecystectomy in 55 patients, cholecystostomy in 5, and transhepatic intubation in 2. Fifty-five patients had septicemic shock before operation; 30 of them were hypotensive at the time anesthesia was induced despite active resuscitation.

Seventeen patients died (20%) and 43 patients had significant postopertive complications. Seventeen patients had more than 1 complication. Univariate analysis of 14 clinical and 11 biochemical parameters identified 10 variables that significantly correlated with postoperative hospital mortality. Postoperative outcomes of the 30 patients who remained in septicemic shock before operation were similar to outcomes in patients who were resuscitated successfully.

Multivariate analysis identified 5 variables with independent predictive value, including the presence of concomitant medical problems, pH of less than 7.4, total bilirubin of more than 90 μmol/L, platelet count of less than 150×10^9/L, and serum level of albumin of less than 30 g/L. Among patients with 3 or more risk factors, postoperative mortality was 55% and postoperative morbidity was 91%. Among patients with 2 or fewer risk factors the postoperative mortality was 6% and postoperative morbidity, 34%.

Because thrombocytopenia appeared even with transient hypotension, timely ductal decompression may improve the postoperative outcome in these patients. In the high-risk population, use of nonoperative biliary drainage by percutaneous or endoscopic approaches as an initial intervention may be of benefit.

▶ After reading this paper 4 times, I finally understood the value of the study. The authors showed that acidosis, thrombocytopenia, hypoalbuminemia, concurrent medical problems, and a total bilirubin above 90 mmol/L were both independent and additive predictive factors for postoperative mortality in severe cholangitis. At first glance, these appear to be so obvious from clinical experience as to be of little interest. Because the morbidity and mortality in patients with 3 or more risk factors is substantial, the authors have interpreted their data to suggest that percutaneous or endoscopic biliary decompression in those patients at greatest risk might improve their survival and hasten their recovery. However, as none of their patients was managed with these preoperative techniques they were not able to test their hypothesis.

This paper lays the groundwork for a study to determine whether preoperative biliary decompression will improve the outcome of patients with severe acute cholangitis. I hope that the authors (or someone else) will undertake that study.—T.P. Bleck, M.D., and J.E. Parrillo, M.D.

Bicarbonate Does Not Improve Hemodynamics in Critically Ill Patients Who Have Lactic Acidosis: A Prospective, Controlled Clinical Study
Cooper DJ, Walley KR, Wiggs BR, Russell JA (Univ of British Columbia, Vancouver)
Ann Intern Med 112:492–498, 1990   9–6

Although sodium bicarbonate is currently used to treat patients with metabolic acidosis, it is controversial whether sodium bicarbonate therapy does in fact improve hemodynamics. Furthermore, serious adverse effects of sodium bicarbonate therapy have been reported, including congestive cardiac failure and hypercapnia. In this prospective study the use of sodium bicarbonate was tested in 14 critically ill patients with metabolic acidosis (bicarbonate less than 17 mmol/L and base excess less than −10) and increased arterial lactate (mean, 7.8 mmol/L). In a randomized, blind, crossover design the effects of infusions of sodium bicarbonate were compared to those of equimolar sodium chloride.

During the 2-hour study there were no differences between the effects of sodium bicarbonate sodium chloride on cardiac output, blood pressure, or pulmonary capillary wedge pressure (Fig 9–3). Acidemia was

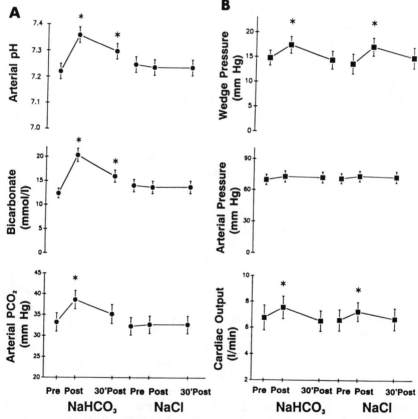

Fig 9–3.—Acid-base (**A**) and hemodynamic (**B**) measurements before (Pre) and after (Post) sodium bicarbonate and sodium chloride infusions in 14 critically ill patients who had lactic acidosis. Increases in pulmonary capillary wedge pressure and cardiac output were not caused by pH correction because identical changes were observed after sodium chloride infusion. All values are mean ± standard error. *P < .01, compared with Pre. (Courtesy of Cooper DJ, Walley KR, Wiggs BR, et al: *Ann Intern Med* 112:492–498, 1990.)

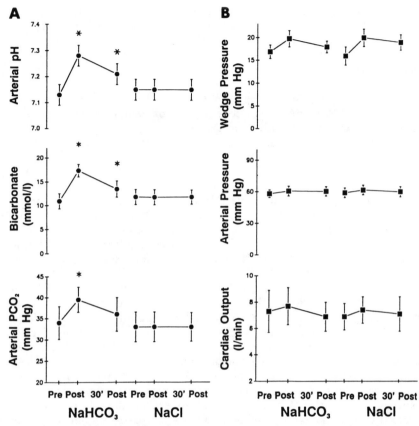

Fig 9–4.—Acid-base (**A**) and hemodynamic (**B**) measurements before (Pre) and after (Post) sodium bicarbonate and sodium chloride infusions in 7 critically ill patients who had severe lactic acidosis (arterial pH less than 7.20). Changes and trends were same as in large group in Figure 9–3. All values are mean ± standard error. *$P < .05$, compared with Pre. (Courtesy of Cooper DJ, Walley KR, Wiggs BR, et al: *Ann Intern Med* 112:492–498, 1990.)

significantly improved by the 2 mmol/kg dose of sodium bicarbonate. Infusion of bicarbonate, but not of sodium chloride, resulted in significant decreases in the plasma level of ionized calcium. Even among the 7 most acidemic patients who had an arterial pH of less than 7.20, increased arterial pH after administration of bicarbonate was not accompanied by increased cardiac output of increased mean arterial pressure (Fig 9–4). These findings provide strong evidence that sodium bicarbonate is an ineffective treatment for severely ill patients with metabolic acidosis.

▶ Here is another study that chisels away at the foundation of the monument erected in the past to sodium bicarbonate therapy in the treatment of circulatory arrest and lactic acidosis. In this blinded crossover trial of patients with metabolic acidosis from lactic acid accumulation, there was no improvement in hemodynamic function after the administration of NaHCO₃ or equimolar NaCl.

The use of bicarbonate did correct the acidosis, but there was also an associated increase in the $Paco_2$ and a decrease in ionized calcium. It now appears that there is only a limited role for $NaHCO_3$ in the treatment of metabolic acidosis, but old habits sometimes change very slowly.— R.A. Balk, M.D., and J.E. Parrillo, M.D.

Metabolic and Hemodynamic Consequences of Sodium Bicarbonate Administration in Patients With Heart Disease
Bersin RM, Chatterjee K, Arieff AI (Univ of California, San Francisco; VA Med Ctr, San Francisco)
Am J Med 87:7–14, 1989   9–7

The use of sodium bicarbonate ($NaHCO_3$) in cardiopulmonary arrest has been questioned, but the effects of $NaHCO_3$ in patients with heart disease are not known. Ten patients with stable congestive heart failure received $NaHCO_3$ and control infusions of equimolar sodium chloride ($NaCl$), and the metabolic and hemodynamic consequences of these infusions were evaluated.

The arterial oxygen tension fell significantly by an average of 10 mm Hg after administration of $NaHCO_3$, but it increased with infusion of $NaCl$. After administration of $NaHCO_3$, consumption of myocardial oxygen decreased significantly by 17% as a result of reduced myocardial oxygen extraction. Systemic oxygen consumption also fell significantly by a mean of 21% as a result of a significant reduction of systemic oxygen extraction. The level of 2,3-diphosphoglyceric acid in red blood cells, which was elevated at baseline, did not change with administration of $NaHCO_3$. The arterial and mixed venous carbon dioxide tensions increased with administration of $NaHCO_3$ but decreased significantly with administration of $NaCl$. Administration of $NaHCO_3$ significantly reduced the partial pressure of oxygen at which 50% of the hemoglobin was saturated and shifted the oxygen-hemoglobin binding curve toward normal (Bohr effect).

The arterial concentration of lactate increased with infusion of $NaHCO_3$. Three patients had net myocardial lactate generation during administration of $NaHCO_3$, and 2 of these had symptoms of angina. The blood glucose concentration fell significantly with administration of $NaHCO_3$. Coronary blood flow did not change with infusion of $NaHCO_3$ but increased with infusion of $NaCl$. Four patients had transient reductions of cardiac output, and 2 had transient pump failure during administration of $NaHCO_3$.

Administration of $NaHCO_3$ to patients with congestive heart failure impairs arterial oxygenation and reduces systemic and myocardial consumption of oxygen. The reduction in utilization of oxygen is associated with anaerobic metabolism, enhanced glycolysis, and elevation of blood levels of lactate, which may lead to transient myocardial ischemia in some patients. Thus the use of $NaHCO_3$ in these patients may have potentially deleterious consequences and warrants reevaluation.

▶ The use of sodium bicarbonate in the acute resuscitation of individuals with circulatory collapse and cardiac arrest has been evaluated critically in the past few years. The result of this evaluation has been the removal of NaHCO$_3$ from the routine treatment algorithms. This study evaluated the use of NaHCO$_3$ and normal saline in patients with congestive heart failure. The patients who received sodium bicarbonate had a lower Pao$_2$, oxygen delivery, arterial oxygen content, and oxygen extraction. This appears to be another nail in the coffin of NaHCO$_3$ in the critical care arena (see Abstract 9–6).—R.A. Balk, M.D., and J.E. Parrillo, M.D.

Refractory Potassium Repletion Due to Cisplatin-Induced Magnesium Depletion
Rodriguez M, Solanki DL, Whang R (Univ of Oklahoma; VA Med Ctr, Oklahoma City)
Arch Intern Med 149:2592–2594, 1989   9–8

Magnesium and potassium are closely related both experimentally and clinically; magnesium is important in maintaining cellular potassium and in cellular repletion of potassium. Cisplatin therapy is a frequent cause of hypomagnesemia and hypokalemia caused by renal losses of magnesium and potassium.

Refractory hypokalemia associated with hypomagnesemia developed in 2 patients after cisplatin therapy for cancer. In both patients potassium supplementation failed to resolve the deficit, and marked hypokalemia persisted until hypomagnesemia was corrected. Hypomagnesemia was not recognized for longer than 1 week in each patient.

This experience indicates that both the serum potassium and magnesium levels should be routinely estimated in patients requiring cisplatin treatment. Repletion of an existing magnesium deficit will allow potassium repletion to take place.

▶ Cisplatin therapy is a well-recognized cause of hypomagnesemia, most likely related to proximal tubular loss of the cation. Other common causes of hypomagnesemia include sepsis, gastrointestinal losses, renal losses, drugs (especially the diuretics), and a host of other uncommon disorders. Less well recognized, yet emphasized by these case reports, is the importance of a normal serum magnesium concentration in helping to maintain normal intracellular potassium homeostasis. The mechanism whereby hypomagnesemia leads to hypokalemia appears to be a reduction in activity of the sodium-potassium adenosine triphosphate pump and alteration in permeability of the renal tubular cell to potassium (1). Regardless of the mechanism, these cases demonstrate the difficulty commonly faced when attempting to achieve adequate potassium repletion without concomitantly replacing magnesium when both ions are depleted.

In addition to refractory hypokalemia, other complications associated with hypomagnesium that are of importance to the intensivist include ventricular and supraventricular arrhythmias, vascular spasm (including that of the epicardial coronary arteries), increased digitalis sensitivity, gastrointestinal symptoms, and neuromuscular irritability. All of these processes, if specifically caused by the hypomagnesemia, can be expected to abate with replacement therapy, thus emphasizing the importance of following magnesium levels in patients at risk for the development of hypomagnesemia or those who demonstrate hypokalemia refractory to replacement therapy.—A.C. Dixon, M.D., and J.E. Parrillo, M.D.

Reference

1. Zaloga GP, Chernow B: Divalent ions: Calcium, magnesium, and phosphorus, in Chernow B (ed): *The Pharmacologic Approach to the Critically Ill Patient*, ed 2. Baltimore, Williams and Wilkins, 1988.

A Comparison of Sclerotherapy With Staple Transection of the Esophagus for the Emergency Control of Bleeding From Esophageal Varices
Burroughs AK, Hamilton G, Phillips A, Mezzanotte G, McIntyre N, Hobbs KEF
(Royal Free Hosp and School of Medicine, London)
N Engl J Med 321:857–862, 1989   9–9

Emergency sclerotherapy in the treatment of acute esophageal variceal bleeding, with or without earlier balloon tamponade, is more effective than balloon tamponade alone. Sclerotherapy is now the treatment of choice in many centers, with operation a second-line treatment. Emergency esophageal transection with a staple gun effectively controls esophageal variceal bleeding and has a mortlity rate similar to that associated with emergency sclerotherapy. A prospective, randomized study was conducted to compare endoscopic sclerotherapy with staple transection of the esophagus in the emergency treatment of esophageal variceal bleeding.

Of 101 patients with cirrhosis of the liver and bleeding esophageal varices, 50 were randomly assigned to emergency sclerotherapy and 51 to staple transection of the esophagus; 4 patients assigned to sclerotherapy and 12 assigned to staple transection did not actually undergo those procedures, but all statistical analyses were made on an intention-to-treat basis.

Sclerotherapy controlled the variceal bleeding in 41 patients and failed in 9. Transection controlled the bleeding in 49 patients and failed in 2. Within 6 weeks of treatment, 22 sclerotherapy patients (44%) and 18 transection patients (35%) died. The difference was not statistically significant. Blood and plasma requirements during the procedures and the first 5 days thereafter were substantially lower in the group having transection. The incidence of rebleeding was also lower in the transection group. A 5-day interval without bleeding was achieved in 88% of the patients assigned to staple transection, whereas only 62% of the patients assigned to sclerotherapy stopped bleeding after a single injection. Staple transection of the esophagus as an emergency treatment for variceal bleeding in patients with cirrhosis of the liver is as safe as sclerotherapy and more effective than a single sclerotherapy procedure.

▶ It must be stressed that the patients in this study were randomly assigned to either sclerotherapy or staple transection of the esophagus only if there was initial failure to control variceal bleeding. The definition of failure was based on the patient's transfusion requirements, as a function of time, as well as on the lack of response to concomitant pharmacologic therapy with vasoactive drugs. Therefore, the data generated from this paper should not be extrapolated to clinical decision making for all patients with acutely bleeding esophageal varices.

It is clear that esophageal varices hemorrhage recurrently, and that the goals of therapy should focus on both the termination of acute hemorrhage as well as the prevention of recurrent hemorrhage. There seems to be a role for both sclerotherapy and staple transection of the esophagus in the first-line management of patients with bleeding varices. The decision of which procedure to perform must be individualized. For example, operative risk may be aggravated by associated organ dysfunction (e.g., renal failure), or there may be contraindications to abdominal surgery. In those situations sclerotherapy would be the logical procedure of choice. However, sclerotherapy should be considered a failure when multiple injections, usually more than 2, fail to control hemorrhage. Until a more definitive form of therapy for the treatment of bleeding esophageal varices is developed, both sclerotherapy and staple transection of the esophagus should be considered the therapeutic options.—F.P. Ognibene, M.D., and J.E. Parrillo, M.D.

Prophylaxis of Upper Gastrointestinal Bleeding in Intensive Care Units: A Meta-Analysis
Lacroix J, Infante-Rivard C, Jenicek M, Gauthier M (Univ of Montreal)
Crit Care Med 17:862–869, 1989   9–10

Cimetidine and antacids appear to be effective in preventing upper gastrointestinal tract bleeding in the intensive care unit, but such prophylaxis is costly. A meta-analysis was conducted of 15 randomized studies on prophylaxis with cimetidine and/or antacids. There were 8 comparisons of cimetidine and 9 of antacids with a control group, and 10 comparisons of cimetidine with antacids.

Rates of upper gastrointestinal tract bleeding in patients given a placebo or no prophylaxis ranged from 3% to 53%. Cimetidine appeared to be significantly more effective than no treatment or a placebo in 5 of 8 comparisons; the typical odds ratio was .32 (Fig 9–5). Antacids were significantly more effective than no treatment or a placebo in 6 of 9 comparisons, with a typical odds ratio of .12. Antacids were significantly better than cimetidine in 2 of 10 comparisons, with a typical odds ratio of 1.61.

Antacids are not significantly better than cimetidine in preventing up-

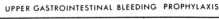

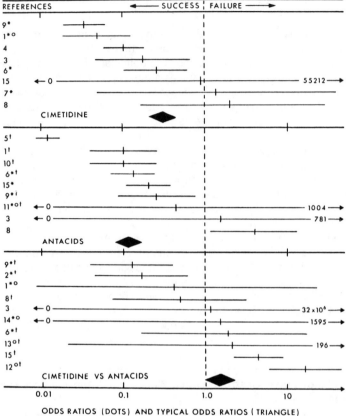

Fig 9–5.—Odds ratio and typical odds ratio with 95% confidence interval limits of studies on the prophylaxis of upper gastrointestinal tract bleeding acquired in the intensive care unit. *Asterisks* marked studies on overt bleeding. A correction factor of .5 is attributed to studies with 0 cells (marked by ⁰). Odds ratios less than 1 *(dashed line)* mean that cimetidine or antacids prevented bleeding, or that cimetidine was more effective than antacids. Results were considered statistically significant if the 95% confidence interval did not override the ratio of 1. Studies where antacids were titrated in increase gastric pH are marked by ᵗ; cimetidine was never titrated in the studies illustrated in this figure. (Courtesy of Lacroix J, Infante-Rivard C, Jenicek M, et al: *Crit Care Med* 17:862–869, 1989.)

per gastrointestinal tract bleeding; both agents are effective. Considering the many weaknesses in study design and the potential biases in many studies, recommendations for systemic prophylaxis cannot be made at present. The cumulative evidence is not very strong, and no measure has been shown to decrease the risk of shock, the need for transfusion, or mortality. Controlled randomized clinical trials will be most informative.

▶ The purpose of a meta-analysis, or overview, is to systematically pool data from the literature following specific guidelines to aid in interpreting the myriad results that often exist. In this particular analysis of studies published before

1986, there was confirmation that antacids are no better than cimetidine in preventing upper gastrointestinal tract hemorrhage (end point of analysis), but that both drugs seem to be effective in limiting bleeding. However, design weaknesses were identified in many studies, and there was significant heterogeneity among the studies. As a result, the conclusions of the meta-analysis may not be as strong as stated.

Because prophylaxis, in one form or another, against upper gastrointestinal hemorrhage is used very commonly in patients in intensive care units, one must carefully weigh the available data before initiating therapy. It makes sound clinical sense that efforts to prevent such hemorrhage should be aggressive; however, additional well-designed, prospective, placebo-controlled studies are necessary to fully confirm what agent(s) to most effective in reducing morbidity and mortality, least costly, and causes the least amount of adverse effects. Until these studies present their results, intensivists will have to decide on therapy based on the existing data and their clinical judgment.—F.P. Ognibene, M.D., and J.E. Parrillo, M.D.

Salutary Effects of Modest Fluid Replacement in the Treatment of Adults With Diabetic Ketoacidosis: Use in Patients Without Extreme Volume Deficit
Adrogué HJ, Barrero J, Eknoyan G (Baylor College of Medicine, Houston)
JAMA 262:2108–2113, 1989   9–11

Fluid therapy is the cornerstone in the management of diabetic ketoacidosis (DKA), yet the optimal rate of fluid administration to correct the volume deficit remains undefined. A prospective study was undertaken to evaluate with DKA 2 regimens of fluid therapy that differed exclusively in the rate of fluid infusion in adult patients. Patients in circulatory shock or with severe renal insufficiency or persistent oliguria were excluded.

In protocol 1, 12 patients were administered normal saline infusion at a rate of 1,000 mL/hr (approximately 14 mL/kg/hr) in the initial 4 hours and 500 mL/hr (approximately 7 mL/kg/hr) during the subsequent 4 hours. In protocol 2, 11 patients received normal saline infusion at half the rates of protocol 1. Insulin therapy and potassium replacement regimens were similar in both groups.

As expected, acid-base parameters showed progressive recovery toward normalcy in both groups. However, the increment in plasma bicarbonate concentration from admission levels at all points of observation was greater with protocol 2, attaining statistical significance at 4 hours and 24 hours after admission. There were no untoward side effects with either protocol.

Relatively modest fluid replacement in the treatment of DKA in adult patients without extreme volume deficit results in prompt recovery and a significant reduction in the overall cost of medical care. The slower recovery from DKA with the high infusion rates is probably caused by the relatively greater acute expansion with a bicarbonate-free solution and sustained loss of bicarbonate precursors in the urine because of continued volume expansion.

▶ This study demonstrates that patients with milder forms of DKA do not have as great an intravascular volume deficit as those with more severe DKA. Historically, however, both groups have often received similar volume replacement regimens, leading to what the authors of this study have demonstrated—a delay in resolution of the metabolic acidosis. This is caused by the development of a dilutional acidosis after the overly zealous administration of bicarbonate-free replacement solutions, which dilute any available bicarbonate buffers in the serum. Additionally, as the authors explain, a sustained volume expansion can promote the urinary loss of bicarbonate precursors, including ketone salts.

Although the regimen used in protocol 2 in this study may be acceptable for most patients with mild to moderate DKA, careful tailoring of the replacement fluids for each patient is advisable rather than applying the "cookbook" approach so commonly used in other disorders. Intravascular hemodynamic monitoring is unwarranted in most patients, but close clinical monitoring of the intravascular volume by noninvasive methods may help prevent the complications seen with excessive replacement therapy.—A.C. Dixon, M.D.,and J.E. Parrillo, M.D.

Pancreatic Carcinoma as a Cause of Unexplained Pancreatitis: Report of Ten Cases
Lin A, Feller ER (Memorial Hosp, Pawtucket, RI; Miriam Hosp, Providence, RI)
Ann Intern Med 113:166–167, 1990   9–12

Data were reviewed on 10 patients seen in 1978–1987 with pancreatic cancer who initially had acute abdominal pain and hyperamylasemia. These patients represented 3% of all patients with pancreatic carcinoma seen in this period, and 1.3% of patients admitted with acute pancreatitis.

Four patients had typical acute pancreatitis and a rapid return of the amylase level to normal as abdominal pain resolved. Obstructive jaundice later developed in 1 of them. Pain persisted and hyperamylasemia did not improve in 4 patients; 2 others had rapidly resolving pancreatitis that recurred after symptom-free intervals of 3 months and 7 months, respectively. All patients had increased serum amylase levels. Laparotomy showed pancreatic adenocarcinoma in 9 patients and an osteoclastic giant cell tumor in 1.

Pancreatitis ranged from clinically mild to severe in these patients. Retrograde cholangiopancreatography may, in the individual patient, fail to distinguish malignant obstruction from inflammation or normal variation. Cancer should be considered in any patient with unexplained acute pancreatic inflammation.

▶ Pancreatic carcinoma develops insidiously, and it is diagnosed typically when the tumor has manifested significant growth and intra-abdominal extension. As a consequence of its late detection, the 5-year survival rate is very low. Clinicians should be alerted to the fact that in a small percentage of patients with pancreatic carcinoma, pancreatitis may be the heralding clinical finding. As a consequence, pancreatic carcinoma should to added to the list of etiologies of pancreatitis, and it should be especially considered in patients with no obvious precipitating reason for the development of pancreatitis.— F.P. Ognibene, M.D., and J.E. Parrillo, M.D.

Management of Severe Hyponatremia: Rapid or Slow Correction?
Cluitmans FHM, Meinders AE (Univ of Leiden, The Netherlands)
Am J Med 88:161–166, 1990   9–13

The management of severe hyponatremia remains controversial. Those who advocate rapid correction fear neurologic damage or death, but this approach has itself been associated with neurologic complications such as central pontine and extrapontine myelinolysis. The literature on this subject was reviewed to identify areas of disagreement, particularly with regard to how fast to correct hyponatremia.

Data on 163 patients with a serum sodium level of less than 121 mM/L were reviewed. In the 38 evaluable patients, morbidity and death occurred only when hyponatremia developed at a rate of .5 mM/L/m or greater. Immediate treatment appears to be necessary, and it should include the removal of causative factors if this is possible. Chronic hyponatremia was most often related to thiazide diuretics and the syndrome of inappropriate antidiuretic hormone secretion. Hyponatremia was corrected at a rate of .5 mM/L/hr or more in 71 of 117 such patients, and 62% of these patients had neurologic sequelae. In only 1 of 46 patients corrected more slowly did central pontine myelinolysis develop.

Immediate and possibly rapid correction can prevent severe morbidity or death in acute hyponatremia. In patients with chronic hyponatremia, however, correction at a rate less than .5 mM/L/hr appears to be indicated. If the rate at which hyponatremia developed is uncertain, rapid correction to a mildly hyponatremic level with hypertonic saline and furosemide probably is the best approach.

▶ Severe hyponatremia is associated with significant morbidity and mortality. However, as noted in this review, methods of correction can also be dangerous, especially if correction to normal serum sodium levels is too rapid. The data suggest that both acute hyponatremia (2–3 days to develop) and too rapid correction of both acute and chronic hyponatremia are associated with the most significantly adverse neurologic sequelae. The first goal of therapy, as outlined, should be to determine the duration of hyponatremia; if it is acute, then rapid sodium correction at a rate of 1 mM/L/hr should occur. If the duration is more chronic, slower correction of serum sodium is warranted. If both the acuteness of the drop in sodium and appropriate rates of correction are addressed, neurologic damage may be limited.— F.P. Ognibene, M.D., and J.E. Parrillo, M.D.

Albumin Supplementation in the Critically Ill: A Prospective, Randomized Trial

Foley EF, Borlase BC, Dzik WH, Bistrian BR, Benotti PN (Harvard Med School)
Arch Surg 125:739–742, 1990   9–14

Hypoalbuminemia is an accurate prognostic indicator of poor outcomes in a variety of clinical settings. Albumin replacement to correct it in critically ill patients is controversial. A prospective, randomized trial of 25% albumin administration was undertaken in 40 hypoalbuminemic, critically ill patients. All had serum albumin levels of less than 25 g/L. Eighteen patients received 25% albumin supplementation to achieve and maintain serum levels of 25 g/L or more, and 22 patients (controls) were given no concentrated albumin. All patients received full parenteral or enteral nutritional support.

No clinical benefit from albumin therapy was observed in the mortality or major complication rate between groups. Mortality in the treatment group was 39% and in the control group, 27%. Major complication rates were 89% and 77%, respectively. There were also no between-group differences in length of hospitalization, stay in the intensive care unit, ventilator dependence, or tolerance of enteral feeding, despite significant increases in the albumin level in the treatment group.

Albumin therapy in hypoalbuminemic critically ill patients has no beneficial impact on a variety of outcome variables, despite its value in raising serum albumin concentrations. Albumin treatment is a costly intervention that does not appear to be justified in this patient population.

▶ The serum albumin level is one of the markers known to predict mortality in severely ill patients. Despite scant supportive evidence and moderate expense associated with albumin administration, the empiric approach of specific albumin supplementation for patients with hypoalbuminemia has become increasingly prevalent.

This study can be criticized because of the small number of patients entered (making potential differences in mortality difficult to detect), but the uniform absence of a significant difference in any of the parameters examined suggests that albumin supplementation is not useful in the critically ill. The possibility that a higher targeted level of serum albumin might have been effective ignores the fact that one would expect the response from the initial increment in serum albumin to be greater than that from later elevations within the physiologic range. Hypoalbuminemia is a marker of the severity of disease but does not cause higher mortality in this context. If nutritional support is utilized, this study argues that albumin supplementation does not appear to be of benefit.—A. Kumar, M.D., and J.E. Parrillo, M.D.

Thiopental Infusion in the Treatment of Intracranial Hypertension Complicating Fulminant Hepatic Failure

Forbes A, Alexander GJM, O'Grady JG, Keays R, Gullan R, Dawling S, Williams R (King's College Hosp; Maudsley Hosp; New Cross Hosp, London)
Hepatology 10:306–310, 1989   9–15

Intracranial hypertension complicating fulminant liver failure is associated with high mortality, especially if accompanied by renal failure. Intravenous thiopental was evaluated in 13 patients with fulminant liver failure, acute oliguric renal failure, and intracranial hypertension refractory to other measures. Eleven patients had taken acetaminophen with suicidal intent, and 2 had presumed non-A non-B viral hepatitis. The dose of thiopental was adjusted until the intracranial pressure was normal or adverse hemodynamic changes occurred.

Intracranial pressure declined in each patient after initial infusion of a median dose of 250 mg of thiopental over 15 minutes. In 8 cases, continued infusion led to stable intracranial and cerebral perfusion pressures. Five patients recovered completely, whereas 3 died of intracranial hypertension. Minor hypotension was readily controlled by lowering the dose of thiopental. One patient had a bullous eruption and hypothermia with the initial infusion.

Thiopental infusion may control otherwise intractable intracranial hypertension in patients with fulminant liver failure. This measure can maintain patients until liver transplantation is possible.

▶ The authors successfully utilized barbiturate infusion to control intracranial pressure during fulminant hepatic failure. It has been well shown that barbiturates decrease cerebral blood flow, cerebral blood volume, and cerebral metabolism in normal brain. It is enlightening to find that the metabolically impaired brain also responds to barbiturates in a similar manner. It is unclear from this report whether the response is quantitatively similar.— R.W. McPherson, M.D.

Ultrapure, Stroma-Free, Polymerized Bovine Hemoglobin Solution: Evaluation of Renal Toxicity

Lee R, Atsumi N, Jacobs EE Jr, Austen WG, Vlahakes GJ (Massachusetts Gen Hosp, Boston; Harvard Med School)
J Surg Res 47:407–411, 1989   9–16

Material developed from stroma-free hemoglobin solutions has shown promise for use as a blood substitute, but renal toxicity has been a problem. This complication was studied when an ultrapure, polymerized bovine hemoglobin solution was used. In Sprague-Dawley rats the material was infused at doses ranging from 25 mL/kg to 100 mL/kg, with or without bicarbonate for alkalinization of urine. Other rats were given this material after it was contaminated with unpurified bovine hemoglobin lysate.

Renal toxicity did not appear until doses of 75 mL/kg were reached; reversible increases in the serum level of creatinine occurred 24 hours after infusion. Bicarbonate significantly diminished the increases in creatinine, even when the dose was 100 mL/kg. Infusion of contaminated solution produced largely irreversible renal toxicity, even at doses of 25 mL/kg. Death followed at higher doses despite the addition of bicarbonate.

Ultrapure, polymerized bovine hemoglobin solution, even at large doses, produces only mild, reversible renal toxicity, which can be diminished by administering bicarbonate. The toxicity apparently occurs by precipitation of hemoglobin or by a direct effect on the renal tubules. The toxicity resulting from hemoglobin lysate-contaminated solution probably results from a different mechanism. Stroma-free hemoglobin solutions with adequate purification of contaminants show potential for use as blood substitutes.

▶ This paper is presented because of increasing concern about our national blood supply and the increasing desire to find effective blood substitutes. Stroma-free bovine hemoglobin solution is one such ultimate potential source. This particular study concentrates on the renal toxicity of this agent, and it is brought to the attention of critical care specialists because of the likelihood that there will be further research and potential clinical implications for this substance.—M.C. Rogers, M.D.

A Randomized, Controlled Trial of Vitamin A in Children With Severe Measles
Hussey GD, Klein M (Univ of Cape Town, South Africa)
N Engl J Med 323:160–164, 1990   9–17

The suggestion that vitamin A may be beneficial in measles appears to be biologically plausible because hyporetinemia occurs almost invariably in children with severe cases of measles, and the reduction in the serum level of retinol is associated with increased mortality. In a randomized, double-blind placebo-controlled trial 189 children with measles who were hospitalized for associated complications such as pneumonia, diarrhea, and croup received either 400,000 international units (IU) of retinyl palmitate or placebo orally beginning within 5 days of onset of the rash. The outcome variables were death and severity of illness.

Baseline characteristics were similar in both the treatment and placebo groups. Although clinically apparent vitamin A deficiency was uncommon in this patient population, serum levels of retinol were markedly low, as were serum levels of retinol-binding protein and albumin. Serum levels of retinol were below .7 μmol/L, which is indicative of hyporetinemia, in 92% of children, and 46% had levels below .35 μmol/L, which placed them at risk for xerophthalmia.

Children who received vitamin A had markedly diminished morbidity and mortality, compared with the placebo group. Vitamin A reduced the death rate by more than half and the duration of pneumonia, diarrhea, and hospitalization by about a third. Vitamin A also reduced the incidence of postmeasles croup and herpes stomatitis, as well as the need for intensive care. The overall risk for an adverse outcome in children treated with vitamin A was half that in the placebo group, particularly in children aged 2 years and older. No adverse effects of vitamin A were noted. All children with severe measles should receive a vitamin A supplement of 400,000 IU.

▶ The decline in immunizations has resulted in epidemics of measles not only in underdeveloped countries but also in the United States. The concept that vitamin A may be useful in decreasing the morbidity and mortality of measles even when there is no nutritional deficiency is an exciting thought that has now been verified in this study. It is worth reading for all individuals who care for patients capable of severe illness with measles.—M.C. Rogers, M.D.

Nutritional Discontinuation: Active or Passive Euthanasia?
Banja JD (Emory Univ)
J Neurosci Nursing 22:117–120, 1990   9– 18

The discontinuation of nutrition from critically ill patients may be as important a bioethical dilemma as abortion. Court decisions on this issue have been contradictory, often with impassioned minority opinions. The moral grounds for differentiating passive from active euthanasia were examined.

According to a 1983 ruling of the Appellate Division of the New Jersey Supreme Court, termination of life-sustaining treatment may occur when a patient is brain dead, irreversibly comatose or vegetative, incurable, terminally ill, and unable to reap any benefit from medical treatment. The Court also considered whether the patient might suffer an unjustifiable degree of invasion of bodily privacy from treatment. These criteria are morally compelling. "Passive euthanasia" is said to occur when death results after termination of treatment for a patient under these conditions. In contrast, an example of active euthanasia would be the injection of air into the patient's veins. The distinction between active and passive is not based on the difference between acts and omissions, however; rather, it is based on the idea that in passive euthanasia the illness is allowed to take its natural course.

It has been argued that discontinuation of nutrition is similar to discontinuation of artificial ventilation or dialysis for dependent patients. However, the predictability of the consequences of these latter actions can never be as certain as the predictability of the consequences of removal of a gastric tube, because no human being can survive without food and fluids. This certainty distinguishes the removal of a feeding tube from the discontinuation of other forms of treatment. The similarity in language between these 2 types of acts does help to argue that nutritional discontinuation for certain patients is a form of passive euthanasia.

Those who care for patients who may desire discontinuation of life-prolonging treatment should learn about the relevant law in their state and prepare a protocol for discontinuation of life-prolonging treatment at their institution. It may be desirable to create a new clinical specialty of euthanatology whose practitioners can assist in a professional way the dying of our increasingly aging population, because it is expected that health care providers will more and more be expected to aid and facilitate the dying of others.

▶ The conception of active or passive euthanasia is at the forefront of ethical issues in intensive care. Nutritional discontinuation is commonly suggested as a way of dealing with critically ill patients who have a poor or no ultimate functional outcome. Because of the ethical dilemmas, however, it is not clear what is an appropriate response to these suggestions. This paper reviews the legal and ethical issues associated with these problems. It should be read by intensivists because these kinds of concerns are likely to become increasingly frequent in our practice.—M.C. Rogers, M.D.

Reconstructive Allotransplantation: Considerations Regarding Integumentary/Musculoskeletal Grafts, Cyclosporine, Wound Coverage in Thermal Injury, and the Immune Response

Hewitt CW, Black KS, Achauer BM, Patel MP (Univ of California, Irvine)
J Burn Care Rehabil 11:74–85, 1990   9–19

With the introduction of cyclosporine, a powerful and selective immunosuppressant, the transplantation of modules of allointegumentary/musculoskeletal tissues or their components for the repair of peripheral tissue defects has been reconsidered. These modules, which are composites of various tissues, are known as composite tissue allografts. Studies have been undertaken to lay the foundation in transplant immunobiology for the clinical use of composite tissue allografts.

The reconstructive surgeon's interest in allotransplantation faded with the dominant success of organ transplants. However, cyclosporine has renewed interest in reconstructive allotransplantation. Cyclosporine appears to exert degree of specificity toward the alloimmune rejection response while sparing important immune functions needed to fight infection. Skin allografts, when used as temporary wound dressings, help to prolong the survival of patients with massive burns. There may be a role for the temporary use of cyclosporine and skin allografts for immediate wound coverage in burn victims not expected to survive. The underlying mechanisms of cyclosporine's actions have not yet been established.

The objective of this continuing research is to induce permanent acceptance of composite tissue allografts. The value of the grafts lies in their potential for complete functional and cosmetic restoration in the surgical reconstruction of tissue in patients with full-thickness burns. The initial results of basic experiments with cyclosporine are encouraging.

▶ When we think of transplants we generally think of heart, lung, kidney, or liver. The use of cyclosporine, however, has allowed increasing numbers of transplants of different kinds of tissues, e.g., allointegumentary/multiple skeletal tissue grafts, as reviewed here. These grafts are useful not only in plastic surgery, but in the functional recovery of muscular skeletal tissue, particularly in burn patients. The purpose of including this paper in the selection is to indicate the kind of unique problems that this special form of transplantation can produce.— M.C. Rogers, M.D.

Management of Nonstaphylococcal Toxic Epidermal Necrolysis: Follow-Up Study of 16 Case Histories
Tegelberg-Stassen MJAM, van Vloten WA, Baart de la Faille H (Zeister Algemeen Ziekenhuis, Zeist, The Netherlands; Univ Hosp of Utrecht)
Dermatologica 180:124–129, 1990   9–20

Toxic epidermal necrolysis (TEN), or scalded skin syndrome, is sometimes but not always caused by *Staphylococcus aureus* infection. Between 1969 and 1987, 14 patients who were suspected of having nonstaphylococcal TEN were treated. Most patients had skin and mucosal eruptions at presentation, and at least 5 had skin tenderness. The extent of skin detachment ranged from 45% to 100%.

The patients were nursed undressed between metallized sheets, and necrotic skin was removed each day. Reversed barrier nursing was used routinely. Broad-spectrum antibiotic coverage began when fever occurred or when extensive bacterial colonization of the skin was confirmed. Steroids were given, orally if possible, when histologic study of the skin confirmed TEN. The daily dose of prednisone was 200 mg in the last 8 patients, and this was tapered as soon as clinical stability was achieved.

The skin began to heal within 1–2 days of the start of treatment, and formation of new bulla ceased. Patients became stable within a week, but mucosal healing sometimes took much longer. One patient died of multibacterial sepsis. Three patients had formation of corneal pannus that impaired their vision. Histologic monitoring showed that a new epidermis began to form 4 or 5 days after blisters appeared.

Steroid therapy, combined with reversed barrier nursing and the timely use of broad-spectrum antibiotics, is an effective approach to nonstaphylococcal TEN. All of the present patients required systemic antibiotics. It would be of interest to determine the effects of other immunomodulators in cases of TEN.

▶ Toxic epidermal necrolysis, or scalded skin syndrome, can be caused by *Staphylococcus aureus* and other organisms. In fact, it also can be caused by drugs or by graft-vs.-host disease. The second-degree burn that results can cause life-threatening complications and a high mortality rate. This paper reviews laboratory data on 14 patients who had nonstaphylococcal TEN and discusses the effective management of these patients. The authors focus on the elements of skin care and the use of antibiotics, and also include an important discussion on the use of steroids in these patients.– M.C. Rogers, M.D.

Reye's Syndrome: A Reappraisal of Diagnosis in 49 Presumptive Cases
Gauthier M, Guay J, Lacroix J, Lortie A (Univ of Montreal)
Am J Dis Child 143:1181–1185, 1989   9–21

The incidence of Reye's syndrome (RS) appears to have decreased dramatically in recent years. This may be because of reappraisal of encephalopathies that would previously have been termed RS. The records of 49 patients with RS seen at 1 Montreal hospital between 1970 and 1987 were evaluated blindly by 3 expert physicians.

Assessments were similar in 86% of the cases; discussion was used to achieve agreement on the remainder. The diagnosis of RS was considered likely in 1 case, probable in 11, unlikely in 21, and excluded in 15.

Therefore, the incidence of RS appears to have been much lower between 1970 and 1987 than examination of the records from that time would indicate. The disappearance of RS in recent times should be reassessed, and RS diagnostic criteria should be reevaluated by the Centers for Disease Control.

▶ Reye's syndrome has virtually disappeared from the listing admission diagnosis in most pediatric intensive care units. Although a large component of this decrease is ascribed to the removal of aspirin from medications given to children, another cause is increasing suspicion that RS is confused with other diseases. This study looks retrospectively at 49 presumed cases and concludes that RS was considered likely in only 1 case. When the 11 probable cases are also included, less than 50% of the patients admitted with the diagnosis of RS were found, in retrospect, to have this disease. This study is likely to reinforce my belief that RS has been a misunderstood and overdiagnosed condition.—M.C. Rogers, M.D.

A Comparison of Ceftriaxone and Cefuroxime for the Treatment of Bacterial Meningitis in Children
Schaad UB, Suter S, Gianella-Borradori A, Pfenninger J, Auckenthaler R, Bernath O, Cheseaux J-J, Wedgwood J (Univ of Berne; Univ of Lausanne; Univ of Geneva, Switzerland)
N Engl J Med 322:141–147, 1990   9–22

The effectiveness and safety of 2 cephalosporin drugs, ceftriaxone and cefuroxime, were compared in 106 children with acute bacterial meningitis. The children were randomized to receive ceftriaxone, 100 mg/kg daily intravenously, or cefuroxime, 240 mg/kg daily intravenously. The latter drug was given in 4 daily doses and the former in a single dose. The mean age was 3 years, and the 2 treatment groups were clinically comparable.

Sterilization of the CSF within 36 hours was more consistently achieved in ceftriaxone-treated patients. All of the patients improved rapidly and were cured, and there were no recrudescences or relapses. Less total treatment time was required with ceftriaxone. Complications were similarly frequent in the 2 groups. Biliary pseudolithiasis occurred in 46% of the ceftriaxone-treated patients but in none of those given cefuroxime. Children given ceftriaxone were less likely to have sensorineural hearing loss.

Ceftriaxone is preferable to cefuroxime in the treatment of children with acute bacterial meningitis. The more rapid sterilization of the CSF and the milder hearing impairment outweigh the problem of reversible biliary pseudolithiasis. Further studies are needed before using dexamethasone routinely to minimize hearing disability.

▶ This important paper compares ceftriaxone to cefuroxime in the treatment of bacterial meningitis in children. Briefly, it concludes unequivocally that ceftriaxone is preferable in that it more rapidly sterilizes the CSF and produces less hearing impairment. An interesting sidelight of this study, however, was the need for further studies before the use of dexamethasone can be recognized as a routine therapy to minimize hearing disability in bacterial meningitis. This article should be of interest to anyone caring for children with bacterial meningitis.—M.C. Rogers, M.D.

Chronic Ethanol Exposure Before Injury Produces Greater Immune Dysfunction After Thermal Injury in Rats
Kawakami M, Meyer AA, Johnson MC, de Serres S, Peterson HD (Univ of North Carolina)
J Trauma 30:27–31, 1990   9–23

Although alcoholic burn patients are known to have a significantly higher rate of death from infection than nonalcoholic patients, the effect of chronic alcohol exposure on immune function in burned patients has not been examined. Immune function was measured in rats with chronic ethanol exposure (EtOH) and burn injury.

Ten animals were in the EtOH plus burn group, 8 in the burn alone group, and 6 in the EtOH alone group. Eight rats served as controls. Immune function was assessed by in vivo chemotaxis and responsiveness of nonadherent splenocytes to both a T cell mitogen, concanavalin A (Con A), and a B cell mitogen, lipopolysaccharide. Measurements were obtained 4 days after the burn injury and/or gavage of 2.4 g/kg/day of ethanol for 14 days.

Both EtOH and burns produced statistically significant suppression in chemotaxis, but only the EtOH plus burn group was significantly different from the control group. The response to lipopolysaccharide was significantly decreased in the EtOH plus burn group but not the response to Con A.

Although the duration of EtOH ingestion used in this study was relatively short and the burn injury small, the size of the burn injury allowed detection of any combined effect of EtOH and injury. Both alcoholics and burned patients had defective leukocyte function. The increased susceptibility to infection in alcoholic burn patients may be a result of chronic alcohol exposure, leading to further impaired immune function after injury.

▶ Because many patients consume alcohol before injury, the additive effect of ethanol exposure on injury is an interesting area of research. This study documents that greater immune dysfunction is produced after thermal injury in rats when the rats are chronically exposed to ethanol. Too often, intensivists concentrate on the acute illness such as a burn without thinking about the background conditions such as chronic ethanol intoxication, which may make the critical care management more difficult.—M.C. Rogers, M.D.

"Endogenous" Benzodiazepine Activity in Body Fluids of Patients With Hepatic Encephalopathy
Mullen KD, Szauter KM, Kaminsky-Russ K (Case Western Reserve Univ)
Lancet 336:81–83, 1990   9–24

An endogenous benzodiazepine-like substance may be involved in hepatic encephalopathy. Benzodiazepine activity was examined in the body fluids of 30 patients with hepatic encephalopathy and in 18 controls. None of those involved in the study had taken synthetic benzodiazepines for at least 3 months.

Benzodiazepine receptor binding was significantly higher in the CSF of patients with hepatic encephalopathy than in controls. The severity of encephalopathy was correlated significantly with benzodiazepine activity by radioreceptor and radioimmunoassay in urine and plasma. In patients with advanced encephalopathy, benzodiazepine activity equivalent to more than 900 ng/mL could be detected.

Hepatic encephalopathy is associated with elevated levels of a substance with benzodiazepine activity. The identity, source, and effects of this substance have yet to be determined. It may have a role in pathogenesis of the neural inhibition seen in hepatic encephalopathy.

▶ This fascinating paper documents endogenous benzodiazepine activity in the body fluids of patients with encephalopathy. The authors are unable to identify the source of this substance but indicate that it may be an important mediator of the neural inhibition associated with hepatic encephalopathy. If this work continues to develop, we will have some new and fascinating insights into the pathogenesis and potential treatment of hepatic encephalopathy.—M.C. Rogers, M.D.

Autoimmune Hypothesis of Acquired Subglottic Stenosis in Premature Infants
Stolovitzky JP, Todd NW (Emory Univ)
Laryngoscope 100:227–230, 1990   9–25

Acquired subglottic stenosis has been reported in 4% of premature infants who receive neonatal intensive care, with prolonged intubation being an important etiologic factor. Not all premature infants acquire subglottic stenosis, and infants with similar characteristics and care have varying laryngeal outcomes. Interestingly, the subglottic stenosis often manifests months after removal of the presumptive causative factors.

It has been hypothesized that an autoimmune mechanism to type II collagen may explain the varying laryngeal outcomes in these premature infants. Trauma to the endotracheal mucosa causes mucosal inflammation and cartilaginous matrix degradation. As a result type II collagen is exposed to the afferent arm of the immune system, becomes immunogenic, and stimulates the synthesis of anticollagen-II antibodies. Activation of the immunoinflammatory cells at the site of trauma may play a role in extending the damage and establishing a chronic process.

To test this hypothesis, a retrospective study was made of premature infants of comparable birth weight, gestational age, and duration of endotracheal intubation. Antibodies to collagen II were found in the serum of 3 of 5 infants who acquired subglottic stenosis but in none of the 8 control infants who did not have subglottic stenosis. The mean onset of subglottis stenosis after removal of the endotracheal tube was 5 months (range, 3–7 months). These findings suggest an autoimmune process in the etiology of subglottic stenosis and warrant further investigation that may lead to new diagnostic and therapeutic measures for these infants.

▶ This paper did a retrospective evaluation of premature infants who had symptoms of airway obstruction on intubation and concluded that subglottic stenosis was associated with serum antibodies to type II collagen. This interesting observation raises the potential for diagnostic evaluation of patients who are at risk for subglottic stenosis and an understanding of the disease.—M.C. Rogers, M.D.

Alteration in Extracellular Amino Acids After Traumatic Spinal Cord Injury
Panter SS, Yum SW, Faden AI (Univ of California, San Francisco; VA Med Ctr, San Francisco)
Ann Neurol 27:96–99, 1990   9–26

The delayed response to impact injuries to the spinal cord may result in part from excitatory amino acids. Recent studies have shown that tissue damage after CNS injury and cell death after extracellular excitatory amino acid exposure are both limited by treatment with N-methyl-D-asparate receptor antagonists. Whether spinal cord trauma alters the concentrations of extracellular amino acids was determined.

A model of traumatic spinal cord injury was produced in male rabbits. Microdialysis was conducted in the spinal cord during and after administration of impact trauma. Amino acids were separated by high-performance liquid chromatography and quantitated via peak areas.

Extracellular concentrations of all amino acids immediately increased after impact trauma, but both the degree and pattern of the increase were related to the severity of injury. Moderate trauma caused an immediate but transient increase (200% to 400%) in the extracellular levels of all amino acids that were measured. A more prolonged and significant increase (400% to 630%) in the concentrations of extracellular amino acids was recorded after severe trauma. After moderate trauma, all amino acids except for alanine returned to pretrauma levels after 20 minutes. Extracellular levels of most amino acids remained significantly elevated for at least 30 minutes after severe trauma.

Disruption of the blood-spinal cord barrier by trauma may result in significant movement of free amino acids from plasma into the extracellular space of the spinal cord. Excitatory amino acids may thus, in part, mediate secondary injury after CNS trauma.

▶ This paper documents experimentally the extracellularization of amino acids after spinal cord injury and develops convincingly the hypothesis that excitatory amino acids contribute to delay tissue injury after CNS trauma. This type of investigation and the potential for receptor blockade of these amino acids remain at the forefront of research and neurologic intensive care. We do need, however, more convincing evidence in humans that this pathogenesis works, and that some treatment modality may alter the outcome.—M.C. Rogers, M.D.

Pralidoxime in the Treatment of Carbamate Intoxication
Kurtz PH (California Dept of Food and Agriculture, Sacramento)
Am J Emerg Med 8:68–70, 1990   9–27

Carbamate insecticides act by inhibiting cholinesterase enzymes that are essential for normal nerve function. Intoxication by cholinesterase inhibitors has been treated with atropine, and the use of enzyme reactivators in such intoxication is controversial.

Without individual testing there is no way to predict whether the toxicity of a specific carbamate compound will be enhanced or antagonized by oxime therapy. With few exceptions, atropine has been found to be superior to oximes in the treatment of carbamate intoxication. Atropine is therefore the antidote of choice. In some cases oxime therapy with atropine therapy is more effective than atropine alone, but the effect is only slight. The use of pralidoxime as an adjunct to atropine is indicated in serious poisonings with unknown cholinesterase inhibitors and in serious mixed poisonings with both organophosphorus and carbamate compounds.

▶ This paper reports a study of the oxime reactivators of inhibited cholinesterase enzymes in carbamate insecticide poisoning, but it actually is a very interesting review of the pharmacology of the disease. It is worth reading in its entirety, as it clearly goes through the steps in treatment recommended for carbamate intoxication.—M.C. Rogers, M.D.

Acute Thyroxine Ingestion in Pediatric Patients

Lewander WJ, Lacouture PG, Silva JE, Lovejoy FH (Rhode Island Hosp, Providence; Brown Univ; Children's Hosp, Boston; Brigham and Women's Hosp, Boston)
Pediatrics 84:262–265, 1989   9–28

During a 1-year period 22 cases of acute ingestion of thyroxine (T_4) were reported in pediatric patients. Fifteen patients (80% boys) younger than age 5 years with documented serum concentrations of T_4 were studied.

The estimated amount of T_4 ingested by 10 patients ranged from 1.5 mg to 8.8 mg (.1–.73 mg/kg). All patients were examined within 6 hours of ingestion and all were asymptomatic. Three patients with initial serum concentrations of T_4 of more than 75 µg/dL had signs and symptoms of toxicity within 12–48 hours after ingestion. These included fever, tachycardia, hypertension, and agitation, all of which resolved within 24–60 hours. The mean elimination half-life of T_4 in 7 patients was 2.8 days, but the mean elimination half-life of triiodothyronine was 6 days, nearly 5 times longer than that observed in physiologic conditions in children.

Acute pediatric overdoses of T_4 are not common and usually result in minimal or no toxicity. The absence of early clinical manifestations, however, does not preclude the delayed onset of toxicity. Initial concentrations of T_4 may help to predict which patients may experience more severe toxicity. Most patients may be managed on an outpatient basis.

▶ Thyroxine overdose is relatively common in infants whose parents take the drug. The authors conclude that the majority of these intoxications are not severe and may be managed on an outpatient basis, but that determination of T_4 concentrations is necessary to predict the ultimate outcome.—M.C. Rogers, M.D.

Vasopressin Antagonist in Early Postoperative Diabetes Insipidus

Seckl JR, Dunger DB, Bevan JS, Nakasu Y, Chowdrey C, Burke CW, Lightman SL (Charing Cross and Westminster Med School, London; John Radcliffe Hosp, Oxford; Radcliffe Infirmary, Oxford)
Lancet 355:1353–1356, 1990   9–29

Pituitary and suprasellar surgery may be complicated by acute postoperative diabetes insipidus, which may be either transient or permanent. In a prospective study to evaluate the pathogenesis of early postoperative diabetes insipidus, plasma concentrations of arginine vasopressin (AVP) were obtained immediately after operation, at the onset of diabetes insipidus, and 24 hours later in 23 patients without preexisting diabetes insipidus who underwent transfrontal (hypothalamic) or transsphenoidal (pituitary) surgery and 12 patients who underwent transsphenoidal surgery but did not have postoperative diabetes insipidus (control). All patients received prophylactic corticosteroid replacement.

The onset of diabetes insipidus occurred between 1 hour and 36 hours after operation. Immediately after transsphenoidal surgery, plasma concentrations of AVP were high, whether or not diabetes insipidus occurred, but then fell to subnormal concentrations with the onset of diabetes insipidus. After transfrontal surgery the onset of diabetes insipidus was significantly earlier and was associated with higher plasma AVP immunoreactivity than after transsphenoidal surgery.

Although plasma AVP immunoreactivity after transfrontal surgery co-eluted with standard synthetic AVP on high-pressure liquid chromatography, the plasma showed no intrinsic antidiuretic bioactivity and greatly attenuated the antidiuretic response to standard AVP.

Early diabetes insipidus after hypothalamic surgery is associated with the release of a substance, presumably an analogue, from the damaged hypothalamo-neurohypophyseal system, which acts as an antagonist to normal AVP activity. Diabetes insipidus after transsphenoidal surgery is associated with failure of neurohypophyseal release of AVP.

▶ In this very interesting study, Seckl et al. compared plasma AVP concentrations in patients with and without diabetes insipidus after transfrontal or transsphenoidal surgery for pituitary and suprasellar lesions. Diabetes insipidus occurred earlier after transfrontal than after transsphenoidal operations. The plasma level of AVP was higher in patients after transfrontal hypothalamic surgery at the onset of diabetes insipidus. In 2 patients, despite high plasma AVP concentrations after transfrontal surgery, this AVP was found to have low biological activity and may actually have antagonistic properties. Unfortunately, the investigators did not present data to answer whether other patients in this or even the transsphenoidal group secreted AVP that was of low biologic activity or had antagonistic properties. Twenty-four hours after onset of diabetes insipidus there was no difference in plasma AVP from patients in the 2 groups. These data suggest that the clinician may need to administer more supplemental synthetic AVP to control diabetes insipidus after transfrontal surgery than after transsphenoidal surgery.—J.R. Kirsch, M.D.

Barbiturate Therapy Reduces Nitrogen Excretion in Acute Head Injury
Fried RC, Dickerson RN, Guenter PA, Stein TP, Gennarelli TA, Dempsey DT, Buzby GP, Mullen JL (Univ of Pennsylvania; Univ of Medicine and Dentistry of New Jersey)
J Trauma 29:1558–1564, 1989   9–30

Pentobarbital lowers energy expenditure in acutely head-injured patients. Nitrogen catabolism and the changes associated with short-term pentobarbital therapy were studied in 7 patients with severe head injuries. A bolus dose of intravenously administered pentobarbital was followed by an infusion adjusted to maintain serum pentobarbital levels of 20–40 mg/L.

The mean Glasgow Coma Scale score at admission was 4.7. Of the patients, 5 survived to be discharged from the hospital. There were no significant differences between the 4 pentobarbital-treated patients and the 3 control patients in Coma Scale scores, peak body temperature, or steroid dose. Caloric and nitrogen intakes also were similar; both groups received a hypocaloric intake. Patients given barbiturates had significantly lower measured energy expenditure than control patients. The barbiturate group had lower urinary total nitrogen excretion and improved nitrogen balance despite a comparable intake of calories and protein. Urinary excretion of 3-methylhistidine was similar in the 2 groups.

Pentobarbital administration may promote nitrogen and energy equilibrium in acutely head-injured patients. Improved survival has not been documented, however, and barbiturates can have hypotensive and myocardial depressant effects.

▶ In general, mean energy expenditure and urinary nitrogen excretion in acutely head-injured patients is much greater than would be predicted. This study, like those of others, has demonstrated that barbiturate therapy is associated with decreased energy expenditure and lower nitrogen excretion with improved nitrogen balance. The mechanism for the nutritional effects of barbiturates remain speculative. All patients in this study received glucocorticoids in addition to pentobarbital. Because glucocorticoids increase urinary nitrogen excretion and augment breakdown of myofibrillar proteins in skeletal muscle, it is not possible from this study to determine what the effects of pentobarbital alone would be on nitrogen excretion. Similarly, although all patients in this study were in negative nitrogen balance, one cannot exclude the possibility that adequate nutrition could be obtained in either group of patients if increased parenteral or enteral nutritional support were provided. Adequate nutritional support should be the goal in all patients regardless of injury and drug therapy. Despite an apparent beneficial effect on nutrition for patients receiving barbiturates after severe head injury, barbiturate therapy is associated with many potential complications, and therapeutic efficacy for control of elevated intracranial pressure is controversial.—J.R. Kirsch, M.D.

Aminophylline and Human Diaphragm Strength In Vivo
Levy RD, Nava S, Gibbons L, Bellemare F (Centre Hosp Toracique de Montréal; Royal Victoria Hosp; McGill Univ)
J Appl Physiol 68:2591–2596, 1990   9–31

Patients with airflow obstruction are often treated with theophylline preparations. This therapy increases central respiratory drive and bronchial smooth muscle relaxation, but controversy exists as to the effect of theophylline on contractility of the normal human diaphragm. The recently developed technique of twitch occlusion with bilateral transcutaneous phrenic nerve stimulation was used to assess the effects of therapeutic concentrations of aminophylline on human diaphragm strength and contractility.

Under carefully controlled conditions, the results of such stimulation closely approximate the diaphragm tension response determined in vitro.

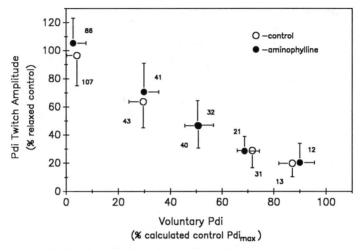

Fig 9–6.—Pooled data from all subjects showing Pdi-twitch amplitude at increasing levels of voluntary diaphragm activation during control conditions and after aminophylline. Error bars represent 1 SD. Numbers beside symbols indicate number of twitches. (Courtesy of Levy RD, Nava S, Gibbons L, et al: *J Appl Physiol* 68:2591–2596, 1990.)

Experiments were carried out on 9 healthy men aged 23–36 years. The transdiaphragmatic pressure (Pdi) twitch response to single shocks from supramaximal bilateral phrenic nerve stimulation was examined before and after acute intravenous infusions of aminophylline. Subjects were in the sitting position against an occluded airway from end expiration.

When compared with control conditions, aminophylline produced no significant difference in peak twitch Pdi from the relaxed diaphragm (Fig 9–6). Other twitch characteristics, including contraction time, half-relaxation time, and maximum relaxation rate, also remained unaltered. No significant change was noted in the mean calculated maximum Pdi between control and aminophylline experiments. Thus the acute administration of therapeutic concentrations of aminophylline does not appear to have significant effects on contractility or maximum strength of the normal human diaphragm in vivo.

▶ This rigorously conducted study suggests that aminophylline has little if any effect on diaphragm strength when administered to normal human volunteers. Aminophylline levels in these subjects were within the therapeutic range (14.9 ± 3.1 mg/mL) but were lower than in vitro concentrations that have been shown to augment rat diaphragm function (about 18 mg/mL). Given the low toxic:therapeutic ratio for aminophylline, it would appear that aminophylline is not likely to be of significant value as a diaphragmatic inotrope. In our intensive care unit, aminophylline is used infrequently because of the high incidence of undesirable tachyarrhythmias. We all await the development of new and safer methylxanthines; perhaps these will be able to be used to augment diaphragm function.—M.J. Breslow, M.D.

Cimetidine Reduces Hyperoxic Lung Injury in Lambs

Hazinski TA, France M, Kennedy KA, Hansen TN (Vanderbilt Univ; Baylor College of Medicine, Houston)
J Appl Physiol 67:2586–2592, 1989   9–32

Pretreatment with endotoxin appears to reduce acute pulmonary oxygen toxicity in lambs. Because endotoxin inhibits cytochrome P-450 mono-oxygenation reactions, it may act by countering oxygen radical production during hyperoxia. Cimetidine, a noncompetitive inhibitor of P-450 activity, was given to lambs before exposure to more than 95% oxygen.

Cimetidine-treated lambs maintained normal gas exchange longer than did control animals and accumulated lung-water more slowly. Microvascular permeability was normal was 72 hours of oxygen exposure. Control animals, in contrast, exhibited increased lung lymph flow and lymph protein clearance. Postmortem levels of oxidized glutathione in lung homogenate samples were significantly lower in treated lambs. Pretreatment with ranitidine, which lacks P-450 inhibitory activity, did not alter the course of oxygen-related injury or postmortem antioxidant levels. Hyperoxia increased the activity of cytochrome P-450 in lung microsomes, an effect not seen in cimetidine-treated animals. These findings are consistent with a role for cytochrome P-450-mediated oxygen metabolism in the pathogenesis of hyperoxic lung injury.

▶ In recent years, several new histamine H_2-receptor antagonists have been introduced. These agents have been touted as being superior to cimetidine because they, unlike cimetidine, do not inhibit the cytochrome P-450 mono-oxygenase system. Although it is true that cimetidine can alter the metabolism of drugs that are normally processed by this enzyme pathway and thus complicate management, this report by Hazinski et al. suggests that there may be benefits from cimetidine-induced P-450 inhibition. Cimetidine substantially reduced hyperoxic lung injury in lambs, presumably by reducing oxygen radical production via a P-450 mechanism. There is considerable uncertainty regarding the extent to which high inspired O_2 concentrations, when appropriately administered to patients with adult respiratory distress syndrome (ARDS), result in lung injury. However, most practitioners are concerned about the problem. If subsequent studies demonstrate that cimetidine can reduce the likelihood of O_2 toxicity in such patients, it could become an important drug in the treatment of ARDS.—M.J. Breslow, M.D.

Outcome of Infants With Cystic Fibrosis Requiring Mechanical Ventilation for Respiratory Failure

Garland JS, Chan YM, Kelly KJ, Rice TB (Med College of Wisconsin, Milwaukee)
Chest 96:136–138, 1989   9–33

A mortality rate of 75% or higher has been reported for infants less than 1 year of age with cystic fibrosis and respiratory failure requiring mechanical ventilation. The outcome of 5 such patients seen between 1980 and 1986 was compared with that of age-matched controls who had cystic fibrosis but not respiratory failure. The study infants underwent ventilation to normalize arterial blood gases.

All study patients were alive 1–6 years after the episode of respiratory failure. Their mean Schwachman score did not differ significantly from a recent mean score for the controls, and the 2 groups had similar numbers of hospitalizations. The mean time of ventilatory support was 7 days. Infants with cystic fibrosis who require mechanical ventilation for respiratory failure may have an outlook as good as those who do not require ventilatory support. Aggressive care of these patients is appropriate.

▶ This report provides yet another piece in the rapidly changing picture of cystic fibrosis. A few years ago many centers considered cystic fibrosis patients with respiratory failure to be inappropriate candidates for admission to an intensive care unit because the disease was irreversible and the outcome almost certainly fatal. Then came the prospect of lung transplantation in cystic fibrosis. Now we are on the threshold of clinical application of gene replacement therapy as a cure for this disease. In that context, it is heartening to know that infants with cystic fibrosis can be supported successfully during an episode of respiratory failure.—D.G. Nichols, M.D.

10 Socioeconomic and Ethical Issues

Age Criteria in Medicine: Are the Medical Justifications Ethical?
Kilner JF (Harvard Univ)
Arch Intern Med 149:2343–2346, 1989   10–1

Because the elderly receive a disproportionately large share of medical resources in the United States, excluding them from treatment would result in considerable savings. Age criteria appear to have broad support as a means of rationing treatment. Four types of possible medical justification for the use of age criteria have been proposed: length of medical benefit, quality of medical benefit, likelihood of medical benefit, and medical benefit for the individual patient.

The first 3 criteria involve patient comparisons and are of questionable value. Because the elderly, as a rule, will not live as long as younger patients, it is assumed that they will not receive the longest benefit from treatment. Prognoses, however, are always uncertain and length of benefit does not take into account the significance of personhood and the importance of each person's life to that person.

The quality of medical benefit also does not justify the use of age criteria. The observers' view of quality of life may not correlate well with the patients' subjective experience. The efforts of medicine should be directed toward making low-quality lives high-quality lives, not toward sacrificing low-quality lives to preserve higher quality lives.

The prospect of medical benefit for 1 group of patients over another is a statistical justification. This results in witholding resources from some patients on grounds that do not apply to them. The fourth form of medical justification identifies the likelihood of significant benefit from treatment for each patient. Because a simple cut-off age is too arbitrary a standard, exclusion from treatment should be based on the inability of an individual patient to benefit medically from that treatment.

► The ability of the United States to support health care is no longer in doubt. Resources are not available to provide unending state-of-the-art care to everyone regardless of their ability to pay for those services. The author quotes a study in which 36% of the respondents favored an age criteria in health care delivery. I suspect that few, if any, of those respondents were of the group that would be excluded from health care because of advanced age. Let's hope that the Golden Rule will prevail as those of us in medicine participate in the evolution of delivery of health care in times of limited resources. We may very well suffer from our own short-sightedness as we grow older.—R.W. McPherson, M.D.

Outcomes of Cardiopulmonary Resuscitation in the Elderly
Murphy DJ, Murray AM, Robinson BE, Campion EW (Beth Israel Hosp; Brigham & Women's Hosp; Massachusetts Gen Hosp, Boston; Harvard Med School; Univ of South Florida, Tampa)
Ann Intern Med 111:199–205, 1989   10–2

The success of cardiopulmonary resuscitation (CPR) (defined as being able to leave the hospital alive) ranges from 0% to 30%. To determine the success rate of CPR in the elderly and to define characteristics of elderly patients for whom such a procedure is effective, data were reviewed on 503 consecutive patients aged 70 years and older who received CPR.

A total of 112 patients survived initially (22%), but only 19 were discharged alive (3.8%). The worst results occurred in patients with unwitnessed arrests, terminal arrhythmias such as asystole and electromechanical dissociation, and those with resuscitation attempts lasting for more than 15 minutes. Only 2 of 244 patients with out-of-hospital arrests were discharged alive. Most of the survivors had ventricular arrhythmias and could be revived within minutes. Patients who survived initially with impaired consciousness or functional impairment had a significantly lower chance of survival than patients who did not have these impairments.

Cardiopulmonary resuscitation is rarely successful in elderly patients with cardiopulmonary arrests that occur out of the hospital, are unwitnessed, or are associated with asystole or electromechanical dissociation. Knowing these facts may make a do-not-resuscitate order less difficult.

▶ Despite great strides in the understanding of the physiology during CPR, the clinical outcome of CPR under real world circumstances is not particularly encouraging. This article reinforces the well-known adage that the sicker the patient, the poorer the outcome. The authors have provided valuable data to help decide when to stop CPR efforts.—R.W. McPherson, M.D.

Ethical Principles in Critical Care
Luce JM (Univ of California, San Francisco)
JAMA 263:696–700, 1990   10–3

Beneficence, or acting to benefit patients by sustaining life, treating illness, and relieving pain, has always been the most compelling principle of medical ethics. Nonmaleficence, or refraining from harm, is closely correlated. Autonomy, or respecting the right of patients to determine much of their medical care, is a third principle of medical ethics that is gaining increasing acceptance in the United States. Disclosure, or providing adequate and truthful information to competent patients to make medical decisions, is closely related to the principle of autonomy. Social justice, or allocating medical resources fairly and according to medical need, is a fifth principle of medical ethics.

The first 4 ethical principles are relatively easy to apply in the primary care setting of community hospitals where physicians have staff privileges and are responsible for their own patients. However, the principles of medical ethics may be more difficult to apply in the intensive care unit (ICU) where physicians often share responsibility for their patients with critical care specialists. Physicians may also have to transfer responsibility for their patients entirely to the ICU staff as they may not have admitting privileges to the ICUs of public hospitals or university medical centers where their patients may have been admitted for trauma care or transplant surgery. Many of the latter facilities are staffed by physicians in training who have had no previous contact with the patient. Physicians who care for critically ill patients should strive to uphold the 5 ethical principles when dealing with common critical care issues, e.g., medical decision making, informed consent, resuscitation, brain death and organ transplantation, withholding or withdrawing of life support, and allocation of medical resources.

▶ Difficulties in meeting ethical responsibilities to the patient and family in the ICU environment are discussed. A source of difficulty is the lack of sole responsibility for patient care. With increasing economic pressures to discontinue support when the outcome is hopeless, clearly defined patient responsibility is imperative. Perhaps hospital ethics committees may assume more responsibilities.—R.W. McPherson, M.D.

Changes in Spinal Reflex Excitability in Brain-Dead Humans

Crenna P, Conci F, Boselli L (Univ of Milan; Hosp Niguarda Ca Granda, Milan)
Electroencephalogr Clin Neurophysiol 73:206–214, 1989   10–4

The process leading to brain death seems to correspond to functional isolation of the spinal cord from the upper centers, representing a state of acute or subacute high spinalization. A longitudinal analysis of this process was attempted to study the excitability of proprioceptive and exteroceptive reflexes, clinically and electrophysiologically, in 8 brain-dead organ transplant donors whose mean age was 47 years. The study took place during the 12-hour monitoring period that is required after brain death and before organ donation.

The soleus H reflex reached a level of steady-state excitability within 2–6 hours after a time of total unresponsiveness. The response regained its normal shape at 10–20 hours. The threshold of the cutaneous reflex that was elicited in the biceps femoris by electrically stimulating the sural nerve became normal within 4–13 hours, but an abnormal multicomponent pattern persisted. Digital responses to mechanical stimulation of the sole of the foot were evident after 6–8 hours. No knee or ankle jerk responses were evoked at any time. The temporal course of changes in excitability did not related directly to the fall in blood pressure that sometimes accompanies brain death.

A state of spinal shock is observed after brain death, followed by the sequential recovery of reflex transmission. Greater vulnerability of polysynaptic pathways to spinal shock might explain why the tendon jerk responses are depressed longer than are H reflexes.

▶ With increasing frequency of organ donation, and a tremendous shortage of donors relative to qualified recipients, improving viability of transplanted organs is imperative. Because clinical criteria are used to determine brain death, understanding the neurologic function that can remain in the brain-dead subject allows the diagnosis to be made earlier and with assurance that the injury to the brain is irreversible.— R.W. McPherson, M.D.

Ethical and Moral Guidelines for the Initiation, Continuation, and Withdrawal of Intensive Care
Bone RC, Rackow EC, Weg JG, and members of the ACCP/SCCM Consensus Panel (Rush-Presbyterian-St Luke's Med Ctr, Chicago)
Chest 97:949–958, 1990   10–5

A Consensus Conference was held to determine how the ethical issues that apply in all medical decision-making relate to the initiation, continuance, and withdrawal of intensive care. Ethically sound decision-making in this area requires the best possible factual basis. Patients should be encouraged to make a treatment plan in advance of potential clinical crises that could render them unable to participate in decision-making. The Conference endorses a presumption to treat initially if there is doubt about the patient's wishes and about the possibility of achieving clinical goals.

The care delivery team must provide coordinated, ongoing support for the psychosocial needs of the patient and family. At the same time, it must take into account the effects of team members' own ethical, social, and religious values. An ethics committee, another physician, or, as a last resort, the court may be necessary if the physician and patient or family disagree about what is to be done. The legal system must respond to societal concerns if the parties involved cannot resolve a conflict. The high costs of critical care are a relevant consideration at all times.

Major religious groups agree that morality is not relative; that there is some flexibility—within limits—in applying religious moral principles; and that human life is of infinite worth. There is wide agreement that age and social worth should not influence the selection of patients for intensive care but, rather, that medical suitability be the sole criterion. Relief of intractable pain is appropriate even if life may be shortened as a result. Intensive measures are inappropriate if there is reasonable medical certainty that the patient is not salvageable. A persistent vegetative state is one factor in deciding whether to withdraw life support, but the patient's expressed wishes and the family's wishes also should be considered.

Educational efforts promoting the use of advance directives should be encouraged. It would be helpful to have regular interdisciplinary forums for discussing these issues.

▶ Ethical, legal, and religious opinion on intensive care has reached a consensus in the United States in a few important areas delineated by this report. There is a much broader landscape of problems in which there is wide diversity of opinion, especially in religious thought. The thorough discussion in this report of this broader landscape should help prepare physicians to participate in the public debate on the moral application of intensive care. Greater physician participation is needed urgently before application of intensive care is driven mainly by legal precedent and economic pressure.—D.G. Nichols, M.D.

Long-Term Outcomes for Elderly Survivors of Prolonged Ventilator Assistance
Elpern EH, Larson R, Douglass P, Rosen RL, Bone RC (Rush-Presbyterian-St Luke's Med Ctr, Chicago)
Chest 96:1120–1124, 1989   10–6

Many resources are needed to care for ventilator-dependent patients, but too little is known of the long-term outcome of this type of care. The posthospital course was evaluated in 95 elderly patients who underwent long-term ventilator-dependent care for 3 days or longer in 1983–1984. Thirty-one patients survived long enough to be discharged. Hemodynamically stable patients had the best chance of surviving to discharge.

The 30 evaluable patients had a median postdischarge survival time of 13½ months. Survival in the total group at 1 year was 16%. Nine patients were alive 3 years after the episode of ventilator dependence. Patients with neurologic disease had the poorest short- and long-term survival. Postdischarage survival was not consistently related to either length of hospitalization or days of mechanical ventilation. All but 4 of the 30 patients were rehospitalized, and 9 spent time in an extended-care facility. More than half of the patients received some type of home nursing support.

Long-term survival of elderly patients who require prolonged ventilator care is quite limited, apart from how long assistance is required. Most survivors require ongoing medical and nursing care. Most patients who are able to survive 3 years after an episode of ventilator dependence, however, are able to function independently.

▶ We are all interested in the cost effectiveness of intensive care services. This article by Elpern et al. documents that few elderly patients requiring mechanical ventilation for more than 3 days recover to full function. However, 10% of this group were alive 3 years after hospital discharge, and quality of life in these long-term survivors was quite good. Additional studies, including many more patients and multiple institutions, are required to determine which patient and disease characteristics are most likely to result in successful long-term survival. Such studies will almost certainly determine public policy regarding institutionalization and continuance of critical care service, and not just for the elderly.—M.J. Breslow, M.D.

Are Elderly People Less Responsive to Intensive Care?

Wu AW, Rubin HR, Rosen MJ (Univ of California, San Francisco; Mt Sinai Med Ctr, New York)

J Am Geriatr Soc 38:621–627, 1990   10–7

When the number of intensive care beds in a hospital is limited, physicians may not admit patients who have an extremely poor prognosis. Because elderly patients are often thought to have a worse prognosis than younger patients, they may be denied access to intensive care. To determine whether advanced age is, in fact, associated with increased mortality after accounting for severity of illness, 2 groups of patients admitted to a medical intensive care unit (ICU) were compared. The first group included 130 patients aged 75 years or older, and the second group, 135 patients between the ages of 55 and 65 years. Severity of illness was based on the Acute Physiology Assessment and Chronic Health Evaluation (APACHE II) system without including points for age (APACHE IIM). The groups had a similar mean APACHE IIM scores and diagnoses, but older patients had more chronic obstructive pulmonary disease.

The overall ICU mortality was 21% and total hospital mortality was 45%. Intensive care unit mortality rates in the 2 groups were similar, although elderly patients had a significantly higher total hospital mortality rate. Logistic regression analysis showed that, after controlling for other variables, older patients were not at a significantly greater risk of dying. Also, older patients with chronic obstructive pulmonary disease did not die at a higher rate than their younger counterparts. Increased mortality was related, however, to higher APACHE IIM scores and the presence of underlying cancer.

Age itself does not predict mortality in patients admitted to medical ICUs. In some diagnostic subgroups, older patients had a similar or even better prognosis than younger patients. Thus elderly patients should not be denied intensive care solely on the basis of their age.

▶ The authors of this article have attempted to determine whether advanced age, by itself, increases the mortality of patients admitted to a medical ICU. Using only 2 age groups and evaluating only those patients who passed some type of a "survivability criteria" for admission to the ICU, Wu et al. report only a very small effect of age on outcome. This type of analysis seems to be contrived; I assume it was selected to yield just this result. Although few would argue with the authors that age alone should not be used to preclude patients from admission to the ICU, their point would be better made by a more rigorous examination of the extent to which age affects outcome.—M.J. Breslow, M.D.

American Association of Critical-Care Nurses Demonstration Project: Patients' Recollections of Critical Care
Simpson TF, Armstrong S, Mitchell P (Univ of Rochester, NY; Univ of Washington; Overlake Hosp Med Ctr, Bellevue, Wash)
Heart Lung 18:325–332, 1989   10–8

The critical care unit (CCU) is a complex physical and interpersonal therapeutic environment. To examine the impact of the critical care experience on patients, 59 patients (mean age, 63 years) were asked to recall their experiences and were assessed for their understanding of critical care within 24–48 hours after discharge from a CCU (35 patients) or a mixed medical-surgical intensive care unit (ICU) (24 patients).

Twenty-two of the 24 ICU patients and 26 of the 35 CCU patients knew accurately why they had been admitted to these units. Patients' responses as to actions recalled were categorized into 4 major conceptual groups: self-care promotion, alleviation of concerns, technical care, and observation. Of all 4 major parameters, patients most often remembered nurses performing actions, and nurses were overwhelmingly associated with activities designed to ease the patients' concerns. On the other hand, physicians were most often cited as the source of information about their condition.

Although most actions recalled by patients were neutral or positive, slightly more than half rated the overall impact of their critical care experience as negative because of a variety of stressors encountered. The stressors identified were consistent with those named by patients in other studies, i.e., pain and discomfort, followed by sleep difficulties. Other stressors were fear and anger, suggesting the patients' sense of loss of control over their physical and emotional well-being. Nursing care should focus on managing stressors that can be alleviated and assisting patients to cope with those stressors that are not reducible.

▶ This paper evaluates the emotional experiences and recollections of patients who were admitted to the ICU. Surprisingly, almost half of the patients who were able to be interviewed described the impact of the experience as positive or neutral. I would have thought that the experience would have been significantly more negative. On the other hand, only half of the patients were able to be interviewed, and perhaps this paper is slightly more optimistic in its observations than would be the case had all of the patients been interviewed.—M.C. Rogers, M.D.

Intensive Care of Status Asthmaticus: A 10-Year Experience
Braman SS, Kaemmerlen JT (Brown Univ; Rhode Island Hosp, Providence, RI)
JAMA 264:366–368, 1990   10–9

Morbidity and mortality rates remain high for hospitalized asthmatic patients, especially those given intensive care. To determine whether the benefits of intensive care outweigh the potential hazards, the outcome of status asthmaticus was examined in 64 patients treated for 80 episodes in a medical intensive care unit (ICU) in a 10-year period.

Respiratory failure with carbon dioxide pressure greater than 50 mm Hg occurred in 50 of 80 episodes of status asthmaticus. Mechanical ventilation was avoided in half of these episodes despite marked acidosis and hypercapnia. Most patients improved rapidly and required only a short stay in the ICU, and there were no deaths. All complications, except for tracheal stenosis in 1 patient, resolved rapidly in the hospital.

These results are ascribed to close monitoring and repeated blood gas analysis. Patients with status asthmaticus in whom respiratory failure develops, or those who have respiratory distress resistant to emergency measures, should go to the ICU. Morbidity can be kept low even in patients who require ventilatory support.

▶ This 10-year review of the intensive care of patients with asthma evaluates 50 episodes of respiratory failure and analyzes how mechanical ventilation was avoided. It is interesting that the criteria for intubation of patients with asthma, particularly younger patients, have gradually changed. It is now considered appropriate in some settings to let the $Paco_2$ rise well above the 50 mm Hg that these authors define as respiratory failure. Regardless of these differences, I agree with the authors that many of the complications seen in patients with asthma are avoidable. This same subject is covered in other abstracts in this edition in which the morbidity and mortality of asthma are discussed.—M.C. Rogers, M.D.

Determinants of Hospital Charges for Coronary Artery Bypass Surgery: The Economic Consequences of Postoperative Complications
Taylor GJ, Mikell FL, Moses HW, Dove JT, Katholi RE, Malik SA, Markwell SJ, Korsmeyer C, Schneider JA, Wellons HA (Southern Illinois School of Medicine, Springfield)
Am J Cardiol 65:309–313, 1990   10–10

Hospital charges for 500 consecutive patients who underwent coronary bypass surgery in a 9-month period during 1985 were related to clinical variables. The mean age was 61 years; 191 patients were aged 65 years and older. An additional procedure was performed on 43 patients, most often valve replacement; 16 patients had emergency surgery. The average hospital stay after surgery was 10 days. The operative mortality was 3.2%. An average of 3.5 bypass grafts were placed.

Only the need for valve replacement and a history of myocardial infarction were significant predictors of a higher average charge on univariate analysis. On multiple regression analysis, higher charges were associated with sternal wound infection, respiratory failure, and left ventricular failure requiring intra-aortic balloon counterpulsation. The absence of all complications predicted a lower average hospital charge.

Surgical complications are the clinical features most likely to increase hospital charges for patients undergoing coronary bypass surgery. Higher-quality surgery may therefore cost less in this setting.

▶ This paper documents a rather obvious conclusion but does it with meaningful data that are useful to contemplate. Hospital charges for coronary artery bypass surgery are influenced by a number of problems that are avoidable. These include sternal wound infection, respiratory and left ventricular failure. Clearly, some of these (e.g., sternal wound infection) are avoidable. As a result of these observations, it is clear that higher-quality surgery reduces morbidity and mortality while it simultaneously lowers hospital costs.—M.C. Rogers, M.D.

Deferred Consent: Use in Clinical Resuscitation Research
Abramson NS, Safar P, and the Brain Resuscitation Clinical Trial II Study Group (Univ of Pittsburgh)
Ann Emerg Med 19:781–784, 1990   10–11

Regulatory constraints on the conduct of clinical research have increased dramatically in recent years. A new approach to the requirement for informed consent in clinical research—deferred consent—was used in a randomized clinical trial of brain resuscitation after cardiac arrest.

Traditional prospective consent usually could not be obtained because the patients were comatose and treatment had to be initiated immediately. In the deferred consent approach, family members were contacted after the first dose of experimental drug or placebo was given and asked for consent for continued participation in the study. Most families were satisfied with the deferred consent approach. The families' main concerns were about the safety of the experimental drug, and whether the drug or placebo was given. Generally, the concepts of randomization, blinding, and placebo-treated controls were not well understood.

To resolve the conflicts between regulatory constraints, ethical considerations, and necessary resuscitation research methodology, a deferred consent approach was used to obtain consent. Although the approach is clearly a compromise, it appears to be a workable solution, striking a balance between patients' rights and the methodologic constraints of resuscitation research.

▶ In this article, Abramson et al. discuss their experience with deferred consent, specifically as encountered during the Brain Resuscitation Clinical Trial II. They suggest that deferred consent is necessary in resuscitation research because therapy must be started early to allow the best chance of it being effective. Because this article simply presents anecdotal reports from individual investigators who would be biased to the importance of deferred consent, the utility of the results are limited. There is no hypothesis tested, and there is no mention of statistical analysis of the results that were obtained. It is not clear from the article whether a standard conversation was used to obtain consent. Family satisfaction may certainly be altered based on how the potential benefits of the proposed therapy are presented. An important issue, which is only transiently discussed, is how to determine whether the risk/benefit ratio of a particular therapy is appropriate. Indeed, many more families may have been unhappy about entering the study had they known prospectively of mixed results of therapeutic efficacy in animal experiments.—J.R. Kirsch, M.D.

Stability of Patient Preferences Regarding Life-Sustaining Treatments
Everhart MA, Pearlman RA (VA Med Ctr, Seattle; Univ of Washington)
Chest 97:159–164, 1990   10–12

Patient preferences are a factor in physicians' decisions to withhold or withdraw medical treatment. Thirty intensive care patients were interviewed concerning their preferences for resuscitation with and without mechanical ventilation, artificial hydration and nutrition, and hospitalization for pneumonia. They were reinterviewed a month later to determine whether their preferences had changes as their health status improved. All had survived an intensive care unit (ICU) or coronary care unit stay of 48 hours or longer.

The patients expressed diverse opinions regarding life-sustaining treatments in the settings of stroke and dementia. Most patients desired resuscitation in the current health situation and hospitalization for pneumonia in the stroke and dementia scenarios. Treatment preferences remained stable despite significant changes in mood and health status between the initial and follow-up interviews. Most patients had consistent preferences regarding all of the life-sustaining treatments.

Patients are willing to discuss their attitudes toward life-sustaining treatments in the ICU, and their responses are likely to remain stable for at least a month. Intensive care unit patients therefore should be actively engaged in making decisions concerning the use of life-sustaining treatment.

▶ We always try to take into account the patient's wishes with regard to life-sustaining treatments. The problem with this approach is that there are no data to indicate that the patient's preferences are sustained over prolonged periods of time. If the patient were to change his or her opinion, then the physician would be hard pressed to take these "new" preferences into account. This study puts this concern to rest by suggesting that patient's preferences for life-sustaining treatments are maintained over long periods of time. This is an interesting insight into the mind set of patients in the ICU.—M.C. Rogers, M.D.

Physicians' Refusal of Requested Treatment: The Case of Baby L
Paris JJ, Crone RK, Reardon F (Univ of Chicago; Harvard Med School; Hassen and Reardon, Boston)
N Engl J Med 322:1012–1015, 1990   10–13

Physicians rarely refuse patients' demands for treatment in life-threatening situations. As a result, the question is rarely reported in the literature and not usually covered in policy statements proposed by ethics committees. One exception is a statement adopted by the Children's National Medical Center in 1988. That policy allows physicians, with approval of the ethics committee, to refuse requested treatments when they are judged to be burdensome and without benefit. Such was the case of Baby L.

The infant was born at 36 weeks, weighing 1,970 g, after a pregnancy complicated by fetal hydronephrosis and oligohydramnios. Resuscitated and stabilized after delivery, the infant showed no responsiveness except to pain. During the first year of life, she experienced intermittent episodes of aspration and uncontrolled seizures. She was discharged after 14 months with 24-hour nursing care but readmitted repeatedly during the second year of life with pneumonia and septic shock. The mother demanded all possible life-saving measures.

The unanimous opinion of hospital staff members, counsel, and chairpersons of the institutional ethics committee was that further medical intervention was not in the patient's best interest. The mother's attorney arranged a hearing in probate court, where a guardian ad litem was appointed for the child. Baby L was subsequently transferred to the care of a pediatric neurologist who was willing to accommodate the parental wishes. Two years later, Baby L remains blind, deaf, quadriplegic, and is fed through the gastrostomy. She averages a seizure a day and has the mental status of a 3-month-old infant.

The denial by the medical team of potentially life-prolonging medical treatment appears to be the first case of its kind. Some argue that the goals of the patient and family should control decision making; others hold that the use of a procedure must be justified by a realistic expectation of prolonged benefit. Several legal decisions have not obliged physicians to order aggressive interventions in futile cases or against their conscience. The issues in such situations are complex and difficult and should remain difficult so that the best interests of the patient are always foremost.

▶ This interesting case revolves around a patient whose family wanted more therapy than the physicians thought was indicated. This is a growing area of conflict in the intensive care unit and was resolved in the case of Baby L by transferring the patient to another physician's care. This is not always possible, and it is clear that institutions must have groups to look prospectively at this potential problem. The "utility or futility" of care is an issue that appears different to physicians and to families, and these distinctions should be thought about long in advance. It is not possible to decide on the care of an individual patient in advance, but it is clear that it is very useful for all concerned to have policies and procedures for confronting these issues when they come up, as they inevitably will do.—M.C. Rogers, M.D.

Stroke Associated With Cocaine Use

Klonoff DC, Andrews BT, Obana WG (Peninsula Hosp, Burlingame, Calif; Univ of California, San Francisco)
Arch Neurol 46:989–993, 1989   10–14

Cocaine abuse is increasing dramatically in the United States. Although the mortality rate related to stroke has declined by about half in the past decade, the number of cocaine-related strokes has increased markedly during the same period. In addition to the 39 cocaine-associated strokes reported previously in the literature, 8 new cases of stroke after cocaine use were encountered.

The mean age of the total 47 patients at the time of stroke was 32.5 years; 76% were men. The incidence of cocaine-related stroke was highest among men in their 20s and declined with each additional decade of life. Stroke occurred after cocaine use whether by the inhalational, intranasal, intravenous, or intramuscular route. The onset of stroke occurred during cocaine use to as long as a day afterward. Cerebral infarction occurred in 10 patients, intracranial hemorrhage in 22, and subarachnoid hemorrhage in 13. In 17 patients intracranial aneurysms or arteriovenous malformations were seen on angiograms or at autopsy. Two patients had cerebral vasculitis. Of the 35 patients with a known outcome, 21 (60%) survived.

The apparent incidence of stroke associated with cocaine use is increasing. Cocaine-associated stroke occurs primarily in young adults and may follow any route of cocaine administration. Stroke after cocaine use is often associated with cerebrovascular abnormalities, and the frequency of intracranial hemorrhage exceeds that of cerebral infarction. Recent cocaine use must be included among the risk factors for stroke in young adults.

▶ This paper adds 8 new cases of stroke to the 39 previously reported in the literature before the time of the study. It appears that cocaine-associated stroke is increasing in incidence and occurs primarily in young adults. It is a sad commentary that as we have tried so hard to make progress in preventing and treating strokes in older patients, we are beginning to see an increasing number of young individuals who have entirely preventable causes of this terrible condition.—M.C. Rogers, M.D.

Cocaine-Related Medical Problems: Consecutive Series of 233 Patients

Brody SL, Slovis CM, Wrenn KD (Emory Univ)
Am J Med 88:325–331, 1990   10–15

Most epidemiologic studies have emphasized the dramatic complications of cocaine use, such as myocardial infarction, stroke, and sudden death, but there has been little information on common cocaine-related medical problems. A retrospective study was made of the characteristics of patients seen in an inner city adult medical emergency department with complaints related to cocaine use.

Between August 1986 and February 1987, 233 consecutive hospital visits were made by 216 cocaine-using patients (165 males and 51 females) aged 16–51 years (mean, 29.5 years). This represented about .6% of the total population seen in the medical emergency department. Cocaine was often used intravenously (50%), but freebase or "crack" use also was common (23%). The use of other intoxicants, particularly alcohol, in combination with cocaine was a common practice (48.5%). Heroin and marijuana were also used with cocaine.

The chief complaints were cardiopulmonary (56%) and neurologic (39%). Thirty-six percent had psychiatric symptoms. The most common complaint was chest pain, but rarely was it believed to be caused by myocardial ischemia. Other common complaints were anxiety, shortness of breath, palpitations, dizziness, and headache. Most patients had acute complaints (80%), and multiple symptoms were common (57.5%).

Short-term pharmacologic therapy was given during 24% of the visits. Only 10% of patients were admitted; admission was primarily because of acute effects or potential complications of cocaine use. Admitted patients were less likely to be cocaine smokers and were significantly older. Only 2 patients died in the emergency department.

Most medical complications of cocaine use are short lived, appear to be related to the drug's hyperadrenergic effects, and are usually not life threatening. Overall, acute morbidity and mortality from cocaine use are low, and only a small minority of cocaine abusers require admission. These data suggest that a major focus in the treatment of cocaine-related emergencies should be referral for drug abuse detoxification and treatment.

▶ This paper is included because it reviews a series of 233 patients and details their cocaine-related medical problems. Clearly, the vast majority of complaints were cardiopulmonary, but it is also clear that neurologic symptoms were nearly as common. As is reported in Abstract 10–14, the frequency of cocaine-induced strokes is increasing dramatically. The authors rightly point out that acute mortality and morbidity rates from cocaine use are very low, but for the patients who do make their way to the intensive care unit, these complications are likely to be major and life threatening.—M.C. Rogers, M.D.

Medication Errors in Neonatal and Paediatric Intensive-Care Units
Raju TNK, Kecskes S, Thornton JP, Perry M, Feldman S (Univ of Illinois, Chicago)
Lancet 2:374–376, 1989   10–16

There are few data on the incidence of medication errors in the neonatal and pediatric intensive care units (ICUs). The frequency of drug-related iatrogenic complications in these ICUs was studied in a 4-year prospective quality assurance study at the University of Illinois Hospital.

Among the 2,147 neonatal ICU and pediatric ICU admissions, 315 iatrogenic medication errors were reported, for an error rate of 1 (14.7%) per 6.8 admissions. Of these, 33 (10.5%) were classified as potentially serious. One patient had acute aminophylline poisoning after receiving 5 doses of aminophylline intravenously at a dosage 10 times higher than prescribed because of an error in calculation during dilution. Mild patient injuries were the result of 32 (10.2%) errors. Errors were most frequent during the day shift, and 60% were attributed to nurses. Only 9 (2.9%) errors were attributed to physicians, but 7 of these were considered potentially serious. Wrong time was the most common type of error.

A longitudinal monitoring system can help to identify iatrogenic complications caused by medication errors and may help in implementing preventive measures. The quality assurance program is a surveillance system that can be used in the ICU.

▶ There have been a number of studies concerning iatrogenic causes of problems for patients in the hospital setting. This study looked at medication errors in neonatal and pediatric ICUs and found an error rate of 1/6.8 admissions (14.7%). More importantly, the frequency of iatrogenic injury of any sort as the result of medication error was 1 injury for every 33 ICU admissions. Some of these errors were serious, and the monitoring of medication errors and their causes should be part of the quality assurance program of all ICUs.—M.C. Rogers, M.D.

Critical Care Education in General Surgery Residencies
Meyer AA, Fakhry SM, Sheldon GF (Univ of North Carolina)
Surgery 106:392–399, 1989   10–17

To determine how much attention has been given to critical care education in general surgery training programs, changes in critical care education consequent to its emphasis by the American Board of Surgery were examined. Directors of 296 approved general surgery residencies were surveyed and 79% participated.

About 90% of the program directors believe that surgical critical care is an essential part of general surgery. More than two thirds believe that a separate intensive care unit (ICU) rotation should be used in critical care education. In about half of the programs, critical care was taught by a separate ICU service. The average ICU rotation was 9 weeks, usually in the second year of training. Seventeen programs presently sponsor critical care fellowships and 25 others were considering them at the time of the survey.

Critical care is a necessary component of general surgery, but many training programs still lack an ICU service for coordinating resident education in surgical critical care. An increased commitment to critical care education in general surgery residencies is appropriate.

▶ This is an enlightening report about the advancements, or lack thereof, made in critical care education in American surgical residency programs in the 9 or 10 years since the last surgery of this kind. Although our knowledge of critical care has advanced significantly, there remains no organized educational agenda in most surgical residency programs. As evidenced in this report, however, attitudes toward critical care by surgical program directors appear to be changing. Most (75%) of program directors would now recommend a career in surgical critical care, up from 47% in 1981 (1). Additionally, roughly 75% of the program directors in this study believe that a separate critical care rotation would best serve the educational interests of their residents; despite this, less than half currently have such a service functioning in their center.

It is hoped that the interest now displayed by the majority of program directors will soon be rewarded by the development of adequate resources for the education of residents in critical care. This step, along with development of the 25 surgical critical care fellowships currently planned, will significantly expand the representation of surgeons in the practice of critical care.—A.C. Dixon, M.D. and J.E. Parillo, M.D.

Reference

1. Machiedo GW, et al: *J Surg Res* 30:223, 1981.

Subject Index

A

Abuse
  drug, inhalational, causing barotrauma, 244
Acidosis
  CPR and, discussion of, 22
  lactic
    bicarbonate in, 283
    effect on hemodynamics and left ventricular function (in dog), 33
  myocardial, associated with CO_2 production during cardiac arrest and resuscitation (in pig), 20
Acquired immunodeficiency syndrome (see AIDS)
Adenosine
  for tachycardia, paroxysmal supraventricular, 156
β-Adrenergic receptor
  regulation, ventricular, in cyanotic heart disease, in newborn (in lamb), 147
Adsorption
  detoxification of plasma containing lipopolysaccharide by, 49
Age
  criteria in medicine, ethical aspects of, 311
AIDS
  patients requiring intensive care, prognosis of, 193
  Pneumocystis carinii pneumonia in
    pentamidine for, 270
    respiratory failure and, improved survival, 192
Airway
  obstruction, mechanisms of pulsus paradoxus in, 239
  reactivity after tumor necrosis factor (in sheep), 78
Albumin
  supplementation in critically ill, 294
Alfentanil
  in septic shock (in dog), 53
Alkalosis
  metabolic, and pulmonary gas exchange, 277
  respiratory, effect of indomethacin on cerebral blood flow during, in newborn (in pig), 208
Allotransplantation
  reconstructive, discussion of, 298
Altitude
  high, causing pulmonary edema, nifedipine for, 235
  intermediate, acute mountain sickness at, 11

Amanita phalloides
  mushroom poisoning, liver transplantation for, 9
Amine
  metabolites, biogenic, in CSF after hypoxia due to cardiac arrest, 26
Amino
  acid alterations, extracellular, after spinal cord trauma, 303
Aminophylline
  diaphragm strength and, in vivo, 307
  effect on organ damage after Escherichia coli sepsis (in guinea pig), 60
Amiodarone
  -induced pulmonary toxicity, clinical features of, 256
  in ventricular arrhythmias, 158
  in ventricular tachycardia, recurrent refractory, 157
Amrinone
  in neonates and infants after cardiac surgery, 231
Anemia
  in acute phase of spinal cord injury, 182
Angina
  rest, angiographic morphology of coronary artery stenosis in, 103
  unstable
    intracoronary thrombus and complex morphology in, 132
    neutrophil elastase release increase in, 106
Angiography
  in angina, unstable, related to intracoronary thrombus and complex morphology, 132
  in coronary artery stenosis in rest angina, 103
Angioplasty
  coronary
    cardiopulmonary bypass during, percutaneous, 101
    after myocardial infarction, anterior, 99
    after myocardial infarction, results of, 121
    after myocardial infarction, in single vessel disease, 98
Anistreplase
  IV, in myocardial infarction, 128
Antacid
  titration in prevention of stress ulcers in surgical patients, 280

Author Index

A

Abrahamson D, 173
Abramson NS, 205, 319
Achauer BM, 298
Acheson A, 154
Adamson RM, 18
Adrogué HJ, 291
Ahmad M, 245
Ahmed S, 46
Ahnefeld FW, 27
Ahuja RC, 133
Akhtar M, 156
Aknin P, 40
Alden PB, 67
Aldrete JS, 230
Alexander GJM, 295
Alexander JP, 9
Alford CA Jr, 220
Allardyce G, 187
Allen JN, 250
Almquist AK, 134, 158
Alpert JS, 197
Amber IJ, 231
Amigoni S, 206
Aminoff MJ, 201
Amirthalingam KN, 245
Anderson JD, 81
Anderson KD, 79
Anderson S, 99
Andrews BT, 322
Andriolo L, 178
Antman EM, 175
Apitz J, 138
Arieff AI, 286
Armitage JM, 149
Armstrong PW, 132
Armstrong S, 317
Artis A, 99
Åsberg A, 86
Ascher NL, 9
Astedt B, 260
Astiz ME, 59
Atsumi N, 295
Auckenthaler R, 300
Austen WG, 295
Auzepy P, 248

B

Baart de la Faille H, 299
Baccini A, 269
Bacharach SL, 167
Balcon R, 96
Ballesteros MA, 278
Banja JD, 297
Barbash GI, 96
Barbey JT, 152
Barbonaglia L, 134
Bardy GH, 153
Barie PS, 263

Barrero J, 291
Barroso-Aranda J, 29
Bärtsch P, 235
Barzilai B, 85
Baskin DS, 181
Bassan S, 96
Bateman TM, 121
Bauer KA, 72
Baum TD, 71
Baumgartner J-D, 51
Beattie C, 17
Becker LC, 109
Becker PJ, 171
Béland MJ, 224
Belenkie I, 238
Bellemare F, 307
Ben Dahan J, 70
Benditt DG, 158
Benhorin J, 90
Benner KG, 9
Bennett ED, 89
Benotti PN, 294
Berko B, 173
Bernath O, 300
Berning J, 157
Bernstein D, 147
Bersin RM, 286
Bersten AD, 80
Bertozzi P, 260
Beskin RR, 13
Beutler B, 219
Bevan JS, 305
Beyar R, 17
Bigorra J, 221
Biondi JW, 166
Bisera J, 19, 20
Bistrian BR, 294
Black KS, 298
Blackey AR, 87
Blanc P-L, 182
Blankenship JC, 134
Bloom BT, 267
Blumhardt R, 120
Boden WE, 137
Bolman RM III, 142
Bone RC, 314, 315
Bonow RO, 167
Booth DC, 148
Borlase BC, 294
Boselli L, 313
Boucher CA, 92, 120
Bourge RC, 230
Bowdler IM, 27
Bracken MB, 181
Braman SS, 272, 317
Brand DA, 114
Braunlin EA, 142
Braunwald E, 118
Bredle DL, 31
Breisblatt WM, 149
Brenner M, 54, 62
Brewster DC, 177
Brigham KL, 78
Brimioulle S, 277

Brody SL, 322
Brower RG, 146
Brown CG, 23
Brown FD, 211
Bruderman I, 254
Brugada P, 112
Brunel W, 234
Brunette DD, 136
Bruscoli G, 269
Brush JE Jr, 167
Buckley MJ Jr, 155
Bulatovic A, 227
Büller HR, 72
Burckart G, 231
Burek K, 102
Burke CW, 305
Burke JF, 73, 252
Burroughs AK, 288
Butler VR Jr, 175
Butt W, 257
Buzby GP, 306
Bysani GK, 49

C

Cafferty PJ, 229
Cahalane SF, 255
Cain SM, 31
Calandra T, 51
Caldwell JE, 251
Cali G, 87
Callahan DB, 153
Calzolari C, 225
Camacho SA, 127
Cammenga R, 223
Campion EW, 312
Caneal D, 46
Cannon JG, 73
Cannon RO III, 167
Canter CE, 142
Capone RJ, 137
Capozzi J, 149
Carbonell A, 221
Caresia L, 206
Carey C, 96
Carosi M, 206
Carroll SF, 66
Carter JM, 247
Cerra FB, 67
Cervenka K, 211
Chaitman BR, 94
Chalmers TC, 113
Chamberlain DA, 105, 128
Chan WWC, 117
Chan YM, 309
Chandra NC, 17, 163
Chang ACK, 41
Chang S-W, 50
Chapekis AT, 102
Chapman HA Jr, 260

349